Mental Health Considerations in the Athlete

Editor

SIOBHÁN M. STATUTA

CLINICS IN SPORTS MEDICINE

www.sportsmed.theclinics.com

Consulting Editor
MARK D. MILLER

January 2024 • Volume 43 • Number 1

ELSEVIER

1600 John F. Kennedy Boulevard • Suite 1800 • Philadelphia, Pennsylvania, 19103-2899

http://www.theclinics.com

CLINICS IN SPORTS MEDICINE Volume 43, Number 1
January 2024 ISSN 0278-5919, ISBN-13: 978-0-443-13091-5

Editor: Megan Ashdown
Developmental Editor: Malvika Shah

Clinics in Sports Medicine (ISSN 0278-5919) is published quarterly by Elsevier Inc., 360 Park Avenue South, New York, NY 10010-1710. Months of issue are January, April, July, and October. Business and Editorial Offices: 1600 John F. Kennedy Blvd., Ste. 1800, Philadelphia, PA 19103-2899. Customer Service Office: 3251 Riverport Lane, Maryland Heights, MO 63043. Periodicals postage paid at New York, NY and additional mailing offices. Subscription prices are $390.00 per year (US individuals), $100.00 per year (US students), $430.00 per year (Canadian individuals), $100.00 (Canadian students), $504.00 per year (foreign individuals), and $235.00 per year (foreign students). For institutional access pricing please contact Customer Service via the contact information below. Foreign air speed delivery is included in all *Clinics* subscription prices. All prices are subject to change without notice. **POSTMASTER:** Send address changes to *Clinics in Sports Medicine*, Elsevier Health Sciences Division, Subscription Customer Service, 3251 Riverport Lane, Maryland Heights, MO 63043. Customer Service (orders, claims, online, change of address): Elsevier Health Sciences Division, Subscription Customer Service, 3251 Riverport Lane, Maryland Heights, MO 63043. **Tel: 1-800-654-2452 (U.S. and Canada); 314-447-8871 (outside U.S. and Canada). Fax: 314-447-8029. E-mail: journalscustomerservice-usa@elsevier.com (for print support); journalsonlinesupport-usa@elsevier.com (for online support).**

Reprints. For copies of 100 or more of articles in this publication, please contact the Commercial Reprints Department, Elsevier Inc., 360 Park Avenue South, New York, NY 10010-1710. Tel.: 212-633-3874; Fax: 212-633-3820; E-mail: reprints@elsevier.com.

Clinics in Sports Medicine is covered in *MEDLINE/PubMed (Index Medicus) Current Contents/Clinical Medicine, Excerpta Medica,* and *ISI/Biomed.*

Contributors

CONSULTING EDITOR

MARK D. MILLER, MD

S. Ward Casscells Professor, Head, Division of Sports Medicine, Department of Orthopaedic Surgery, University of Virginia, Charlottesville, Virginia, USA; Team Physician, James Madison University, Founder, JBJS Deputy Editor for *Sports Medicine*, Director, Miller Review Course, Harrisonburg, Virginia, USA

EDITOR

SIOBHÁN M. STATUTA, MD, FACSM, FAMSSM

Director, Primary Care Sports Medicine Fellowship, Associate Professor, Departments of Family Medicine and Physical Medicine and Rehabilitation, Team Physician, University of Virginia Sports Medicine, University of Virginia Health System, Charlottesville, Virginia, USA

AUTHORS

CINDY MILLER ARON, LCSW

Senior Director of Clinical Services, Ascend Consultation in Healthcare, Chicago, Illinois, USA; Adjunct Professor, Department of Psychiatry, University of Wisconsin-Madison School of Medicine and Public Health, Madison, Wisconsin, USA

SARAH E. BEABLE, MBChB, FACSEP

Sport and Exercise Physician, Axis Sports Medicine Specialists, High Performance Sport New Zealand, Queenstown, New Zealand

JOY CHANG, MD

Assistant Professor, Department of Psychiatry, University of Maryland School of Medicine, Baltimore, Maryland, USA; University of Maryland, College Park Athletic Department, Baltimore, Maryland, USA

HYUNWOO JUNE CHOO, MD, MPH

Fellow, Department of Orthopaedics, Division of Physical Medicine and Rehabilitation, Stanford University, Stanford, California, USA

MARY M. DALEY, MD

Pediatric Sports Medicine Specialist, Department of Orthopaedic Surgery, Division of Sports Medicine, Children's Hospital of Philadelphia, Philadelphia, Pennsylvania, USA; Clinical Assistant Professor of Pediatrics, Perelman School of Medicine, University of Pennsylvania, Philadelphia, Pennsylvania, USA

CARLY DAY, MD

Adjunct Associate Professor, Department of Health and Kinesiology, Purdue University, West Lafayette, Indiana, USA

CARLA D. EDWARDS, MSc, MD, FRCPC
Assistant Clinical Professor, Department of Psychiatry and Behavioural Neurosciences, McMaster University, St. Joseph's Healthcare Hamilton Hamilton, Ontario, Canada

MARCIA FAUSTIN, MD
Assistant Professor, Department of Family and Community Medicine, Department of Physical Medicine and Rehabilitation, University of California, Davis School of Medicine, Sacramento, California, USA

R. SHEA FONTANA, DO
Associate Program Director, Department of Psychiatry and Behavioral Medicine, Prisma Health Greenville, Greenville, South Carolina, USA; Clinical Assistant Professor, University of South Carolina School of Medicine, Greenville, South Carolina, USA

JOSHUA FROST, BSc, MSc
PhD Candidate, The Centre for Youth Mental Health, The University of Melbourne, Melbourne, Australia; Elite Sports and Mental Health, Orygen, Parkville, Victoria, Australia

MICHELLE GARVIN, PhD
Sport Psychologist, Detroit Lions, National Football League, Detroit, Michigan, USA; Owner, Elite Performance Psychology, LLC, Silver Spring, Maryland, USA

ROLANDO GONZALEZ, MD
Clinical Assistant Professor, Department of Family Medicine, Florida State University College of Medicine, Fort Myers, Florida, USA; Pediatric and Sports Psychiatrist, Golisano Children's Hospital of Southwest Florida, Fort Myers, Florida, USA

PAUL GORCZYNSKI, PhD
Senior Lecturer, Psychology and Counselling, School of Human Sciences, University of Greenwich, Old Royal Naval College, Park Row, Greenwich, United Kingdom

BRIAN HAINLINE, MD
Chief Medical Officer, National Collegiate Athletic Association, Indianapolis, Indiana, USA

MARY HITCHCOCK, MA, MS
Senior Academic Librarian, University of Wisconsin-Madison, Ebling Library for the Health Sciences, Madison, Wisconsin, USA

AARON S. JECKELL, MD
Voluntary Professor, Department of Psychiatry and Behavioral Health, Vanderbilt University School of Medicine Nashville, Tennessee, USA

ANDREA KUSSMAN, MD
Associate Professor, Department of Family Medicine, University of Washington, Associate Director of Female Athlete and Bone Health Research Seattle, Washington, USA

COLLIN LEIBOLD, MD, MS
Resident, Department of Family Medicine, University of Virginia, Charlottesville, Virginia, USA

DAVID R. MCDUFF, MD
Clinical Professor, Department of Psychiatry, University of Maryland School of Medicine, Baltimore, Maryland, USA; Sports Psychiatrist, Baltimore Orioles, Major League Baseball, Baltimore, Maryland, USA; Sports Psychiatrist, Maryland Centers for Psychiatry, Ellicott City, Maryland, USA

SARAH MERRILL, MD
Associate Professor, Department of Family Medicine, University of California, San Diego School of Medicine, San Diego, California, USA

MATT MOORE, PhD
Associate Professor, Department of Social Work, Ball State University, Muncie, Indiana, USA; Associate Professor and Department Chair, Department of Family Science and Social Work, Miami University, Oxford, Ohio, USA

TAMMY NG, MD
Resident Physician, Department of Pediatrics, University of California, Davis, School of Medicine, Sacramento, California, USA

NAOYA NISHINO, MD
Postdoctoral Scholar, Sleep and Circadian Neurobiology Laboratory, Department of Psychiatry and Behavioral Sciences, Stanford University School of Medicine, Palo Alto, California, USA

VITA PILKINGTON, BA (Hons)
PhD Candidate, The Centre for Youth Mental Health, The University of Melbourne, Melbourne, Australia; Research Assistant, Elite Sports and Mental Health, Orygen, Parkville, Victoria, Australia

ROSEMARY PURCELL, MPsych, PhD
Professor, The Centre for Youth Mental Health, The University of Melbourne, Melbourne, Australia; Chief of Knowledge Translation, Elite Sports and Mental Health, Orygen, Parkville, Victoria, Australia

CLAUDIA L. REARDON, MD
Professor, Department of Psychiatry, University of Wisconsin-Madison School of Medicine and Public Health, Madison, Wisconsin, USA

SIMON RICE, PhD
Principal Research Fellow, Orygen, Centre for Youth Mental Health, The University of Melbourne, Parkville, Melbourne, Australia

HOWARD SANDERS, MD
Resident Physician, Department of Pediatrics, University of California, Davis School of Medicine, Sacramento, California, USA

RACHEAL M. SMETANA, PSYD
Assistant Professor, Department of Psychiatry and Neurobehavioral Sciences, University of Virginia Health, Charlottesville, Virginia, USA

SIOBHÁN M. STATUTA, MD, FACSM, FAMSSM
Director, Primary Care Sports Medicine Fellowship, Associate Professor, Departments of Family Medicine and Physical Medicine and Rehabilitation, Team Physician, University of Virginia Sports Medicine, University of Virginia Health System, Charlottesville, Virginia, USA

DONALD THOMPSON, MD
Assistant Professor, Department of Psychiatry, University of Maryland School of Medicine, Baltimore, Maryland, USA; Sports Psychiatrist, Baltimore Orioles, Major League Baseball, Baltimore, Maryland, USA

YUKA TSUKAHARA, MD, PhD
Professor, Department of Sports Medicine, Tokyo Women's College of Physical Education, Kunitachi, Tokyo, Japan

Contents

Within elite sport, epidemiological evidence is needed concerning the incidence and prevalence of mental health symptoms and disorders in relation to athlete demographic factors such as (dis)ability, race, ethnicity, sexual orientations, and different genders. Mental health promotion campaigns are often based on mental health literacy strategies. Such strategies aim to increase knowledge of mental health symptoms and disorders, address aspects of self- and public stigma, and promote help-seeking behaviors. Sporting organizations need to take responsibility to ensure that policies, practices, and services reflect organizational values concerning mental health. Organizational mental health literacy ensures that information is culturally competent and responsive, easy to find, straightforward, and offers simple, legitimate opportunities to access support.

Athletes are incredibly motivated and perpetually pursuing dominance in skill, strength, endurance, and execution–often while balancing many additional responsibilities. Despite the appearance of living fun, luxurious, care-free lifestyles, they are vulnerable to exceptional stressors and the same mental health challenges as the general population. The use of screening tools and assessment guided by a biopsychosocial framework can assist in understanding the factors that contribute to the athlete's mental health status. This can facilitate the development of a targeted management approach to mental health challenges.

Athletes and non-athletes experience many anxiety-related symptoms and disorders at comparable rates. Contributory factors may include pressure to perform, public scrutiny, sporting career dissatisfaction, injury, and harassment and abuse in sport. Anxiety may negatively impact sport performance. Specific types of anxiety may have unique presentations in athletes. It is important to rule out general medical and substance-related causes of anxiety symptoms. Psychotherapy and pharmacology treatment options should be considered, bearing in mind athletes' environmental circumstances and physiologies.

Depressive disorders in athletes are thought to be at least as common as the general population. However, athletes have a unique set of risk factors that can affect the likelihood of developing depression. Screening tools have been developed specifically for athletes such as the Sport Mental Health Assessment Tool (SMHAT). The management of the depressed athlete should involve an individualized approach, with methods such as counseling, interpersonal therapy, or cognitive behavioral therapy being used. Some may require antidepressant medication. Depressive disorders are also linked to sucidality in athletes, and the team physician and sporting organisation should have a crisis management plan in place for mental health emergencies. Tackling the stigma that remains in sport is a key part to improving mental wellbeing for all athletes.

Disordered eating (DE) and eating disorders (EDs) are more prevalent in athletes than non-athletes, and can cause devastating health and performance consequences. Although they can affect any athlete, DE/EDs are more common among women and athletes in lean sports, where there is a perceived competitive advantage to being lean. The sports medicine provider plays a crucial role in screening, diagnosis, and treatment of DE/ED. Treatment should involve a multidisciplinary team with a physician, dietitian, and mental health provider. Preventative efforts should seek to educate athletes and their coaches/support staff and should foster a healthy environment, which deemphasizes weight or body image.

Sleep is important for not only general health but also for lowering injury risk and maintaining athletic performance. Sleep disorders are prevalent in athletes, and taking a sleep history, evaluating sleep quality, and addressing other related factors including mental health are essential in diagnosing and understanding sleep disorders. Other methods such as polysomnography, actigraphy, and sheet sensors can also be used. Treatment options for sleep disorders include sleep hygiene, cognitive behavioral therapy, medication, and addressing contributing factors. For athletes, sleep can also be affected by factors such as travel fatigue and jet lag, which should be taken into consideration.

Though research is inconclusive in being able to determine if young athletes are more or less likely to suffer from mental health disorders compared with their non-athlete peers, there are important psychological considerations that are unique to the athletic population. This includes depression in the context of overtraining and burnout, performance anxiety, perfectionism, psychological sequalae of concussion, and injury as an independent risk factor for depression, anxiety, post-traumatic stress, and high-risk behaviors. Optimization of mental health care in youth athletes requires continued efforts to improve mental health literacy, decrease stigma, encourage help-seeking behaviors, and advance the routine implementation of effective screening practices.

CLINICS IN SPORTS MEDICINE

SERIES OF RELATED INTERESTED

Orthopedic Clinics
https://www.orthopedic.theclinics.com/
Foot and Ankle Clinics
https://www.foot.theclinics.com/
Hand Clinics
https://www.hand.theclinics.com/
Physical Medicine and Rehabilitation Clinics
https://www.pmr.theclinics.com/

THE CLINICS ARE AVAILABLE ONLINE!
Access your subscription at:
www.theclinics.com

Foreword
Athletic Mental Health: It's not all in Their Heads!

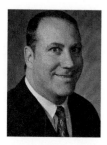

Mark D. Miller, MD
Consulting Editor

Thank you once again to Dr Siobhán M. Statuta for putting together another excellent issue of *Clinics in Sports Medicine*. With all of the recent media attention to this topic (or, in some ways, because of it), and in light of the recent tragedies at our institution and others, we felt that this topic needed to be addressed. Dr Statuta gathered an all-star panel of mental health experts to put together a comprehensive look at how mental health affects athletes, coaches, and even me when I'm staring over that must-make putt at my golf course!

The issue begins with the basics—epidemiology and an overview of the management of mental health. Next, the disorders associated with anxiety, depression, eating, and sleeping are examined. This is followed by a look at mental health in young athletes, substance misuse, attention deficit issues, the media's effect, athlete maltreatment, and finally, coaches and their role.

I would encourage you to carefully read this issue and to have it ready if and when you need it. This problem is real and may become even bigger in your practice.

Mark D. Miller, MD
Division of Sports Medicine
Department of Orthopaedic Surgery
University of Virginia
400 Ray C. Hunt Drive, Suite 330
Charlottesville, VA 22908-0159, USA

E-mail address:
MDM3P@hscmail.mcc.virginia.edu

Clin Sports Med 43 (2024) xiii
https://doi.org/10.1016/j.csm.2023.07.006
0278-5919/24/© 2023 Published by Elsevier Inc.

Preface

Of Sound Mind and Body

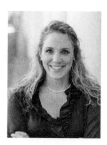

Siobhán M. Statuta, MD, FACSM, FAMSSM
Editor

Those of us in the specialty of "sports medicine" have an intrinsic understanding that we do not simply take care of an athlete's knee meniscal tear. We do not "just" diagnose a concussion and place an athlete on hold until asymptomatic. No. From the moment we pledge the Hippocratic Oath to care for the *entire* individual without doing harm, we consistently strive to identify and diagnose the obvious, all the while considering and anticipating the more obscure. But complete care extends beyond the physical. We must pay close attention to the other crucial component when striving for optimal health: our mental well-being. It is the "yin" to the "yang" for the ideal human body.

The World Health Organization defines mental health as *"a state of well-being in which every individual realizes his or her own potential, can cope with the normal stresses of life, can work productively and fruitfully, and is able to make a contribution to her or his community"*[1] and further declares it a "basic human right." From these tenets, it should be expected, then, that every health care provider worldwide addresses mental health in the quest for injury prevention as well as for the healing of patients. Arguably, athletes need it even more due to the unique and intense stressors they are subject to within the sporting arena: training demands, pressures to perform, financial and social implications, and the eventual retirement from sport, to name a few. These complex, convoluted, and shifting pressures are omnipresent in an athlete and can trigger existing or even create new mental health symptoms. It is incumbent on us, as sports medicine providers, to educate ourselves and to provide the utmost in comprehensive health care for our athletes.

I am honored to have been invited to develop this issue of *Clinics in Sports Medicine* in which assorted topics in mental health are addressed with particular consideration of how they relate to the athlete. The intent is not only for awareness and edification purposes but also to promote literacy and destigmatization surrounding mental health.

Clin Sports Med 43 (2024) xv–xvi
https://doi.org/10.1016/j.csm.2023.06.018
0278-5919/24/© 2023 Elsevier Inc. All rights reserved.

sportsmed.theclinics.com

My sincerest thanks to all contributing authors, who provided invaluable insight while addressing very complicated yet imperative topics relating to mental health. This required even more time and energy from busy schedules and is truly appreciated. It has been an honor to collaborate with true world experts on this vital topic. Last, a heartfelt thank you to Dr Mark Miller for the years of support, encouragement, and the confidence to continue extending me opportunities to further my own professional journey.

Siobhán M. Statuta, MD, FACSM, FAMSSM
Departments of Family Medicine and
Physical Medicine & Rehabilitation
University of Virginia Sports Medicine
University of Virginia Health System
PO Box 800729
Charlottesville, VA 22908-0729, USA

E-mail address:
sms5bb@uvahealth.org

REFERENCE

1. World Health Organization (WHO). Health and Well-Being (who.int). Accessed March 3, 2023.

The Epidemiology of Mental Health Symptoms and Disorders Among Elite Athletes and the Evolution of Mental Health Literacy

Paul Gorczynski, PhD[a,b,*], Cindy Miller Aron, LCSW[b,c],
Matt Moore, PhD[d,e], Claudia L. Reardon, MD[c]

KEYWORDS

- Mental health • Sport • Epidemiology • Mental health literacy • Stigma
- Help seeking

KEY POINTS

- Among elite athletes, strategies are needed to address mental health epidemiological data disparities among different (dis)abilities, races, ethnicities, sexual orientations, and genders.
- Culturally competent mental health literacy strategies are needed to help individuals better understand mental health symptoms and disorders, address stigma, and promote help-seeking behaviors.
- Sporting organizations need to ensure athletes have access to information on mental health and can access services quickly.

INTRODUCTION

A considerable amount of epidemiological research has demonstrated that athletes who compete at elite or professional levels, such as the Olympics, are susceptible to and experience mental health symptoms and disorders.[1–3] Mental health symptoms

[a] Psychology and Counselling, School of Human Sciences, University of Greenwich, Old Royal Naval College, Spinnaker Building, Cambridge Road, Park Row, Greenwich SE10 9LS, UK; [b] Ascend Consultation in Healthcare, 737 North Michigan Avenue #1925, Chicago, IL 60611, USA; [c] Department of Psychiatry, University of Wisconsin School of Medicine and Public Health, 6001 Research Park Boulevard, Madison, WI 53719, USA; [d] Department of Social Work, Ball State University, Health Professions Building, Room 501, Muncie, IN 47306, USA; [e] Department of Family Science and Social Work, Miami University, McGuffey Hall, Room 101C, Oxford, OH 45056, USA
* Corresponding author.
E-mail address: paul.gorczynski@greenwich.ac.uk

Clin Sports Med 43 (2024) 1–11
https://doi.org/10.1016/j.csm.2023.06.001
0278-5919/24/© 2023 Elsevier Inc. All rights reserved.

and disorders can greatly affect not only the training and performance of athletes, but their lives outside of sport as well.[4] At times, mental health symptoms and disorders can cause an individual to exit their chosen sport and end their athletic career.[1] This article will examine the concept of mental health and explore its many facets in relation to sport participation. Epidemiological research of mental health symptoms and disorders among elite athletes will be reviewed with careful attention paid to representation of different population characteristics. Deficits of demographic representation as well as limited research and knowledge of certain populations will be highlighted and accompanied by suggestions for greater rigor in future epidemiological research. Lastly, elements of mental health literacy will be discussed, outlining different areas of knowledge of mental health symptoms and disorders and strategies to address stigma and strengthen pathways to promote help-seeking behaviors among athletes. Suggestions for greater institutional responsibility with respect to mental health literacy will conclude the article.

MENTAL HEALTH

Mental health, as defined by the World Health Organization,[5] is the "state of well-being in which the individual realizes his or her [or their] own abilities, can cope with the normal stresses of life, can work productively and fruitfully, and is able to make a contribution to his or her community." Mental health is best understood as a resource, one that allows individuals to recognize and understand their skills and potential that they may use to pursue their passions and dreams within sport. Mental health allows individuals to work in constructive ways either by themselves or collectively as a group or a community. Social health is an integral component of mental health, where individuals can integrate into society, feel accepted and trusted, contribute to collective efforts, and work toward strengthening their community for the future.[6] Mental health also allows individuals to recognize, understand, and address challenges as they may arise. For athletes, this may mean stressors within sport as well as outside of sport. Holistic life perspectives challenge athletes to critically reflect, explore, and understand their identities and self-concepts.[4] Such perspectives ask athletes to examine the many facets of their lives, including family, friendships, scholastic pursuits, hobbies, leisure activities, and non-athletic jobs and careers, in addition to training for and performing within their chosen sport(s).[7] A holistic life perspective allows individuals to be able to recognize where stressors originate, how they may affect multiple areas of their lives, and how they may be addressed and managed. Overall, mental health is an essential part of one's health.

When individuals experience mental health disorders, they may experience distress and a wide range of clinically significant conditions where areas of functioning are affected.[8] Mental health disorders are characterized by changes that affect an individual's emotional regulations, cognitive processes, and behavior. Broadly, mental health disorders are diagnosed by mental health professionals who have evidenced that mental health symptoms meet diagnostic criteria for duration, frequency, and severity. For athletes, this may mean they are no longer able to train or perform and may need to interrupt their athletic pursuits while they seek treatment.

EPIDEMIOLOGY OF MENTAL HEALTH SYMPTOMS

Athletes who compete or have competed at professional or other elite levels have experienced mental health symptoms and disorders that have stemmed from multiple individual, social, and environmental conditions.[9,10] Epidemiological evidence on the prevalence of mental health symptoms and disorders has shown similar levels among current and retired elite athletes.[2] For instance, mental health symptoms and disorders range between 19% (alcohol use) and 34% (anxiety/depression) for current elite athletes. For retired elite athletes, mental health symptoms and disorders range between 16% ("distress" in general) and 26% (anxiety/depression). Athletes who compete in individual sports have been shown to be at greater risk of certain mental health symptoms and disorders, such as major depressive disorder, than those who compete in team-based sports.[11] This may be related to how individuals view psychological demands of competition, including views of success and failure. Those who compete on teams are more likely to use substances than individuals who compete individually.[1]

Epidemiological research has shown sex differences for certain mental health symptoms. For example, with respect to depressive symptoms, females are twice as likely as males to report such symptoms.[12,13] Female athletes are also more likely than male athletes to report symptoms of anxiety.[3] Research has shown that gender-specific stressors can directly impact the mental health of women, including their overall career satisfaction and longevity in sport.[14] For example, women are more likely than men to experience individual stressors (eg, family planning, caring responsibilities), interpersonal stressors (eg, sexual harassment and violence, abuse, bullying), organizational/structural stressors (eg, disparity in wages, mistrust in leadership roles, sex verification to compete), and socio-cultural stressors (eg, negative and sexualized media coverage, perceptions of less able athleticism). To date, in elite sport, less is known about the epidemiology of mental health symptoms and disorders of women when compared with men. For instance, meta-analytic research by Gouttebarge and colleagues[2] examined the prevalence of alcohol misuse, anxiety, depression, distress, and sleep disturbance among current and retired elite athletes. For current elite athletes, 28% of the participants sampled represented women. For retired elite athletes, 3% of the participants sampled represented women. Greater efforts are needed to recruit diverse samples of women athletes across all sports to better understand epidemiological trends of incidence and prevalence of mental health symptoms and disorders.

Among other demographic characteristics, limited data exist on (dis)ability, race, ethnicity, sexual orientation, and trans or gender non-conforming athletes. A recent study by Olive and colleagues[15] examined psychological distress, mental health caseness, risky alcohol consumption, body weight and shape dissatisfaction, self-esteem, life satisfaction, and problem gambling among 749 Australian para-athletes and athletes. Similar rates of mental health symptoms were found among both groups of individuals, except that para-athletes reported less alcohol consumption and lower levels of self-esteem. Similar findings were reported in another recent comparative cross-sectional study of Australian para-athletes and athletes.[16] Results from a narrative review on mental health symptoms and disorders among para-athletes by Swartz and colleagues[17] have found limited available epidemiological data prompting researchers to issue calls for greater efforts to better understand aspects of descriptive epidemiology (ie, incidence and prevalence of mental health symptoms and disorders) and analytic epidemiology (ie, factors responsible for mental health symptoms and disorders) in para-sport.

Epidemiological research has shown that racial-ethnic minority athletes are at high risk of mental health symptoms and disorders. From a student athlete perspective, although there has been a rise in the number of racial-ethnic minority athletes who compete within the National Collegiate Athletic Association (NCAA) since 2011, few studies have addressed racial and ethnic disparities in mental health.[18,19] Research by Ballesteros and colleagues[18] examined the prevalence of mental health symptoms and mental health service use among African American, Latin(x) American, and Asian American student athletes. Their research found that among African American student athletes, 22% were lonely, 14% were depressed, and 16% were overwhelmingly anxious. Among Latin(x) student athletes, 32% were lonely, 15% were depressed, and 21% were overwhelmingly anxious. Among Asian American student athletes, 26% were lonely, 18% were depressed, 18% were overwhelmingly anxious. Among the 3 groups of athletes, approximately 11% of individuals have received mental health service support. Other mental health studies conducted within the NCAA have shown an increased risk for racial-ethnic minority athletes. For instance, research on suicide has shown that African American student athletes are at greater risk (1.22/100,000) than white student athletes (0.87/100,000).[20] Increased risk of mental health symptoms and disorders may be due to experiences of racism within higher education and athletics.[18] Such disparities have resulted in calls for changes to mental health training including anti-racism and the history of institutional racism in sport, communication enhancements to address mental health symptoms and disorders and how to access services, quality improvement and accountability strategies to report and address racism, and clinical care practices.[21]

Few epidemiological research studies have examined the mental health of athletes where data on sexual orientation, trans identities, and gender non-conformity were collected. Work by Oftadeh-Moghadam and Gorczynski examined the mental health literacy, distress, help-seeking intentions, and well-being of semi-elite rugby players in the UK.[22] In addition to measures of mental health, they collected demographic data on ethnicity, sexual orientation, and whether individuals identified as trans, among other key demographic variables such as age, years of competition, mental health rating, education level, family history of mental health disorders, and previous diagnosis of mental health disorders. Of 208 participants, 195 identified as white (94%), 118 were heterosexual (57%), and no participants identified themselves as trans. With respect to sexual orientation, bisexual individuals were significantly more likely than heterosexual individuals to experience distress. Bisexual individuals also reported lower levels of well-being in comparison to heterosexual individuals. Research by Kroshus and Davoren[23] investigated the mental health and substance use of minority college students and athletes using pre-existing data from the National College Health Assessment administered through the American College Health Association. Their research examined responses from 19,869 varsity athletes and found that sexual minority athletes were at increased risk of experiencing mental health difficulties compared with their heterosexual peers. Substance use was higher among sexual minority athletes when compared with heterosexual individuals. Although no epidemiological data are available on the mental health of trans or gender non-conforming athletes, several researchers have reported that given risks of non-accidental violence and abuse non-athlete trans and gender non-conforming individuals face in society, these athletes are most likely at an increased risk of mental health symptoms and disorders and are also less likely to seek support.[24,25] Although steps are being taken within certain sporting organizations, such as the NCAA, to improve the inclusion and mental health of trans or gender non-conforming athletes,[26] the measurement of mental health symptoms and disorders and demographic data capture practices need to reflect these steps. Overall, research strategies rooted in comprehensive demographic information collection are needed to better understand the mental health needs of sexual and gender minority athletes.[27]

MENTAL HEALTH LITERACY, STIGMA, AND HELP SEEKING

Epidemiological evidence concerning mental health symptoms and disorders within sport provides the foundation for structuring mental health promotion strategies to aid those in greatest need. Such evidence helps not only identify groups who may be at greatest risk of mental health symptoms and disorders, but also helps identify and address potential individual and environmental factors associated with poor mental health and whether individuals will seek support.[28] Mental health promotion strategies within sport are largely designed around the concept of mental health literacy.[29] Mental health literacy refers to how individuals understand and recognize mental health symptoms and disorders, how they address both self- and public stigma with respect to mental health, and how they may make decisions to seek support from mental health professionals or other sources.[30] Within strategies that aim to improve mental health literacy, steps are designed to help individuals identify, question, and adjust their beliefs and perspectives about mental health symptoms and disorders, stigma, and mental health treatment.[29]

Mental health literacy has evolved from health literacy, which largely focused on functional literacy so that individuals could read basic health information often found in pamphlets and prescriptions to help improve their decision-making skills around their health.[31,32] Health literacy has moved on from its early functional literacy focus to incorporate aspects of information sourcing, information quality assessments, cognitive processing, broader social and environmental awareness and engagement around health, and health advocacy, be it for one's own health or the health of a community.[33–36] Health literacy's progressive path forward has fully embraced the social determinants of health as well as aspects of cultural competence, where information is designed and delivered in a specific manner to a particular population to address their unique health needs.

Mental health literacy within an elite sport context is also evolving.[10] Much like strategies to strengthen health literacy, strategies to strengthen mental health literacy have had to incorporate aspects of information dissemination channels, quality, and sources; address aspects of cognitive processing; and address challenges with help seeking, such as availability of treatment and wait times, administrative processes and clinical pathways with accessing treatment, and costs associated with treatment.

A major component of mental health literacy is to address stigma associated with mental health, both self- and public.[30] Stigma, in this context, represents stereotypes or prejudices individuals have toward mental health symptoms and disorders.[37,38] Individuals who hold such stereotypes or prejudices often view individuals living with mental health symptoms and disorders as inferior, when compared with some sort of perceived social norm or expectation. These forms of stereotypes or prejudices are known as public stigma.[39] When an individual begins to apply such stereotypes or prejudices to themselves and internalize these views, thereby altering their self-concept so that it reflects this perceived belief of inferiority of individuals living with mental health symptoms and disorders, this becomes a form of self-stigma.[40] Both self- and public stigma represent some of the greatest challenges that prevent athletes from seeking support or treatment of their mental health symptoms and disorders.[19,41]

It is believed that mental health promotion programs rooted in mental health literacy operate on a premise that through the delivery of information to individuals on mental health symptoms and disorders and treatment options, modifications are possible to stigmatized views individuals hold.[42] Such an approach, based on the Theory of Reasoned Action and the Theory of Planned Behaviour,[43,44] tries to address affective (ie, the emotions or feelings associated with someone or something) and instrumental (ie, whether someone or something serves a valuable or not valuable purpose) components of attitudes associated with stigma and help-seeking behaviors. Additionally, this information also tries to address normative beliefs (ie, what do *we* think *others* think about someone or something) and motivations to comply with others. Both normative beliefs and motivations to comply with others are components of subjective norms (ie, whether others will approve or disapprove of our beliefs or behaviors). Ultimately, changes to attitudes and subjective norms can impact intentions as well as overall behavior. For instance, information that humanizes athletes living with mental health symptoms and disorders and portrays them as valuable members of teams, leagues, and society along with positive roll modeling from others, including athletes and coaches, can begin to address behaviors that stigmatize individuals. This sort of approach can also impact how individuals view mental health services and forms of treatment. This theorical perspective positions mental health literacy as a static and unidirectional transmission of information, moving from information source to information recipient. However, changing behavior is extremely difficult, where recipients of information have established views, are influenced and motivated by individuals around them, and can challenge authority and information sources. As such, mental health promotion strategies based on mental health literacy need to be dynamic and be able to respond to existing held views.[45] For instance, information that comes from a mental health professional rather than a video advertisement can be adjusted and modified based on the recipient's responses and informational needs. However, future research needs to better understand different components within mental health literacy and how information is delivered and how it modifies stigmatized views and help-seeking behavior.[46] Such delivery is not only limited to mental health professionals, per se, but also unique methods currently being promoted using technology to engage individuals online, including the use of responsive chat programs that rely on artificial intelligence.[47]

Research within mental health literacy in sport has shown some positive results from health promotion strategies, including improved mental health symptom awareness and knowledge, increased referral knowledge, reduced stigma, and improved general help-seeking intentions.[48,49] Similar to health literacy, efforts have been made to ensure that mental health promotion strategies rooted in mental health literacy are culturally competent and responsive, meaning they understand the unique and complex mental health needs of a target population, provide information and support in culturally sensitive and appropriate ways, and offer diverse options from a variety of mental health professionals.[10,50,51] Ensuring cultural competence and responsiveness is an ongoing endeavor, one where revision is frequent and constant.

A further evolution to mental health literacy is the need to recognize organizational responsibility with respect to how guidelines, policies, regulations, practices, and systems allow individuals to find, access, use, and understand information about mental health and mental health symptoms and disorders and treatment options in an acceptable and comfortable manner.[52–56] Taking an organizational health literacy perspective to mental health argues that an organization adhere to and enact strategies that are set out in its values and mission statement with respect to mental health.[10,29] In a sense, information, strategies, and services must resemble policies and be inclusive of diverse health needs. Information must be straightforward, offer simple pathways to support, and offer individuals legitimate opportunities to access support. Organizational mental health literacy must be reviewed on a regular basis to ensure that cultural changes and practices as well as evolving mental health needs are identified, recognized, and acted upon. Overall, organizational mental health literacy tries to address and eliminate mental health victim blaming, where individuals blame themselves not only for the causes of their mental health symptoms and disorders, but also inabilities to address them. Further research is required to ensure that sporting organizations that have set out policies to address mental health symptoms and disorders measure overall organizational capacity to enact policies, including financial resources, appropriately trained staff, access to training and professional development, and opportunities for interprofessional collaboration.[57] Ultimately, organizations must embrace change, examine and address areas of individual resistance to change, and help design and create cultural climates that support the mental health of athletes.

DISCUSSION

Mental health symptoms and disorders present risks to athletes that threaten their time in and outside of sport. Much of the epidemiological evidence collected has demonstrated that elite athletes are as likely as those outside of sport to experience mental health symptoms and disorders.[1,3,12] Deficits within the epidemiological evidence collected so far has shown that little information is currently available concerning (dis)ability, race, ethnicity, sexual orientation, and trans or gender non-conforming athletes. These deficits in knowledge unfortunately limit the creation of culturally competent and responsive mental health promotion programs and services.[28] Both descriptive and analytic epidemiological evidence is needed concerning diverse and representative populations. Such research will not only render a better understanding of trends of mental health symptoms and disorders across time in different geographic locations, but it will also provide an identification of risk factors and determinants associated with mental health symptoms and disorders.[28] Collection of such demographic information is needed within future research programs as well as part of good clinical record keeping. Lastly, nearly all epidemiological research studies that have examined the mental health symptoms and disorders of elite athletes have taken place in developed economies of the world.[2] Geographic diversity and representation of data is also needed for a better understanding of the incidence and prevalence of mental health symptoms and disorders around the world.[10]

With respect to mental health literacy within sport, research has shown positive outcomes with respect to increased knowledge of mental health symptoms and disorders, increased referral knowledge, reduced stigma, and improved general help-seeking intentions.[48,49] Mental health literacy needs to be a priority for sport organizations who have a responsibility to ensure that information concerning mental health and service provisions is easy to find, access, use, and has a simple pathway to support.[10,29] Researchers need to ensure that future research helps create theoretically driven and culturally competent information and services that support the unique mental health needs of diverse populations. Much like the future of epidemiological practice within the mental health of sport, culturally competent demographic design that addresses aspects of (dis)ability, race, ethnicity, sexual orientation, and trans or gender non-conforming athletes needs to be applied to work within mental health literacy evaluation. Unique strategies to disseminate information, including methods that use artificial intelligence, need further evaluation.[47] Measures of organizational capacity among sports organizations are also needed to ensure that enacted policies concerning mental health are being followed and that information and services are accessible.

SUMMARY

Although there is a great deal of data about the incidence and prevalence of certain mental health symptoms and disorders, much of the current knowledge is limited to men. Strategies are needed to better understand the epidemiology of mental health symptoms and disorders in relation to (dis)ability, race, ethnicity, sexual orientations, and genders. Mental health promotion strategies rooted in mental health literacy can help improve knowledge of mental health, address stigma, and enhance help-seeking behaviors. Organizational responsibility is needed to ensure mental health promotion programs that are designed around mental health literacy principals ensure individuals receive information that is easy to understand, accessible, and provides a clear path to timely support.

CLINICS CARE POINTS

- Ensure diverse representation of athletes in epidemiological research.
- Collect demographic data concerning (dis)ability, race, ethnicity, sexual orientation, and gender.
- Clinical pathways to seeking mental health support needs to be easy to find, access, simple, and offer individuals access in a timely, acceptable, and comfortable manner.

DISCLOSURE

The authors have nothing to disclose.

REFERENCES

1. Reardon CL, Hainline B, Aron CM, et al. Mental health in elite athletes: international olympic committee consensus statement (2019). Br J Sports Med 2019; 53(11):667–99.
2. Gouttebarge V, Castaldelli-Maia JM, Gorczynski P, et al. Occurrence of mental health symptoms and disorders in current and former elite athletes: a systematic review and meta-analysis. Br J Sports Med 2019;53(11):700–6.
3. Rice SM, Gwyther K, Santesteban-Echarri O, et al. Determinants of anxiety in elite athletes: a systematic review and meta-analysis. Br J Sports Med 2019;53(11): 722–30.
4. Stambulova NB, Wylleman P. Athletes' career development and transitions. In: Papaioannou A, Hackfort D, editors. Routledge companion to sport and exercise psychology. Oxforshire, UK: Routledge; 2014. p. 605–21.
5. World Health Organization. Strengthening mental health promotion. In World Health Organization Fact sheet, No. 220. 2001. Available at: https://www.euro.who.int/__data/assets/pdf_file/0017/348011/Fact-sheet-SDG-Mental-health-UPDATE-02-05-2018.pdf. Accessed March 20, 2023.
6. Keyes CLM. Social well-being. Soc Psychol Q 1998;61(2):121–40.
7. Walsh DW, Ferrara M, Arlinghaus KR, et al. Sport: a holistic approach to lifestyle medicine. Am J Lifestyle Med 2022;16(4):439–42.
8. American Psychiatric Association. Diagnostic and statistical manual of mental disorders (DSM-5). Washington, DC, USA: American Psychiatric Publishing; 2013.
9. Purcell R, Gwyther K, Rice SM. Mental health in elite athletes: increased awareness requires an early intervention framework to respond to athlete needs. Sports Med Open 2019;5(1):46.
10. Gorczynski P, Currie A, Gibson K, et al. Developing mental health literacy and cultural competence in elite sport. J Appl Sport Psychol 2021;33(4):387–401.

11. Schaal K, Tafflet M, Nassif H, et al. Psychological balance in high level athletes: gender-based differences and sport-specific patterns. PLoS One 2011;6(5): e19007.
12. Gorczynski PF, Coyle M, Gibson K. Depressive symptoms in high-performance athletes and non-athletes: a comparative meta-analysis. Br J Sports Med 2017; 51(18):1348–54.
13. Gorczynski P. Major depressive disorder and depressive symptoms. In: Reardon CL, editor. Mental health care for elite athletes. Berlin, Germany: Springer; 2022. p. 51–9. https://doi.org/10.1007/978-3-031-08364-8_6.
14. Pascoe M, Pankowiak A, Woessner M, et al. Gender-specific psychosocial stressors influencing mental health among women elite and semielite athletes: a narrative review. Br J Sports Med 2022;56:1381–7.
15. Olive LS, Rice S, Butterworth M, et al. Do rates of mental health symptoms in currently competing elite athletes in paralympic sports differ from non-para-athletes? Sports Med Open 2021;7(1):62.
16. Olive LS, Rice SM, Gao C, et al. Risk and protective factors for mental ill-health in elite para- and non-para athletes. Front Psychol 2022;13:939087.
17. Swartz L, Hunt X, Bantjes J, et al. Mental health symptoms and disorders in paralympic athletes: a narrative review. Br J Sports Med 2019;53:737–40.
18. Ballesteros J, Tran AGTT. Under the face mask: racial-ethnic minority student-athletes and mental health use. J Am Coll Health 2020;68:169–75.
19. Moreland JJ, Coxe KA, Yang J. Collegiate athletes' mental health services utilization: a systematic review of conceptualizations, operationalizations, facilitators, and barriers. J Sport Health Sci 2018;7(1):58–69.
20. Rao AL, Asif IM, Drezner JA, et al. Suicide in national collegiate athletic association (NCAA) athletes: a 9-year analysis of the NCAA resolutions database. Sports Health 2015;7:452–7.
21. Kroshus E, Coakley S, Conway D, et al. Addressing mental health needs of NCAA student-athletes of colour: foundational concepts from the NCAA Summit on Diverse Student-Athlete Mental Health and Well-Being. Br J Sports Med 2023; 57:137–45.
22. Oftadeh-Moghadam S, Gorczynski P. Mental health literacy, help-seeking, and mental health outcomes in women rugby players. WSPAJ 2021;30(1).
23. Kroshus E, Davoren AK. Mental health and substance use of sexual minority college athletes. J Am Coll Health 2016;64:371–9.
24. Kamis D, Glick ID. Improving competition and mental health for transgender athletes. Phys Sportsmed 2021. https://doi.org/10.1080/00913847.2021.1949250.
25. Jones BA, Arcelus J, Bouman WP, et al. Sport and transgender people: a systematic review of the literature relating to sport participation and competitive sport policies. Sports Med 2017;47:701–16.
26. Kroshus E, Ackerman KE, Brown M, et al. Improving inclusion and well-being of trans and gender nonconforming collegiate student–athletes: foundational concepts from the national collegiate athletic association summit on gender identity and student–athlete participation. Br J Sports Med 2023. https://doi.org/10.1136/bjsports-2022-106392.
27. Gorczynsk P, Reardon CL, Miller Aron C. Lesbian, gay, bisexual, trans, and queer mental health in elite sport: a review. Advances in Psychiatry and Behavioral Health 2022;2(1):9–16.
28. Gorczynski P, Webb T. Developing a mental health research agenda for football referees. Soccer Soc 2021;22(6):655–62.

29. Gorczynski P, Gibson K, Thelwell R, et al. The BASES expert statement on mental health literacy in elite sport. The Sport and Exercise Scientist 2019;59:6–7.
30. Jorm AF, Korten AE, Jacomb PA, et al. "Mental health literacy": a survey of the public's ability to recognise mental disorders and their beliefs about the effectiveness of treatment. Med J Aust 1997;166(4):182–6.
31. Kutcher S, Wei Y, Coniglio C. Mental Health Literacy: Past, Present, and Future. Can J Psychiatry 2016;61(3):154–8.
32. American Medical Association Ad Hoc Committee on Health Literacy. Report of the Scientific Council on Health Literacy. JAMA 1992;281(6):552–7.
33. Canadian Alliance on Mental Illness and Mental Health (CAMIMH). National integrated framework for enhancing mental health literacy in Canada: Final report. CAMIMH 2008.
34. World Health Organization. Health promotion glossary. 1998. Available at: https://www.who.int/publications/i/item/WHO-HPR-HEP-98.1. Accessed March 20, 2023.
35. Jorm AF. The concept of mental health literacy. In: Okan O, Bauer U, Levin-Zamir D, et al, editors. International handbook of health literacy: research, practice and policy across the life-span. Policy Press; 2019. p. 53–66.
36. Jorm AF. Mental health literacy: empowering the community to take action for better mental health. Am Psychol 2012;67(3):231–43.
37. Ahmedani BK. Mental health stigma: society, individuals, and the profession. J Soc Work Values Ethics 2011;8(2):41–416.
38. Dudley JR. Confronting stigma within the services system. Soc Work 2000;45:449–55.
39. Parcesepe AM, Cabassa LJ. Public stigma of mental illness in the United States: a systematic literature review. Adm Policy Ment Health 2013;40(5):384–99.
40. Corrigan PW, Rao D. On the self-stigma of mental illness: stages, disclosure, and strategies for change. Can J Psychiatry 2012;57(8):464–9.
41. Castaldelli-Maia JM, Gallinaro JGDME, Falcão RS, et al. Mental health symptoms and disorders in elite athletes: a systematic review on cultural influencers and barriers to athletes seeking treatment. Br J Sports Med 2019;53:707–21.
42. Adams C, Gringart E, Strobel N. Explaining adults' mental health help-seeking through the lens of the theory of planned behavior: a scoping review. Syst Rev 2022;11:160.
43. Ajzen I. The theory of planned behavior. Organ Behav Hum Decis Process 1991;50(2):179–211.
44. Ajzen I, Fishbein M. Understanding attitudes and predicting social behavior. Englewood Cliffs: Prentice-Hall; 1980.
45. Bamgbade BA, Harrison TC, Barner JC. Mental health literacy theory: a critical evaluation. Value Health J 2014;17(3):PA33.
46. Spiker DA, Hammer JH. Mental health literacy as theory: current challenges and future directions. J Ment Health 2019;28(3):238–42.
47. Graham S, Depp C, Lee EE, et al. Artificial intelligence for mental health and mental illnesses: an overview. Curr Psychiatry Rep 2019;21(11):116.
48. Breslin G, Shannon S, Cummings M, et al. An updated systematic review of interventions to increase awareness of mental health and well-being in athletes, coaches, officials and parents. Syst Rev 2022;11(1):99.
49. Breslin G, Shannon S, Haughey T, et al. A systematic review of interventions to increase awareness of mental health and well-being in athletes, coaches and officials. Syst Rev 2017;6:177.
50. Moore MA, Gorczynski P, Miller Aron C. Mental health literacy in sport: the role of the social work profession. Soc Work 2022;67(3):298–300.

51. Moore M, Gorczynski P, Aron C, et al. Leaving professional competition on the field: professional collaboration in promoting college athlete mental health. Front Psychiatry 2022;13:1079057.
52. Farmanova E, Bonneville L, Bouchard L. Organizational health literacy: review of theories, frameworks, guides, and implementation issues. Inquiry 2018;55. https://doi.org/10.1177/0046958018757848. 46958018757848.
53. Brach C, Keller D, Hernandez LM, et al. Ten attributes of health literate healthcare organizations. Washington, DC, USA: Institute of Medicine; 2012. Available at: https://nam.edu/wp-content/uploads/2015/06/BPH_Ten_HLit_Attributes.pdf. Accessed March 20, 2023.
54. Brega AG, Hamer MK, Albright K, et al. Organizational health literacy: quality improvement measures with expert consensus. Health Lit Res Pract 2019;3(2): e127–46.
55. Sentell T, Foss-Durant A, Patil U, et al. Organizational health literacy: opportunities for patient-centered care in the wake of COVID-19. Qual Manag Health Care 2021;30(1):49–60.
56. Smith CN, Gorczynski P, Thomas JD. The ever-evolving nature of health literacy in organizations: a commentary on the 2021 JPHMP article "updating health literacy for healthy people 2030". J Public Health Manag Pract 2022;28(6):E804–7.
57. Lombardi MM, Spratling RG, Pan W, et al. Measuring organizational capacity to accelerate health care innovation in academic health centers. Qual Manag Health Care 2018;27(1):1–7.

Management of Mental Health Challenges in Athletes
Screening, Pharmacology, and Behavioral Approaches

Carla D. Edwards, MSc, MD, FRCPC

KEYWORDS

• Athlete • Sport • Mental health • Treatment • Mental illness • Formulation

KEY POINTS

- Athletes are vulnerable to exceptional stressors and the same mental health challenges as the general population.
- Pre-participation screening with single- or multi-tool instruments provides an opportunity to detect and address the presence of mental health symptoms in athletes.
- Comprehensive systems supporting athlete mental health include screening, assessment, referral, management, and return to play pathways.
- Biopsychosocial formulation with cultural considerations helps the clinician to develop an individualized comprehensive management plan.
- Clinical practice guidelines for pharmacologic and non-pharmacological management of mental illnesses should be applied to athletes, with consideration for adverse effects that could compromise sport performance such as sedation, weight gain, activation, and prohibited drug lists.

INTRODUCTION

Athletes are an incredibly motivated group that is perpetually engaged in training for dominance in skill, strength, endurance, and execution often while balancing many additional responsibilities. Although high-profile athletes are sometimes assumed to live fun, luxurious, care-free lifestyles, they are vulnerable to exceptional stressors and the same mental health challenges as the general population.[1,2] The use of a biopsychosocial framework can assist in understanding the factors contributing to the

Department of Psychiatry and Behavioural Neurosciences, McMaster University, St. Joseph's Healthcare Hamilton West 5th Campus, Administration B3, 100 West 5th Street, Hamilton, Ontario L8N 3K7, Canada
E-mail address: edwardcd@mcmaster.ca
Twitter: @Edwards10Carla (C.D.E.)

Clin Sports Med 43 (2024) 13–31
https://doi.org/10.1016/j.csm.2023.06.006
0278-5919/24/© 2023 Elsevier Inc. All rights reserved.

mental health challenges and facilitate the development of a targeted management approach.

This article navigates through essential aspects of mental health assessment and management for athletes, beginning with an overview of common challenges faced by athletes.

BACKGROUND
The Role of Adversity

There are many common sources of adversity that can be experienced by anyone, including deaths, relationship losses, economic hardship, and job loss. Abuse, neglect, mental illness, suicide, and exposure to domestic violence are additional stressors that can impact a person's function and long-term well-being.[3] Racial and ethnic disparities are well described across several types of adversity, including economic hardship, parental divorce or separation, living with someone experiencing mental illness, parental incarceration, and experiencing discrimination.[4] Many of these elements are referred to as adverse childhood experiences.

Athletes have several unique stressors that can compromise their capacity for resilience and subsequent mental health and performance. Challenges faced by athletes, defined as elements that can distract, cause stress, test resilience, and ultimately impact performance and quality of life, are summarized in **Box 1** and described below.

1. *Finances*: Although many believe that athletes live a glamorous life—free of financial stressors—there are many financial challenges that they face.
   - *Sponsorship*: May be the main source of income for athletes at early stages of their careers, or if they compete in sports that are not associated with team-based contracts, for example, tennis, triathlon, and athletics. Even well-established athletes can receive substantial income from sponsorships. Sponsorship deals are often contingent on performance, image, and behavior; and athletes often feel "under the microscope" when trying to impress sponsors.

Box 1
Unique stressors that can compromise athlete resilience, mental health, and performance

Challenges faced by athletes that can distract, cause stress, test resilience, and impact performance and quality of life

1. Finances
   - Sponsorship
   - Supporting families
   - Supporting the elite athlete lifestyle
   - Supporting the athlete social lifestyle
   - Wealth management

2. Performance pressure

3. **Balancing demands of the elite athlete lifestyle and family**

4. Injuries/illness

5. Transitions
   - Career stage
   - Role
   - Trades
   - Life after sport

6. **Commodification**

- *Supporting the family:* Sport provides many athletes with an opportunity to leave states of poverty, unstable housing, and family adversity (including unemployment, single parents, incarceration, and domestic violence). When athletes start to be paid as a professional, they either feel obligated, or are expected, to financially support their immediate and extended families.
- *Supporting the elite athlete lifestyle:* High-performance, elite, and professional athletes need a team around them to keep them on top of their training, physical treatment, media interviews, social media guidance, and travel. For some sports, athletes have to pay their coaches and training support staff themselves. Athletes who have multimillion dollar contracts also need help managing that income, finding appropriate/desired housing, and "keeping up" with that lifestyle, including vehicles and personal possessions.
- *Supporting the athlete social lifestyle:* Athletes sometimes need to maintain a "persona" that is associated with their position in the sports world. Culture in professional sports establishes expectations for standards to meet, including social events, appearances (for sponsors), social media engagement, and parties.
- *Wealth management:* Professional athletes can find themselves having to manage substantial amounts of money, usually without any relevant experience. With a good advisor, athletes can develop a sound approach to financial management. Without appropriate guidance, vast amounts of wealth can be lost or stolen. Athletes can also become targets of people who try to manipulate them and funnel money away into their own pockets.

2. *Performance pressure:* Pressure for optimal performance comes from all sides— family, friends, spouses, teammates, coaches, organizations, sponsors, the media, communities, countries, and within the athlete themselves.
3. *Balancing demands of the elite athlete lifestyle and family:* Competing in high-performance sport requires many sacrifices, which begin early in childhood with dozens of hours training, weeks and months traveling, and training occurring throughout the calendar year. Most Olympic and professional athletes reach the peaks of their careers during times in their lives when their friends are in school, getting married, or having children—while they are busy playing lengthy seasons, traveling to international competitions, or living their lives according to Olympic "quads." Some athletes live away from their spouse and children during their seasons, which can become extremely challenging for everyone. Others sacrifice "everything" to fully immerse themselves in the elite athlete lifestyle. Well-known athletes can also struggle to engage in "normal society" without having people follow them, take their pictures, and invade their personal lives.
4. *Injuries/illness:* Athletes depend on their brains and bodies to be healthy to perform. Injuries that lead to prolonged absences from training or competition can lead to mental health challenges such as anxiety, depression, and insomnia. The nature and severity of the injury, timing in the season, reinjury status, potential impact on contract/role on team/future career, and prognosis for recovery are important factors.
5. *Transitions:* Transition points in an athlete's career can create challenges, depending on the context and timing:
   - *Career stage:* An athlete's elite or professional career is time limited. As the athlete navigates toward the latter stages in their careers, it is important for them to have support in exploring their readiness to retire and build other skills or interests to ease the transition out of their sport.
   - *Role:* The natural transition for an athlete through their careers flows from being a relative unknown, to a contributor, to "star" status (for some), and then the other

side when younger athletes become the latest headlines and the future of the sport. This change in role may be difficult for some athletes.

- *Trades:* The business side of sports creates an environment in which athletes can be traded—often without choice and with little notice.
- *Life after sport:* Many athletes worry about what life will look like when their careers have ended, and they leave the sport. Some athletes prepare for this transition by meeting with advisors, building skills and knowledge before leaving their sport, and having a plan well in advance. Leaving a life of elite or professional sports can create a significant void in postretirement athletes, which they will need to learn to fill as they form a new relationship with sports and physical activity.

6. *Commodification*: Athletes may be treated like assets as opposed to individuals with rights, which increases the risk of their personal needs and rights being neglected or invalidated.[5]

Additional Potentially Contributing Elements

Other elements that may lead to mental health challenges in athletes include maltreatment,[5] genetics, sport-related environmental factors, performance failure, success at a young age, fame, and traumatic brain injury.[6] Pressure and challenging lifestyle conditions for high-achieving youths in sport, performing arts, or academics may also place them at risk of maltreatment and its subsequent effects on mental health.[7]

SCREENING

Screening tools are instruments that can be used at contact points of care to explore the presence of symptoms; however, questionnaires alone are insufficient to support the mental health needs of athletes. A clearly identified pathway for interpretation of results and subsequent actions based on those results must be established.

Screening tools are validated, free and easy to access, and simple to administer. Incorporating them into pre-participation screening is a simple way to detect problems and initiate support. Administering screening tools following injury or adversity can also capture evolving struggles before they develop into severe illness or impairment.

Screening Tool Types

Good screening tools should be easy to administer, straight-forward to interpret, and validated to identify potential challenges early enough to facilitate intervention. The purpose of these tools is to identify individuals at risk of having specific illnesses, which should then prompt further referral or exploration to establish diagnoses. Screening tools may assess for symptoms of specific areas of difficulty (ie, depression) or more general struggles (ie, psychological distress). Although research into athlete mental health is burgeoning, only a small number of screening tools have been studied and validated in the athlete population. Screening tools that are commonly used with athletes can be found in **Table 1**.

In 2019, the International Olympic Committee Mental Health Working Group (IOC MHWG) published a consensus statement on the mental health of elite athletes, which identified the importance of early identification and management of mental health challenges in athletes.[25] This was followed by the release of the Sport Mental Health Assessment Tool (SMHAT-1) and Sport Mental Health Recognition Tool (SMHRT-1) in 2020.[26] Although the SMHAT-1 has several screening tools embedded in the three-stage assessment,[8] the SMHRT-1 serves as a guide that can be used by athletes, coaches, family members, and all other health professionals and members of the athlete's entourage to recognize mental health problems and understand when to seek support.

Table 1	
Tools commonly used to screen for mental health symptoms in athletes	
Screening Tool	**Target Symptoms/Disorders**
SMHAT-1[8]	Embedded tools screen for psychological strain, depression, anxiety, sleep problems, disordered eating/eating disorder, bipolar disorder, attention-deficit hyperactivity disorder, post-traumatic stress disorder, psychotic disorder
PHQ-9[9]	Depression
GAD-7[10]	Anxiety
ASSQ[11]	Sleep problems
CAGE-AID[12]	Substance misuse (alcohol)
AUDIT-C[13]	Substance misuse (drugs)
BEDA-Q[14]	Disordered eating/eating disorder
BDSA[15]	Depression (validated in athletes)
MDQ[16]	Bipolar disorder
Mini-SPIN[17]	Social anxiety
SAPAS[18,19]	Personality disorders
CET-A[20,21]	Compulsive exercise (adapted for athletes)
YBOCS[22,23]	Obsessive compulsive disorder
CCAPS-34[24]	Depression, generalized anxiety, social anxiety, academic distress, eating concerns, frustration/anger, and alcohol use

Combined Screening Tool

Sport Mental Health Assessment Tool-1: The SMHAT-1 is a three-stage tool that can be completed on paper or online. [8] It can be used by sports medicine physicians and other licensed/registered health professionals, but the clinical assessment (and related management) within the SMHAT-1 should be conducted by sports medicine physicians and/or licensed/registered mental health professionals.

In Step 1, all athletes complete the Athlete Psychological Strain Questionnaire which has a defined threshold. If this threshold is surpassed, the athlete is then directed to complete Step 2, which consists of six additional embedded screening tools. These embedded screens include tools that assess for symptoms of depression (Patient Health Questionnaire-9 [PHQ-9]),[9] anxiety (Generalized Anxiety Disorder [GAD-7]),[10] sleep problems (Athlete Sleep Screening Questionnaire [ASSQ]),[11] alcohol use disorders (Alcohol Use Disorders Identification Tool [AUDIT-C]),[13] other substance misuse (Cut Down/Annoyed/Guilty/Eye-opener Adapted to Incude Drugs [CAGE-AID]),[12] and disordered eating (Brief Eating Disorder Assessment Questionnaire [BEDA-Q]).[14,27] Each of these embedded screens also have thresholds that define severity of symptoms, which guide subsequent clinical decisions. The SMHAT-1 features an algorithm that outlines interventions (Step 3) given specific scoring outcomes. Additional screening tools are embedded for athletes registering scores beyond a specified level, which further evaluate for Attention Deficit Hyperactivity Disorder (ADHD) (Adult ADHD Self-Report Scale: ASRS-v1.1),[28,29] bipolar disorder (BD; Mood Disorder Questionnaire),[30,31] post-traumatic stress disorder (PTSD),[20,21] gambling,[32,33] and psychosis.[34,35]

Individual Screening Tools

Individual tools can be used on their own or as part of a collection of tools for a more comprehensive screen. Each of the individual tools embedded in the SMHAT-1 are available online and have clearly defined thresholds (other than the BEDA-Q). The threshold for the BEDA-Q was assigned by the IOC MHWG for the SMHAT-1 based on articles that were available for review.

Patient Health Questionnaire-9: This depression screening tool can assess for the presence and severity of depressive symptoms. Threshold values are defined as none-minimal (0–4), mild (5–9), moderate (10–14), moderate–severe (15–19), and severe (20–27).[9]

Generalized Anxiety Disorder: This tool screens for the presence and severity of symptoms of anxiety. Threshold values are defined as minimal (0–4), mild (5–9), moderate (10–14), and severe (15–21).[10]

Athlete Sleep Satisfaction Questionnaire: This tool was developed to detect clinically significant sleep disturbances and daytime dysfunction and to provide interventions based on the type and severity of the problem that is identified in an athlete population. The SMHAT-1 contains a new five-item version of the ASSQ that categorizes athlete sleep problems as none (0–4), mild (5–7), moderate (8–10), and severe (11–17).[11]

AUDIT-C: This tool is a brief screening instrument that identifies individuals who are engaging in hazardous drinking patterns or have active alcohol use disorders (including alcohol abuse or dependence). Each AUDIT-C question has five answer choices valued from 0 to 4 points. In men, a score of four or more is considered positive, whereas in women, a score of three or more is considered positive. Positive scores are considered optimal for identifying hazardous drinking or active alcohol use disorders. Higher scores suggest more unsafe drinking patterns.[13]

CAGE-AID: This tool was adapted from the CAGE questionnaire, which was originally developed to assess for alcohol use disorders. Scores of 1 or more should prompt consideration of referral for further assessment by mental health or addictions professionals. The version of the CAGE-AID embedded in the SMHAT-1 contains examples of illicit substances listed on the form for easy identification of substances used by the athlete.[12]

Brief Eating Disorder Assessment Questionnaire: This tool is a brief questionnaire that can be used to distinguish between female athletes with or without an eating disorder.[14]

Baron Depression Screener for Athletes (Baron): This screener was developed for, and validated in, the athlete population. Higher scores represent more severe depressive symptoms across elements including mood, fatigue, sport-related anhedonia, self-image, suicidal ideation, and substance abuse.[15]

Mood Disorder Questionnaire: This brief questionnaire has a high rate of accuracy in identifying the presence of symptoms consistent with BD types 1 and 2 as well as BD not otherwise specified.[16]

Mini-Social Phobia Inventory: Mini-SPIN (social anxiety disorder): This three-item screener is a brief questionnaire that is used to identify individuals who are at risk of having social anxiety disorder.[17]

Standardized Assessment of Personality: Abbreviated Scale: This is a brief tool to screen for the presence of personality disorders in a general clinical setting.[18,19]

Compulsive Exercise Test: Athlete version: This tool was designed to assess for the core features of problematic exercise in the eating disorder population.[36–38]

Yale-Brown Obsessive-Compulsive Scale: This questionnaire assesses for historic and current obsessions and compulsions, degree of symptom severity, time consumed by symptoms, and magnitude of distress experienced.[22,23]

Counseling Center Assessment of Psychological Symptoms: The Counseling Center Assessment of Psychological Symptoms (CCAPS-34) is a remotely managed 34-item multidimensional assessment instrument that contains seven subscales. The assessment provides percentile scores in the domains of depression, generalized anxiety, social anxiety, academic distress, eating concerns, frustration/anger, and alcohol use in addition to an overall distress index (CCAPS Web site).[24]

Pathways Beyond Screening

Screening tools are useful not only for identifying presence of symptoms but also for indicating severity of symptoms. This can be used to determine next steps in the athlete support pathway. Mild to moderate severity can sometimes be managed very appropriately in the sports medicine physician's office, depending on knowledge base, skill set, and comfort level. Athletes who demonstrate mild to moderate depression or anxiety symptoms may also benefit from referral to a mental health clinician such as a social worker, registered psychotherapist, or psychologist. Athletes who score in the high-moderate to severe range in any of these tools should be referred to a psychiatrist for further assessment and treatment. A sports psychiatrist would be able to provide a sport-informed assessment and work with the sports medicine physician, interdisciplinary support team, coaches, and the athletes to develop a comprehensive approach to balancing treatment and sport.

DIAGNOSING MENTAL ILLNESS

Comprehensive mental health assessment for diagnostic purposes entails a full clinical interview by a qualified mental health professional such as a psychiatrist, with collateral information from partners or family members as available and appropriate. In the sport setting, collateral information may also be provided by coaches or members of the interdisciplinary support team (either solicited, with consent, or unsolicited). Additional structured diagnostic instruments may be used in the assessment process. Medical evaluation, including laboratory investigations and diagnostic imaging, may be included in the diagnostic workup to explore potential medical causes for psychiatric symptoms.

The key elements that should be included in the mental health clinical interview for diagnostic assessment of an athlete are listed in **Box 2**.

Select medical conditions associated with psychiatric symptoms are listed in **Table 2**.

BIOPSYCHOSOCIAL FORMULATION

To facilitate an understanding of the multifactorial elements that lead to the athlete's present struggles as well as the features that contribute to ongoing challenges, balanced with the athlete's inherent strengths, a biopsychosocial formulation is a valuable tool to use. Effective comprehensive mental health care of athletes should consider and incorporate biopsychosocial and cultural factors in the context of the athlete.[40]

The biopsychosocial formulation is built on information collected during the clinical assessment process, which can be organized in a grid format for more facile interpretation and synthesis. Biological, psychological, and social elements populate the column headings, whereas predisposing, precipitating, perpetuating, and protective factors demarcate the rows of the grid.[41] The biopsychosocial grid model with elements to consider for each domain can be found in **Table 3**.

Cultural elements should be considered during diagnostic assessment and formulation.[44] A standardized approach to cultural formulation was adopted by the American Psychiatric Association in the *Diagnostic and Statistical Manual of Mental Disorders*, Fifth Edition,[45] which provides a systematic outline for incorporating

---

Box 2
Key elements that should be included in the clinical mental health interview for diagnostic assessment of an athlete

Recommended components of the mental health assessment of athletes

1. *Identification:* including name, age, living situation (type of residence, who they live with)

2. Primary complaint/reason for referral

3. *History of presenting illness:* including primary symptom cluster, associated symptoms, exploration of diagnostic criteria, current comorbidities

4. *Sport history:* including influence of sport on mental health challenges or vice versa. Explore current sport, support system, primary care providers, history of maltreatment, dynamic in sport environment, response to sport-related adversity

5. *Screening:* explore previous/recurrent/comorbid psychiatric diagnoses

6. *Past psychiatric history:* including previous diagnoses, hospitalizations, self-harm, suicide attempts, previous assessments, or therapeutic relationships with mental health professionals

7. *Past medical history:* including thyroid disease, traumatic brain injury, iron deficiency, low energy availability, vitamin B12 deficiency, sleep apnea, previous surgeries

8. *Medications:* including past medications, optimization of trials, adherence, adverse effects; present prescribed and over the counter medications, adherence, and response; herbal supplements, vitamins, minerals, workout supplements, homeopathic preparations

9. Allergies and adverse reactions to medications or substances

10. *Substance use:* including caffeine, alcohol, cannabis, unprescribed medications, stimulants, illicit drugs, performance enhancing drugs (including anabolic steroids)

11. *Family psychiatric history:* including mood, anxiety, or psychotic disorders, psychiatric hospitalizations, suicide, violence, ADHD, learning disorders, substance misuse, and undiagnosed (but suspected) psychiatric illness

12. *Social history:* including cultural elements, relationship development, academic and employment history, family sport history, influence of family on sport experience and identity

13. *Forensic history:* including history of Involvement with the legal system, incarceration, aggression, and anger management difficulties

14. *Mental status examination:* including descriptions of appearance, eye contact, speech patterns, orientation to person, place and time, thought content and formation, mood (subjective), affect (objective, including range and congruence with behavior and content being discussed), intellectual resources, insight, judgment, suicidal and homicidal ideation

---

culturally relevant information when conducting a diagnostic assessment. These elements are outlined in **Table 4**.

MANAGEMENT OF MENTAL HEALTH CHALLENGES

After exploration of the athlete's mental and physical health has been completed and the mental health challenge has been diagnosed or characterized, a comprehensive individualized management approach can be developed. Addressing medical challenges that have been identified may lessen or resolve some symptoms, if they were caused by the underlying medication condition. Persistent mental health challenges should be approached in a multidimensional fashion, considering elements identified in the biopsychosocial exploration as well as cultural contexts. Foundational wellness components such as sleep, nutrition, balance, self-care, relationships,

Table 2	
Select medical conditions associated with psychiatric symptoms[39]	
Medical Condition/Symptom	**Potential Psychiatric Symptoms**
Iron Deficiency	Depression
Vitamin B12 deficiency	Low energy
Hypothyroidism	Amotivation
Low energy availability	Poor concentration
Traumatic brain injury	Insomnia or hypersomnia
Obstructive sleep apnea	
Overtraining syndrome	
Chronic fatigue syndrome	
Infection	
Delirium	
Epilepsy	
Hypoxemia	
Autoimmune disorder	
Intoxication or withdrawal	
Medication side effects	
Hyperthyroidism	Anxiety
Traumatic brain injury	Hyperactivity
Delirium	Psychosis
Intoxication or withdrawal	Confusion
Medication side effects	Insomnia

spirituality, leisure activities, and healthy outlets should be reviewed regularly. Activities such as meditation, yoga, mindfulness, relaxation, journaling, and focused interests such as photography, painting, knitting, and cooking can provide additional opportunities for healthy social or individual endeavors. Specific therapeutic approaches may be recommended to address moderate to severe mental health challenges. These are classified as non-pharmacological or pharmacologic approaches.

Non-Pharmacological Approaches

Non-pharmacological approaches to mental health challenges can include foundational wellness components as well as psychotherapy. Although athletes represent a highly motivated group that regularly engages in goal setting and practice, they may be reluctant to engage in psychotherapy due to stigma, minimization of symptoms, and less positive attitudes toward mental health services than the general population.[48] Various types of psychotherapy have been found to be efficacious in treating mental health challenges and illnesses. Psychotherapy is delivered by trained professionals in a specified format that is typically offered in a defined number of sessions. Select types of psychotherapy and the challenges and illnesses they commonly target are listed in **Table 5**.

Cognitive behavior therapy (CBT) is founded on a model in which psychological challenges are based in part on distorted or unhelpful thought patterns and linked to learned patterns of unhelpful behavior.[57–59] Through the process of therapy, new ways of thinking (cognitive) and behaving (behavior) facilitate symptom relief. CBT has been shown to have large effect sizes for illnesses such as unipolar depression, panic disorder, and PTSD.[49] A specific type of CBT, exposure and response prevention, is the first-line psychotherapy for obsessive-compulsive disorder (OCD) and has been associated with large treatment effects.[58,59]

Dialectical behavior therapy was adapted from CBT and humanism to support suicidal and self-injuring individuals through skills including validation, mindfulness,

Table 3
Biopsychosocial formulation grid

	Biological	Psychological	Social
Predisposing factors	• Early temperament • Personality features • Family psychiatric history • Toxic exposures in utero • Birth complications • Developmental disorders • Medical illnesses (including traumatic brain injury) • Substance misuse • Neurodevelopmental history	• Attachment style[42] • Family behavior styles and structure • Emotional dysregulation • Cognitive style (eg, negative, rigid, inflexible, adaptable) • Self-image, self-esteem • Internalizing/externalizing tendencies	• Poverty • Low socioeconomic status • Teenage parenthood • Access to health care • Adverse childhood experiences[43]
Precipitating factors	• Medical illness or injury • New or increasing substance use • Treatment nonadherence • Hormonal changes • Sleep deprivation	• Any stressor that may trigger one or more psycho-emotional processes, including: • Cognitive: core beliefs, cognitive distortions • Dialectical: emotional dysregulation and dysfunction • Interpersonal: grief, loss, disagreement, change/transitions • Psychodynamic: unconscious conflicts, defenses; unconscious repetition of early relationship patterns	• Loss of significant relationship (eg, close family, partner, or friend) • Interpersonal violence • Work, academic, or financial stressors • Recent immigration, loss of home, loss of a supportive service • Recurrence of a previous stressful situation
Perpetuating factors	• Chronic illness • cognitive deficits • learning disorder • Suboptimal medication management • Suboptimal treatment or follow-up • Current substance misuse • Chronic medical problems, pain, cr disability	• Psychological processes that maintain the unwell state: • Cognitive: chronic negative thoughts • Dialectical: tendencies for seeking or rejecting help, chronic emotional dysregulation, poor distress tolerance • Interpersonal: Chronic or unresolved dysfunctional relationships, interpersonal conflict, role transition	• Chronic relationship discord • Lack of empathy or support from family/friends • Dangerous or hostile neighborhood • Trans-generational problems of immigration • Lack of culturally competent services • Ongoing transitions and stressors • Economic hardship

	• *Psychodynamic*: recurring themes, chronic primitive defenses • Beliefs about self, others, and the world • Internalized concepts • Maladaptive coping mechanisms • Limited or lack of insight • Personality traits • Attachment style	• Reflective capacity • Emotional regulation skills • Adaptive coping mechanisms • Positive sense of self • Psychological mindedness • Cognitive flexibility • Previous positive response to psychotherapy • Good insight • Good coping skills	• Positive relationships • Supportive community, including family/friends • Religious/spiritual beliefs • Good interpersonal supports • Financial resources/disability support • Treatment team
Protective factors	• Good health • Absence of family psychiatric history • Good response to treatment (including medication) • Previous remission • Average or above average intellectual resources • Resilience • Talents/abilities • Absence of substance misuse		

Table 4
Systematic outline for incorporating culturally relevant information when conducting a multiaxial diagnostic assessment

Cultural Elements	Clinically Relevant Features[44–47]
Cultural identity of the person	• The person's ethnic or cultural reference groups • For immigrants and ethnic minorities, note the degree of involvement with their culture of origin and host culture (where applicable) • Language ability, use, and preference (including multilingualism).
Cultural explanations of the person's illness, including cultural concepts of distress	• The predominant idioms of distress through which symptoms or the need for social support are communicated (eg, "nerves," possessing spirits, somatic complaints, inexplicable misfortune) • The meaning and perceived severity of the individual's symptoms in relation to norms of the cultural reference group • Local illness category used by the individual's family and community to identify a condition (eg, ataque de nervios in the Caribbean population, Latin American and Latin Mediterranean populations, Dhat in the Asian Indian population, nervios in the Latin American population, shenjing shuairuo in the Chinese population, susto in the Latino American, Mexican, Central and South American populations, and taijin kyofusho in the Japanese population.[47] The perceived causes or explanatory models that the individual and the reference group use to explain the illness • Current preferences for and past experiences with professional and popular sources of care
Cultural factors related to psychosocial environment and level of functioning	• Culturally relevant interpretations of social stressors, available social supports, and levels of functioning and disability • Include stresses in the local social environment and the role of religion and kin networks in providing emotional, instrumental, and informational support
Cultural elements of the relationship between client and clinician	• Differences in culture and social status between client and clinician • Identify any problems these differences may cause in diagnosis and treatment (for example, difficulty communicating in the client's first language, eliciting symptoms or understanding their cultural significance, negotiating an appropriate relationship or level of intimacy, determining whether a behavior is normative or pathologic
Overall cultural assessment for diagnosis and care	• Discuss how cultural considerations specifically influence comprehensive diagnosis and care

Adapted from McKee J, Brahm N. Medical mimics: Differential diagnostic considerations for psychiatric symptoms. Ment Health Clin. 2016 Nov 3;6(6):289-296. doi: 10.9740/mhc.2016.11.289. PMID: 29955484; PMCID: PMC6007536.

distress tolerance, and emotional regulation. It has been validated for symptoms of depression, anxiety, PTSD, substance use disorders, self-harm, borderline personality disorder, suicidal behavior, bulimia, and binge eating disorder.[51]

Predominantly behavioral interventions are effective treatments for certain disorders. *Habit reversal training* is an effective intervention for body-focused repetitive behaviors such as nail biting, skin picking, and hair pulling.[60,61]

Table 5
Select types of psychotherapy and targeted mental health challenges

Psychotherapy Type	Targeted Symptoms and Illnesses
Cognitive behavior therapy[49]	Unipolar depression Generalized anxiety disorder Social anxiety disorder Panic disorder (with and without agoraphobia) Post-traumatic stress disorder Marital distress Anger Chronic pain Eating disorders Schizophrenia Bipolar disorder Obsessive-Compulsive Disorder
Interpersonal psychotherapy[50]	Grief and bereavement Depression Role dispute Role transition
Dialectical behavior therapy[51]	Depression Anxiety PTSD Substance use disorders Bulimia and binge eating disorder Borderline Personality Disorder Self-injurious behavior Suicidal thoughts and behaviors
Psychodynamic psychotherapy[52]	Depression Anxiety Social anxiety disorder Eating disorders Pain Relationship difficulties
Solution-focused therapy[53]	Goal development Solution construction
Supportive psychotherapy[54]	Flexible Can fit a wide range of diagnoses
Acceptance and commitment therapy[55]	Transdiagnostic Skills: Cognitive flexibility, mindfulness, broad perspective, clarification of goals, cultivating commitment, acceptance of unwanted feelings, and defusion
Mindfulness-based stress reduction[56]	Mindfulness meditation Chronic diseases Debilitating conditions Anxiety Depression

Pharmacologic Approaches

Comprehensive review of pharmacologic treatments for psychiatric disorders experienced by athletes is beyond the scope of this article. Consideration for pharmacologic treatment should include the symptom complex, diagnosis, severity of illness/symptoms, extent of functional impairment, and athlete willingness to take medications.

In general, clinical practice guidelines for pharmacologic treatment of psychiatric disorders should be followed with the athlete population, with special consideration for undesirable side effects such as weight gain and sedation.[25,62,63] The clinician must also be mindful of medications and substances found on the World Anti-Doping Agency prohibited list,[64] and those which require a therapeutic use exemption form to be permitted for use during competition.[65] Many national psychiatric associations have published practice guidelines for treatment of mood, anxiety, and psychotic disorders.

Major Depressive Disorder: A survey of practicing sports psychiatrists identified Bupropion as the preferred treatment of major depressive disorder (MDD) without anxiety or BD.[62] Bupropion is an activating medication from the norepinephrine-dopamine-reuptake inhibitor family that is not associated with weight gain and does not impair performance.[25,63,66] Bupropion should not be prescribed for athletes with eating disorders with restrictive or purging features due to the increased risk of seizures.[67] Other preferred medications prescribed for MDD in athletes include selective serotonin reuptake inhibitors (SSRIs such as fluoxetine, sertraline, and escitalopram) and serotonin-norepinephrine reuptake inhibitors (such as venlafaxine and duloxetine).[25,62,63]

Bipolar disorder: Although there is no cure for BD, treatment may reduce the morbidity and mortality associated with the disorder.[68] Assessment of safety and impairment can guide the decision around optimal treatment setting. Screening for the presence or history of manic or mixed features, or a family history of BD, is important before prescribing an antidepressant for any individual. Ensuring thorough diagnostic evaluation for BD before initiating treatment is also important as the recommended agents can have significant side effects and safety concerns.[69] Agents of choice by sports psychiatrists are lithium (which targets both depressive and manic phases) and lamotrigine (which is more reliable in preventing and treating the depressed phase).[62] Lithium levels are influenced by hydration status; thus, serum levels should be monitored closely when there is extensive sweating and dehydration.[25,70] Other medications (including atypical antipsychotic agents and valproic acid) used to treat BD can cause weight gain, sedation, and other unwanted side effects.[62] Because aripiprazole, lurasidone, and ziprasidone are relatively less likely to cause weight gain and sedation, they may be preferable for use with athletes.

Anxiety disorders: Pharmacotherapy may be used alone or in combination with psychotherapy for athletes with moderate to severe anxiety and those for whom psychotherapy has not been effective or suitable. Antidepressant medications, specifically the SSRIs fluoxetine, escitalopram, and sertraline, are preferred agents for this population[66] given their efficacy and positive side effect profiles.[66] Benzodiazepines should be used with caution as they are associated with side effects such as sedation, which may impair athletic performance[71] and pose a risk of dependence.

Psychotic disorders: Early identification and treatment may favorably influence the trajectory of these disorders (in terms of minimizing impairment and duration of illness). Many first and second generation antipsychotic agents are associated with sedation, weight gain, metabolic side effects, and tremor, which would negatively impact anthropometrics and athletic performance. Owing to its tendency to have less negative side effects, aripiprazole was identified as the preferred agent by sports psychiatrists to treat psychotic disorders.[62,72]

SUMMARY

Identification and management of mental health challenges in athletes is important not just for athletic performance, but for overall health, quality of life, and long-term wellness. An organized and comprehensive approach to mental health support includes screening, diagnostic assessment (including medical work up), and development of an individualized management plan based on a biopsychosocial understanding of the athlete's unique circumstances and cultural considerations. Implementation of the management plan should include the diverse expertise available within an interdisciplinary support team, when available. Symptoms or illnesses with mild to moderate severity can sometimes be managed very appropriately in the sports medicine physician's office, and athletes may also benefit from referral to a mental health clinician for specialized mental health support. Athletes with significant impairment or challenges in the high-moderate to severe range should be referred to a psychiatrist for further assessment and treatment. A sports psychiatrist would be able to provide a sport-informed assessment and work with the sports medicine physician, interdisciplinary support team, coaches, and the athletes to develop a comprehensive approach to balancing treatment and sport.

CLINICAL CARE POINTS

- Comprehensive screening should be incorporated into pre-participation assessments and after performance interruption due to illness or injury.
- Diagnostic assessment of mental illness should include screening, comprehensive history, and formulation (with consideration of cultural contexts).
- Management of mental health challenges can include pharmacologic and non-pharmacological treatment approaches (after medical illness has been ruled out).
- Pharmacologic athletes can be safely and effectively used with athletes, with consideration of undesired side effects such as excessive sedation, weight gain (or loss), negative impact on fine motor function, and prohibited lists.
- There are a myriad of psychotherapies that can be aligned with the nature of the athlete's psychological challenges, readiness for change, and therapist fit.

DISCLOSURE

The author has nothing to disclose.

Abbreviation: BDSA, Baron Depression Screener for Athletes; MDQ, Mood Disorder Questionnaire; SAPAS, Standardized Assessment of Personality: Abbreviated Scale; CET-A, Compulsive Exercise Test: Athlete version; YBOCS, Yale-Brown Obsessive-Compulsive Scale.

REFERENCES

1. McDowell E. 12 athletes who've spoken about their mental health struggles. Jun 6, 2021. https://www.insider.com/athletes-mental-health-struggles-depression-2021-6. Accessed March 15, 2023.
2. Asmelash L. Why mental health matters for athletes – even as they give their all to win. July 26, 2022. https://www.cnn.com/2022/07/22/us/athlete-mental-health-united-shades-wellness-cec/index.html. Accessed March 15, 2023.
3. Centers for Disease Control and Prevention. Adverse Childhood Experiences Prevention Strategy. Atlanta, GA: National Center for Injury Prevention and Control, Centers for Disease Control and Prevention, 2021. https://www.cdc.gov/injury/pdfs/priority/ACEs-Strategic-Plan_Final_508.pdf.

4. Novoa C and Morrissey T. Adversity in Early Childhood. August 27, 2020. https://www.americanprogress.org/article/adversity-early-childhood/. Accessed March 15, 2023.

5. Mountjoy M, Brackenridge C, Arrington M, et al. International Olympic Committee consensus statement: harassment and abuse (non-accidental violence) in sport. Br J Sports.Med 2016;50:1019–29.

6. Edwards CD. Depression Assessment: Challenges and Treatment Strategies in the Athlete. Psychiatr Clin North Am 2021;44(3):381–92.

7. Tofler IR, Knapp PK, Lardon MT. Achievement by proxy distortion in sports: A distorted mentoring of high-achieving youth. Historical perspectives and clinical intervention with children, adolescents and their families. Clin Sports Med 2005;24:805–28.

8. SMHAT-1: https://bjsm.bmj.com/content/bjsports/55/1/30/DC2/embed/inline-supplementary-material-2.pdf?download=true. Accessed March 17, 2023.

9. Patient Health Questionnaire-9: www.depression_patient_health_questionnaire.pdf (gov.bc.ca). Accessed March 17, 2023.

10. Generalized Anxiety Disorder-7 : GAD-7_Anxiety-updated_0.pdf (adaa.org). Accessed March 17, 2023.

11. Athlete Sleep Satisfaction Questionnaire : ASSQ+tool+and+scoring.pdf (squarespace.com) Accessed March 17, 2023.

12. CAGE-AID : https://www.hopkinsmedicine.org/johns_hopkins_healthcare/downloads/all_plans/CAGE%20Substance%20Screening%20Tool.pdf.   Accessed March 18, 2023.

13. AUDIT-C : AUDIT-C (nih.gov) Accessed March 17, 2023.

14. BEDA-Q: MSS13987 1666. 1675 (sportsmedicinebroadcast.com). Accessed March 18, 2023.

15. Baron DA, Baron SH, Tompkins J, et al. Assessing and treating depression in athletes. In: Baron DA, Reardon C, Baron SH, et al, editors. Clinical sports psychiatry: an international perspective. Chichester. West Sussex: Wiley; 2013. p. 65–78.

16. MDQ: https://www.sadag.org/images/pdf/mdq.pdf.

17. Mini-SPIN: https://www.verywellmind.com/mini-social-phobia-inventory-mini-spin-3024440. Accessed March 18, 2023.

18. Ball L, Tully RJ, Egan V. The SAPAS, Personality Traits, and Personality Disorder. J Pers Disord 2017;31(3):385–98.

19. Moran P, Leese M, Lee T, et al. Standardized Assessment of Personality-Abbreviated Scale (SAPAS): Preliminary valiation of a brief screen for personality disorder. The British journal of Psychiatry 2003;183(3):228–32. https://doi.org/10.1192/bjp.183.3.228.

20. Prins A, Ouimette P, Kimerling R, et al. The primary care PTSD screen (PC–PTSD): development and operating characteristics. Prim Care Psychiatr 2004; 9:9–14.

21. Spoont MR, Williams JW, Kehle-Forbes S, et al. Does this patient have posttraumatic stress disorder?: rational clinical examination systematic review. JAMA 2015;314:501–10.

22. Yale-Brown Obsessive Compulsive Scale. https://pandasnetwork.org/wp-content/uploads/2018/11/y-bocs-w-checklist.pdf. Accessed November 23, 2022.

23. Storch EA. Measuring Obsessive-Compulsive Symptoms: Common Tools and Techniques. International OCD Foundation. Summer 2005. https://iocdf.org/expert-opinions/expert-opinion-measuring-oc-symptoms/YBOCS-SR https://static1.squarespace.com/static/58cab82ff5e231f0df8d9cad/t/60945b3af4680c68037f8188/1620335418443/YBOCS-II-SR.pdf.

24. Counseling Center Assessment of Psychological Symptoms (CCAPS) Instruments https://ccmh.psu.edu/ccaps-34-62. Accessed March 17, 2023.
25. Reardon CL, Hainline B, Aron CM, et al. Mental health in elite athletes: International Olympic Committee consensus statement: 2019. Br J Sports Med 2019; 53:667–99.
26. Gouttebarge V, Bindra A, Blauwet C, et al. International Olympic Committee (IOC) Sport Mental Health Assessment Tool 1 (SMHAT-1) and Sport Mental Health Recognition Tool 1 (SMHRT-1): towards better support of athletes' mental health. Br J Sports Med 2021;55:30–7.
27. Martinsen M, Holme I, Pensgaard AM, et al. The development of the brief eating disorder in athletes questionnaire. Med Sci Sports Exerc 2014;46(8):1666–75. PMID: 24504432.
28. Kessler RC, Adler L, Ames M, et al. The world Health organization adult ADHD selfreport scale (ASRS): a short screening scale for use in the general population. Psychol Med 2005;35:245–56.
29. Ustun B, Adler LA, Rudin C, et al. The world Health organization adult attention-deficit/hyperactivity disorder self-report screening scale for DSM-5. JAMA Psychiatr 2017;74:520–6.
30. Dodd S, Williams LJ, Jacka FN, et al. Reliability of the mood disorder questionnaire: comparison with the structured clinical interview for the DSM-IV-TR in a population sample. Aust N Z J Psychiatry 2009;43:526–30.
31. Hirschfeld RM, Williams JB, Spitzer RL, et al. Development and validation of a screening instrument for bipolar spectrum disorder: the mood disorder questionnaire. Am J Psychiatry 2000;157:1873–5.
32. Holtgraves T. Evaluating the problem gambling severity index. J Gambl Stud 2009;25:105–20.
33. Sharp C, Steinberg L, Yaroslavsky I, et al. An item response theory analysis of the problem gambling severity index. Assessment 2012;19:167–75.
34. Loewy RL, Bearden CE, Johnson JK, et al. The prodromal questionnaire (PQ): preliminary validation of a self-report screening measure for prodromal and psychotic syndromes. Schizophr Res 2005;77:117–25.
35. Ising HK, Veling W, Loewy RL, et al. The validity of the 16-item version of the prodromal questionnaire (PQ-16) to screen for ultra high risk of developing psychosis in the general help-seeking population. Schizophr Bull 2012;38:1288–96.
36. Plateau, Carolyn, Caroline Meyer, and Jon Arcelus. 2021. Compulsive Exercise Test (athlete Version; CET- A). Loughborough University. https://doi.org/10.17028/rd.lboro.14465541.v1. Accessed March 18, 2023.
37. Taranis L, Touyz S, Meyer C. Disordered eating and exercise: Development and preliminary validation of the compulsive exercise test (CET). Eur Eat Disord Rev 2011;19(3):256–68.
38. Plateau CR, Shanmugam V, Duckham RL, et al. Use of the Compulsive Exercise Test with athletes: Norms and links with eating psychopathology. J Appl Sport Psychol 2014;26(3):287–301.
39. McKee J, Brahm N. Medical mimics: Differential diagnostic considerations for psychiatric symptoms. Ment Health Clin 2016;6(6):289–96.
40. Stull T, Glick I, Kamis D. The Role of a Sport Psychiatrist on the Sports Medicine Team, Circa 2021. Psychiatr Clin North Am 2021;44(3):333–45.
41. Formulation: https://www.psychdb.com/teaching/biopsychosocial-case-formulation. Retrieved March 19, 2023.
42. Attachment : Attachment Theory - PsychDB https://www.psychdb.com/child/attachment/1-theory. Accessed March 19, 2023.

43. ACES: Adverse Childhood Experiences (ACEs) - PsychDB https://www.cdc.gov/vitalsigns/aces/pdf/vs-1105-aces-H.pdf. Accessed March 19, 2023.
44. Center for Substance Abuse Treatment (US). Improving Cultural Competence. Rockville (MD): Substance Abuse and Mental Health Services Administration (US); 2014. (Treatment Improvement Protocol (TIP) Series, No. 59.) Appendix E, Cultural Formulation in Diagnosis and Cultural Concepts of Distress. Available from: https://www.ncbi.nlm.nih.gov/books/NBK248426/.
45. American Psychiatric Association. Diagnostic and statistical manual of mental disorders. In: DSM-5). Fifth Edition. Washington, DC: American Psychiatric Publishing; 2013. p. 749–59.
46. Culture: Glossary - Improving Cultural Competence - NCBI Bookshelf (nih.gov). Accessed March 19, 2023.
47. Cultural Concepts of distress: Cultural Formulation in Diagnosis and Cultural Concepts of Distress - Improving Cultural Competence - NCBI Bookshelf (nih.gov): https://www.ncbi.nlm.nih.gov/books/NBK248426/#appe.s2. Accessed March 19, 2023.
48. Stillman MA, Glick I, McDuff D, et al. Psychotherapy for mental health symptoms and disorders in elite athletes: a narrative review. Br J Sports Med 2019;53(12):767–71.
49. Butler AC, Chapman JE, Forman EM, et al. The empirical status of cognitive-behavioral therapy: a review of meta-analyses. Clin Psychol Rev 2006;26(1):17–31.
50. Markowitz JC, Weissman MM. Interpersonal psychotherapy: principles and applications. World Psychiatr 2004 Oct;3(3):136–9. PMID: 16633477; PMCID: PMC1414693.
51. DBT: https://psychotherapyacademy.org/dbt/history-of-dialectical-behavioral-therapy-a-very-brief-introduction/Accessed April 1, 2023.
52. https://www.psychologytoday.com/us/therapy-types/psychodynamic-therapy Accessed April 1, 2023.
53. https://solutionfocused.net/what-is-solution-focused-therapy/#:~:text=Solution%2DFocused%20Brief%20Therapy%20(SFBT)%20is%20a%20short%2D,rather%20than%20focusing%20on%20problems. Accessed March 20, 2023.
54. Grover S, Avasthi A, Jagiwala M. Clinical Practice Guidelines for Practice of Supportive Psychotherapy. Indian J Psychiatry 2020;62(Suppl 2):S173–82.
55. Dindo L, Van Liew JR. Arch JJ. Acceptance and Commitment Therapy: A Transdiagnostic Behavioral Intervention for Mental Health and Medical Conditions. Neurotherapeutics 2017;14(3):546–53.
56. MBSR: https://www.apa.org/topics/mindfulness/meditation.
57. CBT: https://www.apa.org/ptsd-guideline/patients-and-families/cognitive-behavioral.pdf Accessed April 1, 2023.
58. Ost LG, Havnen A, Hansen B, et al. Cognitive behavioral treatments of obsessive-compulsive disorder. A systematic review and meta-analysis of studies published 1993-2014. Clin Psychol Rev 2015;40:156–69.
59. McGuire JF, Piacentini J, Lewin AB, et al. A meta-analysis of cognitive behavior therapy and medication for child obsessive-compulsive disorder: moderators of treatment efficacy, response and remission. Depress Anxiety 2015;32:580–93.
60. Azrin NH, Nunn RG. Habit-reversal: a method of eliminating nervous habits and tics. Behavior Research and Therapy 1973;11:619–28.
61. Morris SH, Zickgraf HF, Dingfelder HE, et al. Habit Reversal training in trichotillomania: guide for the clinician. Expert Rev Neurother 2013;13:1069–77.

62. Reardon CL, Creado S. Psychiatric medication preferences of sports psychiatrists. Phys Sports Med 2016;44(4):397–402. https://doi.org/10.1080/00913847.2016.1216719.
63. Reardon CL. Managing psychiatric disorders in athletes. In: Hong E, Rao AL, editors. Mental health in the athlete. London: Springer; 2020. p. 57–67.
64. World Anti-Doping Agency. List of prohibited substances and methods. 2021. Available from https://www.wada-ama.org/sites/default/fles/resources/fles/2021list_en.pdf. Accessed March 20, 2023.
65. U.S. Anti-Doping Agency. Apply for a therapeutic use exemption (TUE). Available from https://www.usada.org/substances/tue/apply/. Accessed 11 May 2021.
66. Reardon CL, Factor RM. Sport psychiatry: a systematic review of diagnosis and medical treatment of mental illness in athletes. Sports Med 2010;40:961–80.
67. Davidson J. Seizures and bupropion: a review. J Clin Psychiatry 1989;50(7): 256–61.
68. American Psychiatric Association Practice Guidelines for Bipolar Disorder: https://psychiatryonline.org/pb/assets/raw/sitewide/practice_guidelines/guidelines/bipolar.pdf. Accessed March 20, 2023.
69. Currie A, Gorczynski P, Rice S, et al. Bipolar and psychotic disorders in elite athletes: a narrative review. Br J Sports Med 2019;53(12):746–53.
70. Reardon CL. The sports psychiatrist and psychiatric medications. Int Rev Psychiatry 2016;28(6):606–13.
71. Johnston A, McAllister-Williams RH. Psychotropic drug prescribing. In: Currie A, Owen B, editors. Sports psychiatry. Oxford: Oxford University Press; 2016. p. 133–43.
72. Macleod AD. Sport psychiatry. Aust N Z J Psychiatry 1998;32(6):860–6.

Anxiety Disorders in Athletes

Claudia L. Reardon, MD[a],*, Paul Gorczynski, PhD[b],
Brian Hainline, MD[c], Mary Hitchcock, MA, MS[d], Simon Rice, PhD[e,f]

KEYWORDS

- Anxiety • Athletes • Sport • Performance anxiety • Psychiatry • Psychology
- Generalized anxiety • Panic disorder

KEY POINTS

- Athletes experience many anxiety symptoms and disorders, including generalized anxiety disorder, panic disorder, and social anxiety disorder, at rates approximating those in the non-athlete population.
- Athletes may experience the anxiety-related disorders of obsessive-compulsive disorder and post-traumatic stress disorder at rates exceeding those in the non-athlete population.
- Sport- and non-sport factors may precipitate or worsen anxiety symptoms and disorders in athletes.
- Clinicians should take into account athletes' psychosocial context and physiology when treating athletes for anxiety symptoms and disorders.

INTRODUCTION

Athletes experience a wide variety of mental health symptoms and disorders.[1] Among these are anxiety and related disorders, including generalized anxiety disorder (GAD), panic disorder, social anxiety disorder, obsessive-compulsive disorder (OCD), post-traumatic stress disorder (PTSD), separation anxiety disorder, specific phobia, and, while not specifically a diagnosis in the Diagnostic and Statistical Manual of Mental Disorders, competitive performance anxiety.[1] Anxiety disorders are among the most common mental health disorders around the world,[2] with earlier onsets than a majority of other mental health disorders.[3] A multitude of biopsychosocial factors incite and

[a] Department of Psychiatry, University of Wisconsin School of Medicine and Public Health, 6001 Research Park Boulevard, Madison, WI 53719, USA; [b] Psychology and Counselling, School of Human Sciences, University of Greenwich, Old Royal Naval College, Park Row, Greenwich SE10 9LS, UK; [c] National Collegiate Athletic Association, 700 West Washington Street, PO Box 6222, Indianapolis, IN 46206, USA; [d] University of Wisconsin-Madison, Ebling Library for the Health Sciences, 2339 Health Sciences Learning Center, 750 Highland Avenue, Madison, WI 53705, USA; [e] Orygen, 35 Poplar Road, Parkville, Melbourne, Australia; [f] Centre for Youth Mental Health, The University of Melbourne, Locked Bag 10, Parkville, Melbourne, Australia
* Corresponding author.
E-mail address: clreardon@wisc.edu

Clin Sports Med 43 (2024) 33–52
https://doi.org/10.1016/j.csm.2023.06.002
0278-5919/24/© 2023 Elsevier Inc. All rights reserved.

sportsmed.theclinics.com

perpetuate anxiety in this population.[4] Athletes with anxiety symptoms and disorders may present differently than other cohorts such that there are important considerations when it comes to diagnosing these conditions in this group.[1] Treatment mandates careful consideration of relevant psychosocial and physiologic factors as well. This paper provides a clinical review of GAD, panic disorder, social anxiety disorder, OCD, PTSD, separation anxiety disorder, specific phobia, and competitive performance anxiety in athletes across competitive levels.

METHODS

An experienced academic librarian (MH) searched Cochrane, PsycINFO, PubMed, Scopus, and SportDiscus databases from inception until January 2023. Authors reviewed reference lists of the original articles for possible inclusion as well. They selected studies that were written in English and included clinical information on athletes and anxiety-related symptoms or disorders. Resources and manuscripts describing anxiety in non-athlete populations were included where sport-based research was unavailable.

RESULTS
General Information on Anxiety in Athletes

According to Schaal,[5] whose research involves a large sample of athletes with mental health disorders diagnosed by licensed clinicians, anxiety disorders across types affect athletes in a combined past 6-month prevalence of approximately 9%.This is comparable to rates reported in the general population (11%–12%).[6,7]

Other research has examined comparative rates of anxiety in different categories of sports. *Individual* sport athletes may be at relatively greater risk for anxiety than are *team* sport athletes.[8–10] Starting at younger ages, motivations for athletes to join individual sports tend to include goal-oriented reasons such as winning scholarships or controlling weight.[8] Conversely, athletes joining team sports tend to trace the origins of their participation to a desire to have fun with friends.[8] The former reasons may be more associated with an underlying anxious temperament or may be more prone to contribute to the development of anxiety. Individual sport athletes may also be relatively more perfectionistic, set extreme personal goals, internalize failure after loss, experience less social support, train in a single sport throughout the year (increasingly common in childhood sports), and suffer injuries, all of which may lead to anxiety.[11,12] Among specific individual sports, those in which judges score athletes (eg, gymnastics, figure skating, diving) are most highly correlated with anxiety.[5] These athletes experience pressure to distinguish themselves from their competition as they pursue flawlessness and judges' approval.[5]

Several other factors have been associated with higher risk for anxiety in athletes (**Table 1**).

Anxiety symptoms and disorders impact performance in sport. Anxiety affects attention, executive functioning, information selection, muscle tension, and stimulus processing—all of which are involved in sport.[4] Elite athletes reporting higher anxiety experience more skill errors and negative performance outcomes.[24–26] For example, anxiety impacts balance among youth and young adults participating in gymnastics and is associated with worse performance.[27] Additionally, an athlete's interpretation of stress and anxiety pre-competition may mediate the functional impact on performance.[28] That is, if the athlete interprets the feelings as helpful in getting "pumped up" for competition, that may be functionally adaptive. However, if the athlete perceives the feelings as detrimental, then behavioral responses are unhelpfully

Table 1 Factors associated with higher risk for anxiety in athletes	
Domain of Factors Associated with Higher Risk for Anxiety in Athletes	**Specific Factors**
Sport specific	• Sense of pressure to perform[13] • Public scrutiny[13] • Sporting career uncertainty or dissatisfaction[14,15] • Injury[16–18] (concussion and musculoskeletal injury reportedly equal risk)[19] • Harassment and abuse in sport[20]
Non-sport specific	• Female[4,9,21] • Younger age[4] • Recent experience of adverse life events (eg, recent death of a close friend or change in financial state)[4] • Behavioral inhibition[22] • Social withdrawal or avoidance[22] • Rumination[22] • Less religiosity[23]

Reprinted with permission in edited form from Advances in Psychiatry and Behavioral Health, Vol 1, Reardon CL, Gorczynski P, Hainline B, Hitchcock M, Purcell R, Rice S, Walton CC, Anxiety disorders in athletes: a clinical review, pages 149-160, Copyright Elsevier (2021).

avoidance-based, and performance negatively affected.[29–31] Finally, anxiety in athletes is one of the factors most consistently associated with sport injury occurrence[31,32] and severity.[33] After injury occurs, recovery from and return to sport can be negatively impacted by anxiety as well.[34] Notably, though, higher levels of satisfaction with social support received while injured are associated with *decreases* in post-injury anxiety symptoms.[35]

Generalized Anxiety Disorder

Although the above research described non-specific "anxiety" in athletes, some research has examined specific anxiety-related disorders. For example, GAD is characterized by persistent and excessive worry about a number of different topics.[36] GAD in athletes appears to occur at similar rates (6.0% per clinician diagnosis[5] and 14.6% per self-report) as in the general population.[37] Like in non-athlete samples, female athletes report GAD more often than do male athletes.[38–44] Aesthetic sports (eg, artistic swimming, figure skating, gymnastics) across genders are associated with a higher risk for GAD among elite athletes.[5] Athletes in these sports have described feeling a lack of control over the outcome of their performances, which are judged by others.[45] Conversely, "high-risk sports," which include aerial sports, motor sports, and sliding sports (eg, luge), are associated with relatively lower risk for GAD among elite athletes.[5] These sports have a relatively high risk of fatalities. Their athlete participants have been described as "thrill seekers,"[46,47] and they may cope better with stressful circumstances.[48] Other risk factors for GAD as reported in a study of collegiate athletes from China may include sport injury, attention-deficit/hyperactivity disorder, and a high level of fear of failure.[49] In that same population, satisfaction in sport was significantly protective against GAD.[49]

Panic Disorder

Panic disorder is characterized by unexpected and recurrent episodes of intense fear accompanied by other symptoms such as a racing heartbeat or shortness breath, with fear of future such episodes.[36] Approximately 4.5% of athletes self-report panic disorder symptoms,[50] approximating rates in the general population.[51] Exercise is known to be anxiolytic, but conversely, exercise can precipitate acute anxiety and panic attacks, with nearly one-third of patients with panic disorder and/or the related condition of agoraphobia (fear of open/crowded places, of leaving one's home, or of being in places from which escape is difficult) reporting increased anxiety while exercising.[52] Consequently, panic disorder sufferers may avoid exercise.[53] The relationship between exercise and panic attacks may owe to the physical experiences of exercise (eg, increased heart rate, shortness of breath, sweating), which resemble those of panic. The athlete with panic disorder may worry they are experiencing a panic attack, which perpetuates further panic symptoms.[54] Conversely, one study suggests that participation in adolescent sport might *decrease* the risk of panic disorder (more so than other anxiety disorders) in adulthood.[55] The authors of the latter hypothesize that sports participation acts as a form of exposure therapy such that youth learn not to fear symptoms such as increased heartbeat, rapid breathing, and sweating via desensitization to those symptoms.

Social Anxiety Disorder

Social anxiety disorder (social phobia) is characterized by fear of being judged or negatively evaluated in a social or performance situation.[36] Those with the disorder avoid such situations or endure them with significant distress. By self-report, symptoms of social anxiety disorder impact 14.7% of athletes,[50] which is similar to the rate of 13% in the general population.[51] Significant fear of social evaluation, especially if extending to contexts beyond sport, warrants evaluation for this disorder.[56] It can be challenging in some cases to discern whether symptoms represent competitive performance anxiety or social anxiety disorder. In competitive performance anxiety, the symptoms are limited to sport participation, with fear of scrutiny by others not a driving factor, compared to social anxiety disorder, in which fears relate to negative evaluation by and interaction with others.[57] It is possible that encouragement of sports participation for socially reticent children and young adults may provide opportunities for repeated exposure to feared social situations, resulting in a reduction in social anxiety as they desensitize to those situations.[58] For others, pressure to perform in sports may perpetuate fears of being negatively evaluated in social settings.[58] The net "average" effect of sports participation on social anxiety is thus unknown.

There may be a correlation between social anxiety and avoidance of *individual* sports (where athletes may feel that they as an individual are being watched by many people), but not *team* sports (where spectator viewing is distributed across multiple athletes).[58] Athletes with social anxiety disorder may avoid meals and meetings with the team, media interviews, and rehabilitation exercises in the athletic training room where they may perceive that they are too much the center of attention. Some cases of social anxiety disorder, especially in youth, may be associated with selective mutism, where there is consistent failure to speak in specific social situations in which there is an expectation for speaking[36] (eg, during team sports participation). In all of these situations, the athlete tends to be focused on self rather than sport-related task, with potential resultant negative impact of social anxiety on performance.[59]

Obsessive-Compulsive Disorder

OCD is characterized by recurring, unwanted thoughts, ideas or sensations (obsessions) that make the person feel driven to do something repetitively (compulsions).[36] By self-report, OCD has been found to impact 5.2% of collegiate athletes across 13 sports,[60] which is higher than general population rates (2.3%).[61] Moreover, in that same self-report study, nearly 35% of athletes endorsed OCD *symptoms* without meeting full OCD criteria,[60] compared to 28% in the general population.[62] Similarly, a small study of professional tennis players carried out via self-report and clinical interview demonstrated rates of OCD symptoms higher in both active and retired players compared to controls.[63] In contrast, in the yearly psychiatric evaluations of French elite athletes, relatively fewer (1.6%) received an OCD diagnosis compared to the general population.[5] Despite the somewhat conflicting findings, researchers have hypothesized that perfectionism and the compliance to strict daily routines that sport mandates,[63] along with superstitions and rituals that can be taken to extremes,[60] may confer athlete vulnerability to OCD.

Dysfunction from OCD can ensue in sport if intrusive thoughts interfere with present moment attention or if the athlete cannot stop the obsessive-compulsive rumination or routine to engage in sport performance.[59] For example, an endurance runner may log more miles than proscribed if they feel compelled to repeatedly run back to a certain spot in the road to confirm that they did not inadvertently kick a rock into the way of forthcoming runners. A swimmer may need to repeat a lap unnecessarily if it took an odd (vs even) number of seconds to complete it.

It is imperative not to overdiagnose OCD in athletes who may engage in superstitious rituals. Such rituals are common in sport,[59,60,63] and seemingly peculiar routines in themselves do not warrant a diagnosis of OCD if they do not cause significant distress or dysfunction.[1] These behaviors may serve to offer a sense of predictability and routine to athletes, for whom other aspects of their sport environment (eg, how their opponent will perform, whether they become ill before competition, the weather, whether spectators will cheer or boo, how officials will call the competition) are unpredictable.[56] However, if rituals surrounding competition gradually become more time-consuming or extend beyond sport, clinicians should screen for OCD.[56] For example, if an athlete develops a routine of tying his shoelaces in a particular way before races, that may be a harmless and reassuring superstitious ritual. However, if it starts to take up increasing amounts of time before each race, to the point that warmups and actual races are missed because the shoelaces never feel "just right," then OCD may be present. Ultimately, to be diagnosed as OCD, there is often an hour or more per day of obsessions and/or compulsions.[36]

Post-Traumatic Stress Disorder

PTSD is a disorder that may occur in someone who has experienced or witnessed a traumatic event and who then has intrusive thoughts and feelings and associated behavioral changes related to that event.[36] Rates of this disorder in athletes have been reported to be approximately 13%,[64] exceeding the 6% to 9% lifetime prevalence in the general population.[65,66] Major injury during sports participation is increasingly described as an inciting traumatic event,[67] and devastating humiliation, bullying, or harassment/abuse are among other events in sports that may lead to trauma-related symptoms. Female athletes, adolescent athletes (ie, those aged 15–21 years as compared to younger athletes), and those who have a stronger athletic identity may experience greater emotional trauma following injury.[68] Athletes with pre-existing trauma exposure who then suffer traumatic sports injury may also be at greater risk for PTSD.[69]

In athletes, symptoms of PTSD may include inconsistencies in athletic performance, increased somatic complaints, and avoidance symptoms specific to sport (eg, avoidance of rehabilitation exercises, of a return to the site where an injury occurred, of engagement in the type of activity being done when an injury occurred, or of training to full intensity), particularly where the inciting event involved athletic participation.[67,70]

The common approach of encouraging the athlete to "toughen up and get back out there" is unlikely to help if the symptoms go clinically unaddressed.

Separation Anxiety Disorder

Separation anxiety disorder is a relatively common anxiety disorder, particularly in youth, diagnosed when anxiety about separation from attachment figures is excessive for developmental age and interferes with school or other daily activities.[36] In affected athletes, the normal separation anxiety that exists in toddlers becomes *more* rather than *less* pervasive as the child becomes older. They often worry that harm will befall their attachment figure while they are separated.[36] This disorder has been little researched in athletes. However, when present, it can make it difficult for athletes to separate from their caretakers to attend sports practices or competition. They may be distracted at practice (if caregivers do not remain on site), step out of practice to send texts or place calls to caregivers to make sure they are okay, or experience somatic symptoms such as headaches or stomachaches, worrying that something will happen to their caregivers during that time. Typically, there will be a generalization of separation anxiety to multiple settings (eg, the athlete is fearful about leaving caregivers not only to attend sport-related activities but also to attend school, play dates, and birthday parties),[36] thereby distinguishing it from anxiety related to particular events happening in a single setting (eg, bullying at sports practice).

Specific Phobia

Specific phobia involves marked fear or anxiety about a specific object or situation.[36] The phobic object or situation is actively avoided or endured with intense fear or anxiety. Although rates of this condition in athletes are unknown, when present, it commonly develops prior to the age of 11 years.[36] Sport participation may present situations where specific phobias become particularly apparent, for example, in the case of sport-related travel involving airplanes or elevators, both of which are common specific phobias.[36] Loud sounds and costumed characters (such as mascots) are additional relatively common specific phobias[36] that may manifest in sport contexts. Finally, fear of vomiting or choking—also frequent phobias[36]—may result in insufficient dietary intake to support high levels of physical activity in sport.

Competitive Performance Anxiety

Competitive performance anxiety in sport is defined as fear an athlete has occurring around the time of sport participation, especially competition, that they will not be able to perform in the desired manner, that the situation will be too challenging, and/or that it will be dangerous or harmful.[71] This results in physiologic arousal, anxious cognitive appraisals, and/or anxious behavioral responses. It is important but often challenging to differentiate competitive performance anxiety, normal competition-induced hyperarousal, and full anxiety disorders.[71] Clinicians can distinguish among these 3 possibilities via observation of patterns of symptom onset, source(s) of the worry, duration, and severity of symptoms (**Table 2**).[71] Importantly, specific anxiety disorders such as GAD can co-exist and/or overlap with competitive performance anxiety.[24,71,72] Thus, suspicion for competitive performance anxiety should generate careful evaluation for overt anxiety disorders.

Competitive performance anxiety—like other types of anxiety—frequently brings with it several general physical symptoms. These symptoms include the typical "fight-flight-freeze" response symptoms such as dry mouth, flushed or pale skin, increased heart and respiratory rates, shakiness, and sweaty hands.[71] Additionally, numerous reports have been published describing how gastrointestinal disturbances

Table 2
Differentiation between normal competition-induced hyperarousal, competitive performance anxiety, and anxiety disorders[1,56,59,71]

	Normal Competition-Induced Hyperarousal	Competitive Performance Anxiety	Anxiety Disorder (eg, GAD)
Pattern of symptom onset	Mild hyperarousal symptoms (eg, feeling mildly nervous) typically starting during the day before/of or during sport performance	Hyperarousal symptoms starting any time before or during sport performance	Anxiety symptoms present most days irrespective of performance times (though symptoms might become even worse before/during performance). In GAD, symptoms have been present at least 6 mo[36]
Source of worry	Performance in sport	Performance in sport	Worries that are often multiple (in the case of GAD) and that are not solely sport related
Duration	Typically <24 h	Variable; can be up to a week or more before performances	Ongoing
Severity	No negative impact on functioning or significant distress, and arousal to a certain degree may *improve* performance according to the "inverted-U" hypothesis[73]	Detrimental impact on sport performance and/or significant distress	Detrimental impact on life functioning outside of (and sometimes within) sport and/or significant distress

including cramping, diarrhea, nausea, regurgitation/reflux, urges to defecate, and emesis are fairly common around times of competition and even training, especially among endurance athletes.[74] These disturbances may relate to competitive performance anxiety[74,75] and/or trait (longstanding and not just situational) anxiety.[76]

Competitive performance anxiety can be distressing and highly dysfunctional for athletes. This type of anxiety may contribute to a "slump" (an extended period of performance at a level less than capability) or a "choke" (acute performance—especially in high stakes circumstances—at a level less than capability).[77] "The yips" describe a variant of a choke in which there is an involuntary movement during a sport task, especially in sports that require fine motor control such as bowling, cricket, darts, golf, or shooting.[78] For example, a golfer may experience a problematic jerk, posture, or tremor during chipping, full swing, or putting.[79] Research on the yips is minimal, but it may be relatively common and underdiagnosed.[79] A spectrum of etiologies may exist for the yips, ranging from competitive performance anxiety to a focal dystonia, with a continuum between the 2.[78,79] The 2 etiologies may be distinguishable based on if the involuntary movement occurs in low-stakes settings (eg, when the athlete is hitting the golf ball by themselves), with focal dystonia a more prominent factor if it occurs even in these low-key settings.[78] Another variant of the yips may be the "twisties"—a potentially dangerous phenomenon in which gymnasts lose their sense of control in the air; it has been minimally studied but reportedly sometimes considered a dissociative symptom and related to stress and anxiety.[80] Regardless of how competitive performance anxiety manifests in a particular athlete, it can result in losses that are important to this population,[57,81] including loss of continued sport participation, ability to progress to the next competitive level, financial/scholarship/sponsorship support, and medals/championships.

Risk factors for competitive performance anxiety in athletes have been reported to include female gender,[82] younger age,[82,83] lower athletic experience,[82] away versus home competitions (exception being playing at home against nearby teams who are historic rivals),[82] athlete perception of coaching behaviors as controlling versus autonomy-supporting,[84] a sport environment in which athletes perceive that they are being rewarded only for being the best performer (vs for personal learning and improvement),[85] and individual versus team sports.[82,86] The reason younger age may be a risk is that athletes with greater experience appear to have more ability to control their distress and more effective coping strategies to deal with criticism from self and others.[8,82] Additionally, social media use shortly before or during competition, especially if push notifications are activated, is associated with competitive performance anxiety.[87] This type of media use may be a marker for baseline anxious traits, may increase comparisons to others, and/or may interfere with mental preparation for (which is important for confidence during) competition.[87]

Other Anxiety-Related Disorders

We found no research on other anxiety or related disorders, including adjustment disorder with anxiety or obsessive-compulsive personality disorder, in athletes. Adjustment disorder with anxiety may be common in this population owing to many temporary, sport-related stressors such as injury or competitive failure[88]

General Principles of Diagnosis and Management

There are no known athlete-specific, comprehensive, validated screening tools for anxiety-related disorders. The International Olympic Committee (IOC) published its Sports Mental Health Assessment Tool 1 (SMHAT-1), which includes several screening tools presented together for use in athlete populations.[89] The SMHAT-1 incorporates the GAD-7—which appears to be an acceptable choice for athletes—as its general anxiety screening tool.[89] Clinicians may incorporate the entire SMHAT-1, or the GAD-7 if singularly wishing to screen for anxiety, into preparticipation physical examinations. Additionally, the IOC advises that screening with the SMHAT-1 be repeated after injury/illness or suspected harassment/abuse, if there are unexplained performance concerns, at the end of competitive cycles, during other adverse life events, and upon retirement from sport.[89] The Sport Anxiety Scale-2 may be used to screen specifically for competitive performance anxiety.[90]

Clinicians should always consider general medical and substance-related conditions that may contribute to anxiety symptoms (**Table 3**).[56,71,91] In the presence of such conditions, it is imperative to address these underlying contributors, in addition to managing the manifesting anxiety symptoms.

The primary treatment for mild to moderate anxiety in athletes—just as in the general population—is often psychotherapy.[1,103,104] Athletes may be more wary than nonathletes of potential medication side effects, thereby further leading them to psychotherapy as the first treatment option.[1] Psychotherapy providers who are familiar with

Table 3
Common general medical and substance-related conditions that may contribute to anxiety symptoms in athletes[56,71,91]

General Medical or Substance-Related Condition	Signs/Symptoms that May Mimic Anxiety in Athletes	Relevance to Athletes	Typical Initial Evaluation	Typical Management
Anemia	• Shortness of breath • Tachycardia • Fatigue	• Endurance athletes and athletes with unintentional underfueling or eating disorders may be at risk for anemia	• Hemoglobin and ferritin laboratory tests	• Increased dietary iron intake • Iron supplementation
Asthma	• Shortness of breath that may contribute to a sense of anxiety, panic, or impending doom • Tachycardia	• Asthma may be exercise-induced • Athletes in certain sports (eg, swimming) may have relatively high rates of asthma[92]	• Lung auscultation • Pulmonary function testing	• Beta-agonists (some are prohibited at higher levels of competition without therapeutic use exemptions)[93] • Other daily controller medications
Caffeine use	• Nervousness • Restlessness • Jitteriness • Insomnia • Tachycardia	• Athletes may use caffeine to increase energy or enhance performance[94,95]	• Clinical interview	• If caffeine is causing problems, taper it (athletes consuming large doses may experience short-term withdrawal effects that may temporarily exacerbate anxiety)
Concussion[96]	• Nervousness • Irritability • Trouble concentrating • Insomnia • Fatigue	• Athletes experience sport-related concussion (SRC) • Anxiety symptoms may be multifactorial post-SRC • Athletes who have an anxious profile at baseline are likely to experience greater concussion symptom burden following SRC[97] • Negative, anxiety-related perceptions about concussions are prevalent in collegiate athletes[98]	• Immediate clinical neurologic assessment • Serial symptom assessment • Possible neuropsychological testing • Possible neuroimaging	• Gradual return-to-sport and return-to-learn protocols. Having an accurate understanding of baseline anxiety levels for these athletes may help to inform return-to-learn and return-to-play decisions and may prevent athletes from being withheld from activity unduly[99] • Symptom-targeted pharmacology as needed • Psychotherapy if mental health symptoms are persistent or severe

(continued on next page)

Table 3
(continued)

General Medical or Substance-Related Condition	Signs/Symptoms that May Mimic Anxiety in Athletes	Relevance to Athletes	Typical Initial Evaluation	Typical Management
Exercise-induced laryngeal obstruction (EILO)[100]	• Episodic shortness of breath that can lead to acute anxiety/panic	• Symptoms occur during exercise, resolve within minutes of stopping exercise, and are especially common in adolescent female athletes	• Referral to otolaryngology • Spirometry before/after bronchodilator and bronchoprovocation challenge, with confirmation via continuous laryngoscopy during exercise	• Behavioral management with speech-language pathologist • Management of psychosocial stressors related to EILO episodes
Hypoglycemia[101]	• Acute episodes of nervousness, jitteriness, irritability, and/or sweating	• High training demands with insufficient or poorly timed caloric intake may occur in athletes • Unintentional underfueling or eating disorders may be associated with hypoglycemia	• Glucose laboratory test while symptomatic	• Improved timing and composition of meals and snacks
Thyroid dysfunction[102]	• Palpitations • Tremors • Restlessness • Insomnia • Fatigue	• Overtraining in female athletes is associated with thyroid dysfunction • Iron deficiency (common in some athlete populations) is commonly comorbid with hypothyroidism • Athletes may use exogenous thyroid hormone to attempt to improve performance	• Thyroid function laboratory tests	• Medication • Sometimes radioactive thyroid ablation or thyroidectomy

Reprinted with permission in edited form from Advances in Psychiatry and Behavioral Health, Vol 1, Reardon CL, Gorczynski P, Hainline B, Hitchcock M, Purcell R, Rice S, Walton CC, Anxiety disorders in athletes: a clinical review, pages 149-160, Copyright Elsevier (2021).

the psychosocial context of sport are usually most equipped to meet athletes' needs and preferences.[105]

There is a dearth of empirical evidence on the effectiveness of psychotherapeutic interventions for most mental health symptoms and disorders, including anxiety, in athletes.[106] Studies on therapeutic approaches have generally focused on performance enhancement rather than treatment of psychopathology, and between-subject designs and healthy athlete samples have disproportionately been included.[106] However, athletes with anxiety may do well with cognitive-behavioral therapy (CBT), given its structural components that are similar to sport: completion of homework, following of rules, and receiving instruction.[103] Elements may include arousal reduction for GAD or panic disorder, graded exposure and behavioral experimentation for social anxiety, separation anxiety, PTSD, and specific phobia, and response prevention for OCD.[107] For panic attacks exacerbated by general physical sensations during exercise, treating the panic symptoms via exposure—and discouraging phobic avoidance of exercise—is the recommended course.[56] Specific mental factors that are deemed important for success in sport—affect regulation, healthy coping mechanisms, maintenance of motivation and of supportive relationships, and self-confidence,[4,108]—simultaneously help in anxiety management.[2] Thus, focus on these factors can be high yield.

Other therapies may be beneficial as well. Mindfulness-based programs have demonstrated efficacy for anxiety symptoms in the general population,[109] and are increasingly popular among athletes.[110] A systematic review and meta-analysis demonstrated reduced symptoms of anxiety in elite athletes participating in these programs, though adequately powered trials are required in the future.[111] Nutritional support may be helpful for athletes experiencing gastrointestinal manifestations of anxiety during sport.[75] Finally, a meta-analysis has demonstrated an anxiolytic effect of exercise for people with anxiety and related disorders.[112] Although presumably athletes are getting adequate exercise such that there would be no room for anxiolytic gain in this regard, it is one factor (of many) to consider if their anxiety increases during times of break from sport. Moreover, location of exercise matters regarding degree of anxiolytic (possibly moreso than for antidepressant) impact.[113] Outdoor exercise appears more beneficial than indoor exercise, and specifically a systematic review and meta-analysis that included 16 studies reporting outcomes for anxiety has demonstrated that exercise undertaken in outdoor *green natural* environments versus outdoor *urban* environments is significantly more anxiolytic.[113]

Medications may be necessary to treat anxiety in athletes—either as monotherapy or added to psychotherapy—especially when symptoms are moderate to severe.[1] However, prescribers should be aware of side effects that could compromise sport performance or safety.[114] Selective-serotonin reuptake inhibitors (SSRIs) are antidepressants that tend to be first choice of medications for athletes across anxiety disorders.[115] Specifically, a survey study has shown that the top choices of sports psychiatrists for anxiety in athletes are escitalopram, sertraline, and fluoxetine.[115] Of these, fluoxetine has received modest study in exercising subjects and has not been found to have a negative performance impact.[116,117] However, performance measures that may not be fully translatable to competitive sport, short study duration, lack of subject diversity, and small sample size were limitations in these studies. Escitalopram and sertraline have not been studied in athletes, but anecdotally they are frequently used in this population.[115] Tricyclic antidepressants (TCAs) are also used for anxiety-related disorders (especially clomipramine for OCD) in general populations, but they have been even less studied in athletes than have SSRIs. Clinicians should monitor blood levels of these medications in anyone taking them, as blood levels that are too high can be dangerous and cause severe side effects.[1] This may be especially important for athletes, as cardiac consequences of toxic blood levels may be dire in this heavily exercising cohort. Furthermore, eating disorders are generally considered contraindications to use of TCAs, and given the overrepresentation of eating disorders among athletes, this is another reason that these medications would not be used in this popuation.[118]

Another medication, buspirone, is a partial agonist of serotonin receptors that is used for its anxiolytic effects. One small study suggested impaired performance in recreational athletes.[119] However, only a single 45 mg dose was tested—far from duration and dose used in the real world—such that translation to use in actual athletes is not possible.[119]

Medications are rarely indicated for competitive performance anxiety.[1] Benzodiazepines, which can be used as fast-acting, as-needed options for acute anxiety in the general population, are prone to impair sport performance. They may cause sedation or muscle relaxation and decrease reaction time.[57,120–122] Propranolol and other beta-blockers may decrease cardiopulmonary capacity[123] and lower blood pressure (and thus cause dizziness) in athletes who may already have low blood pressure.[1] Additionally, the World Anti-Doping Agency prohibits beta-blockers both *out-of-competition* and *in-competition* in archery and shooting, and *in-competition* in automobile, billiards, darts, golf, some skiing/snowboarding, and some underwater sports.[93] The National Collegiate Athletic Association prohibits beta-blockers in rifle.[124] In these sports, beta-blockers may be performance enhancing by reducing physiologic tremor and thus improving fine motor control.[1] As a result, psychotherapy is the preferred choice for management of competitive performance anxiety,[57] and it has been demonstrated to be effective per meta-analysis and systematic review.[125] Athletes need practice in modulating and interpretating the feelings of being "psyched up" during competition just as they need practice in the other physical aspects of sport. Additionally, while sometimes used, pharmacologic options including benzodiazepines and botulinum toxin have been minimally studied in the treatment of the yips.[79] Behavioral approaches to address the yips, depending on sport, may include development of a new biomechanical sequence while engaging in the problematic motion, change in grip technique or length/type of golf club or other implement used, or hypnosis.[79] For the twisties, training on soft surfaces until the problem passes has been suggested, but none of these strategies have been rigorously evaluated.[80]

Athletes at higher levels of competition (especially collegiate and beyond) must exercise caution if using any non-regulated supplements to manage anxiety. Athletes sometimes prefer "natural" products, but high levels of competition enforce strict prohibitions of certain substances.[93,124] There is no regulatory body that approves the accuracy of supplement labels or the safety of supplement contents before they are sold. Dietary supplements may thus be contaminated—unbeknownst to the athlete—with prohibited substances.[1] Inaccurate labeling of supplements and ignorance of ingredients are not recognized as valid excuses for adverse analytical findings on drug tests.[1] Therefore, if supplements are taken, they should be obtained from a reputable company and ideally certified by a third-party program that tests for substances prohibited in sport.[1] Beyond the concern about contamination, several supplements marketed for anxiety (eg, kava, valerian) may cause sedation,[91] which could impact sports performance. Recently, cannabidiol (CBD) has been marketed to athletes as helpful for anxiety, among other conditions, but there is inadequate research to encourage its use for this purpose.[126] Moreover, athletes consuming CBD risk ingesting a relatively small amount of associated tetrahydrocannabinol (THC), which is prohibited by several governing bodies.[93,124] In the rare instance athletes have been included as the target population when studying the impact of supplements on anxiety, sample sizes have generally been low.[127]

DISCUSSION

Athletes may suffer from the full complement of anxiety symptoms and disorders that manifest in the general population, albeit often with nuanced precipitating and perpetuating factors and symptom presentations. If providers are aware of the risk factors and sometimes subtle presentations of anxiety in this population, they can intervene sooner. For example, the athlete in an individual, aesthetic, judged sport who is suffering from an injury, has a known eating disorder, and receives much pressure from family to maintain full scholarship support is likely at high risk for anxiety, and screening for such disorders should be undertaken liberally. Intervention as soon as possible may help prevent progression from mild symptoms to full, disabling disorders that make continued participation in sport—and life—difficult.

Clinicians should consider athletes' unique biopsychosocial contexts when making treatment recommendations. Anecdotally, athletes sometimes worry that treatment of anxiety might negatively impact sport performance via lessening of their anxiety-driven conscientiousness and strong work ethic; however, the authors found no evidence to justify this concern. On the contrary, there is ample evidence that ongoing anxiety negatively impacts sport performance in a variety of ways. Nonetheless, clinicians should be aware of the potential relevance of medication side effects in sport. Preliminary research on performance impacts of daily SSRI controller medication is reassuring, but limitations in study methods are substantial. Clinicians should thus solicit input from individual athletes about how they perceive medications to be impacting them and should take such reports seriously, as athletes are generally highly attuned to any changes in how their bodies are functioning.

Clinicians who provide mental health care to athletes who are suffering from anxiety ideally should be well-versed in the anxiogenic aspects of sport culture. They should not need their athlete patients to educate them about the stressors unique to life as an athlete. Their providers should not glamorize or idolize their athlete patients; in contrast, they should appreciate that the reality of their lives is demanding and full of pressures from many angles. At the same time, athletes do not necessarily want to be advised by their psychotherapist that their sport is too stressful and that they should simply quit. Clinicians should strive to find an adequate balance between being alert for problematic circumstances in sport (eg, abuse, playing through severe pain or injury) that warrant intervention (and possibly help exiting that particular sport context), while not rushing to a stance of, "Well then just quit if it's so bad." Additionally, clinicians should be aware of the relative mental health benefits of sport when pursued for the enjoyment it affords, versus the more negative impacts when associated with demanding, pressure-filled, lonely pursuits of individual perfection. It may be appropriate to help an athlete develop insight into their anxious tendencies, how their chosen sport may perpetuate those tendencies, and how such tendencies can be managed.

SUMMARY

Athletes are susceptible to the full spectrum of anxiety symptoms and disorders. Manifestations of such symptoms are varied, and there should be a low index of suspicion for their presence. Effective treatment should be employed promptly to optimize functioning in sport and in life.

CLINICS CARE POINTS

- Clinicians should ask all athletes if they spend a lot of time feeling anxious or worried, with use of more formal screening if possible.
- If a clinician suspects an anxiety-related disorder in an athlete, they should seek to confirm the diagnosis, discuss treatment (specifically psychotherapy and medications) and referral options with the athlete, and make an intervention promptly.

DISCLOSURE

The authors have nothing to disclose.

REFERENCES

1. Reardon CL, Hainline B, Aron CM, et al. Mental health in elite athletes: International Olympic Committee consensus statement (2019). Br J Sports Med 2019; 53(11):667–99.
2. Whiteford HA, Ferrari AJ, Degenhardt L, et al. The global burden of mental, neurological and substance use disorders: an analysis from the of Disease Study 2010. PLoS One 2015;10:e0116820.
3. Kessler RC, Berglund P, Demler O. Lifetime prevalence and age-of-onset distributions of DSM-IV disorders in the national comorbidity survey replication. Arch Gen Psychiatry 2005;62(6):593–602.
4. Rice SM, Gwyther K, Santesteban-Echarri O, et al. Determinants of anxiety in elite athletes: a systematic review and meta-analysis. Br J Sports Med 2019; 53:722–30.
5. Schaal K, Tafflet M, Nassif H, et al. Psychological balance in high level athletes: gender-based differences and sport-specific patterns. PLoS One 2011;6: e19007.
6. Somers JM, Goldner EM, Waraich P, et al. Prevalence and incidence studies of anxiety disorders: a systematic review of the literature. Can J Psychiatry 2006; 51:100–13.
7. Wittchen H-U, Jacobi F. Size and burden of mental disorders in Europe—a critical review and appraisal of 27 studies. Eur Neuropsychopharmacol 2005;15: 357–76.
8. Pluhar E, McCracken C, Griffith KL, et al. Team sport athletes may be less likely to suffer anxiety or depression than individual sport athletes. J Sports Med Sci 2019;18(3):490–6.
9. Correia M, Rosado A. Anxiety in athletes: gender and type of sport differences. Int J Psychol Res 2019;12(1):9–17.
10. Gligor S, Oravitan M, Pantea C. Anxiety of students practicing competitive sports: part of a vicious circle, or not? South Afr J Res Sport Phys Educ Recr 2021;43(2):47–58.
11. Nixdorf I, Frank R, Hautzinger M, et al. Prevalence of depressive symptoms and correlating variables among German elite athletes. J Clin Sport Psychol 2013; 7(4):313–26.
12. Nixdorf I, Frank R, Beckmann J. Comparison of athletes' proneness to depressive symptoms in individual and team sports: research on psychological mediators in junior elite athletes. Front Psychol 2016;7:893.

13. Hodge K, Smith W. Public expectation, pressure, and avoiding the choke: a case study from elite sport. Sport Psychol 2014;28:375–89.
14. Brown CJ, Webb TL, Robinson MA, et al. Athletes' retirement from elite sport: A qualitative study of parents and partners' experiences. Psychol Sport Exerc 2019;40:51–60.
15. Gustafsson H, Hassmén P, Kenttä G, et al. A qualitative analysis of burnout in elite Swedish athletes. Psychol Sport Exerc 2008;9:800–16.
16. Lavallée L, Flint F. The relationship of stress, competitive anxiety, mood state, and social support to athletic injury. J Athl Train 1996;31(4):296–9.
17. Ivarsson A, Johnson U. Psychological factors as predictors of injuries among senior soccer players. A prospective study. J Sports Sci Med 2010;9(2):347–52.
18. Kilic Ö, Aoki H, Goedhart E, et al. Severe musculoskeletal time-loss injuries and symptoms of common mental disorders in professional soccer: a longitudinal analysis of 12-month follow-up data. Knee Surg Sports Traumatol Arthrosc 2018;26:946–54.
19. Sabol J, Kane C, Wilhelm MP, et al. The Comparative Mental Health Responses Between Post-Musculoskeletal Injury and Post-Concussive Injury Among Collegiate Athletes: A Systematic Review. Int J Sports Phys Ther 2021;16(1):1–11.
20. Mountjoy M, Brackenridge C, Arrington M, et al. International Olympic Committee consensus statement: harassment and abuse (non-accidental violence) in sport. Br J Sports Med 2016;50:1019–29.
21. Weber ML, Dean J-HL, Hoffman NL, et al. Influences of mental illness, current psychological state, and concussion history on baseline concussion assessment performance. Am J Sports Med 2018;46:1742–51.
22. Leach LS, Christensen H, Mackinnon AJ, et al. Gender differences in depression and anxiety across the adult lifespan: the role of psychosocial mediators. Soc Psychiatry Psychiatr Epidemiol 2008;43:983–98.
23. Guntoro TS, Putra MFP. Athletes' religiosity: How it plays a role in athletes' anxiety and life satisfaction. HTS Theolog Stud 2022;78(1):8.
24. Halvari H, Gjesme T. Trait and state anxiety before and after competitive performance. Percept Mot Skills 1995;81(3_suppl):1059–74.
25. Morgan WP, O'Connor PJ, Ellickson KA, et al. Personality structure, mood states, and performance in elite male distance runners. Int J Sport Psychol 1988;19:247–63.
26. Turner PE, Raglin JS. Variability in precompetition anxiety and performance in college track and field athletes. Med Sci Sports Exerc 1996;28:378–85.
27. Ariza-Vargas L, Dominguez-Escribano M, Lopez-Bedoya J, et al. The effect of anxiety on the ability to learn gymnastic skills: a study based on the schema theory. Sport Psychol 2011;25(2):127–43.
28. Rice SM, Purcell R, De Silva S, et al. The mental health of elite athletes: a narrative systematic review. Sports Med 2016;46:1333–53.
29. Hatzigeorgiadis A, Chroni S. Pre-competition anxiety and in-competition coping in experienced male swimmers. Int J Sports Sci Coach 2007;2:181–9.
30. Jones G, Hanton S, Swain A. Intensity and interpretation of anxiety symptoms in elite and non-elite sports performers. Pers Individ Dif 1994;17:657–63.
31. Ford JL, Ildefonso K, Jones ML, et al. Sport-related anxiety: current insights. Open Access J Sports Med 2017;8:205–12.
32. Garit JR, Surita YP, Dominguez EF, et al. Anxiety and psychological variables of sports performance related to injuries in high-performance sportsmen. Apunts Sports Med 2021;56:211.

33. Pal S, Kalra S, Awasthi S. Influence of Stress and Anxiety on Sports Injuries in Athletes. J Clin Diag Res 2021;15(4):YE01–5.

34. Coronado RA, Bley JA, Huston LJ, et al. Composite psychosocial risk based on the fear avoidance model in patients undergoing anterior cruciate ligament reconstruction: Cluster-based analysis. Phys Ther Sport 2021;50:217–25.

35. Sullivan L, Ding K, Tattersall H, et al. Social support and post-injury depressive and anxiety symptoms among college-student athletes. Int J Environ Res Public Health 2022;19(11):6458.

36. American Psychiatric Association. Diagnostic and statistical manual of mental disorders (DSM-5). Washington, DC: American Psychiatric Publishing; 2013.

37. Du Preez EJ, Graham KS, Gan TY, et al. Depression, anxiety, and alcohol use in elite rugby league players over a competitive season. Clin J Sport Med 2017;27: 530–5.

38. Junge A, Feddermann-Demont N. Prevalence of depression and anxiety in top-level male and female football players. BMJ Open Sport Exerc Med 2016;2: e000087.

39. Brand R, Wolff W, Hoyer J. Psychological symptoms and chronic mood in representative samples of elite student-athletes, deselected student-athletes and comparison students. School Mental Health 2013;5:166–74.

40. Yang J, Peek-Asa C, Corlette JD, et al. Prevalence of and risk factors associated with symptoms of depression in competitive collegiate student athletes. Clin J Sport Med 2007;17:481–7.

41. Lancaster MA, McCrea MA, Nelson LD. Psychometric properties and normative data for the brief symptom Inventory-18 (BSI-18) in high school and collegiate athletes. Clin Neuropsychol 2016;30:321–33.

42. Weber S, Puta C, Lesinski M, et al. Symptoms of anxiety and depression in young athletes using the hospital anxiety and depression scale. Front Physiol 2018;9:1–12.

43. Gerber M, Holsboer-Trachsler E, Puhse U, et al. Elite sport is not an additional source of distress for adolescents with high stress levels. Percept Mot Skills 2011;112:581 00.

44. Ivarsson A, Johnson U, Podlog L. Psychological predictors of injury occurrence: a prospective investigation of professional Swedish soccer players. J Sport Rehabil 2013;22:19–26.

45. Kerr G, Goss J. Personal control in elite gymnasts: the relationships between locus of control, self-esteem and trait anxiety. J Sport Behav 1997;20:69–82.

46. Carton S, Morand P, Bungenera C, et al. Sensation-seeking and emotional disturbances in depression: relationships and evolution. J Affect Disord 1995;34: 219–25.

47. Michel G, Carton S, Jouvent R. Sensation seeking and anhedonia in risk taking. Study of a population of bungy jumpers. Encephale 1997;23:403–11.

48. Larkin M, Griffiths M. Dangerous sports and recreational drug-use: rationalizing and contextualizing risk. J Commun & Appl Soc Psychol 2004;14:215–32.

49. Li C, Fan R, Sun J, et al. Risk and protective factors of generalized anxiety disorder of elite collegiate athletes: a cross-sectional study. Front Public Health 2021;9:607800.

50. Gulliver A, Griffiths KM, Mackinnon A, et al. The mental health of Australian elite athletes. J Sci Med Sport 2015;18:255–61.

51. Bandelow B, Michaelis S. Epidemiology of anxiety disorders in the 21st century. Dialogues Clin Neurosci 2015;17:327–35.

52. Cameron OG, Hudson CJ. Influence of exercise on anxiety level in patients with anxiety disorders. Psychosomatics 1986;27:720–3.

53. Broocks A, Meyer TF, Bandelow B, et al. Exercise avoidance and impaired endurance capacity in patients with panic disorder. Neuropsychobiology 1997;36:182–7.

54. Strohle A, Graetz B, Scheel M, et al. The acute antipanic and anxiolytic activity of aerobic exercise in patients with panic disorder and healthy control subjects. J Psychiatr Res 2009;43:1013–7.

55. Ashdown-Franks G, Sabiston CM, Jewett R, et al. The association between adolescent socioeconomic status, sport participation and early adulthood anxiety. London, ON: Presented at Canadian Society for Psychomotor Learning and Sport Psychology; 2014.

56. Reardon CL. Psychiatric comorbidities in sports. Neurol Clin 2017;35:537–46.

57. Patel DR, Omar H, Terry M. Sport-related performance anxiety in young female athletes. J Pediatr Adolesc Gynecol 2010;23:325–35.

58. Northon PJ, Burns JA, Hope DA. Generalization of social anxiety to sporting and athletic situations: gender, sports involvement, and parental pressure. Depress Anxiety 2000;12:193–202.

59. Chang CJ, Putukian M, Aerni G, et al. Mental health issues and psychological factors in athletes: detection, management, effect on performance, and prevention: American Medical Society for Sports Medicine Position Statement. Clin J Sport Med 2020;30(2):e61–87.

60. Cromer L, Kaier E, Davis J, et al. OCD in college athletes. Am J Psychiatr 2017; 174:595–7.

61. Goodman WK, Grice DE, Lapidus KAB, et al. Obsessive-compulsive disorder. Psychiatr Clin North Am 2014;37:257–67.

62. Ruscio AM, Stein DJ, Chiu WT, et al. The epidemiology of obsessive- compulsive disorder in the National Comorbidity Survey Replication. Mol Psychiatry 2010; 15:53–63.

63. Marazziti D, Parra E, Amadori S, et al. Obsessive-compulsive and depressive symptoms in professional tennis players. Clin Neuropsychiatry 2021;18(6): 304–11.

64. Thomson P, Jaque S. Visiting the muses: creativity, coping, and PTSD in talented dancer and athletes. Am J Play 2016;8:363–78.

65. Goldstein RB, Smith SM, Chou SP, et al. The epidemiology of DSM-5 posttraumatic stress disorder in the United States: results from the National Epidemiologic Survey on Alcohol and Related Conditions-III. Soc Psychiatry Psychiatr Epidemiol 2016;51:1137–48.

66. Van Ameringen M, Mancini C, Patterson B, et al. Post-traumatic stress disorder in Canada. CNS Neurosci Ther 2008;14:171–81.

67. Aron CM, Harvey S, Hainline B, et al. Post-traumatic stress disorder (PTSD) and other trauma-related mental disorders in elite athletes: a narrative review. Br J Sports Med 2019;53(12):779–84.

68. Padaki AS, Noticewala MS, Levine WN, et al. Prevalence of posttraumatic stress disorder symptoms among young athletes after anterior cruciate ligament rupture. Orthop J Sports Med 2018;6(7). 2325967118787159.

69. Cloitre M, Stolbach BC, Herman JL, et al. A developmental approach to complex PTSD: childhood and adult cumulative trauma as predictors of symptom complexity. J Traum Stress 2009;22:399–408.

70. Lynch JH. Posttraumatic Stress Disorder in Elite Athletes. Curr Sports Med Rep 2021;20(12):645–50.

71. Reardon CL, Gorczynski P, Hainline B, et al. Anxiety disorders in athletes. Adv Psych Behav Health 2021;1(1):149–60.

72. Guillén F, Sánchez R. Competitive anxiety in expert female athletes: sources and intensity of anxiety in national team and first division Spanish basketball players. Percept Mot Skills 2009;109:407–19.

73. Yerkes RMD, Dodson JD. The relation of strength of stimulus to rapidity of habit formation. J Comp Neurol Psychol 1908;18(5):459–82.

74. Wilson PB, Russell H, Pugh J. Anxiety may be a risk factor for experiencing gastrointestinal symptoms during endurance races: An observational study. Eur J Sport Sci 2021;21(3):421–7.

75. Wilson PB, Fearn R, Pugh J. Occurrence and impacts of gastrointestinal symptoms in team-sport athletes: a preliminary survey. Clin J Sport Med 2022;33(3): 36476634.

76. Wilson PB. The psychobiological etiology of gastrointestinal distress in sport: a review. J Clin Gastroenterol 2020;54(4):297–304.

77. Diotaiuti P, Corrado S, Mancone S, et al. An Exploratory Pilot Study on Choking Episodes in Archery. Front Psychol 2021;12:585477. https://doi.org/10.3389/fpsyg.2021.585477.

78. Adler CH, Temkit M, Crews D, et al. The yips: methods to identify golfers with a dystonic etiology/golfer's cramp. Med Sci Sports Exerc 2018;50(11):2226–30.

79. Dhungana S, Jankovic J. Yips and other movement disorders in golfers. Mov Disord 2013;28(5):576–81.

80. Yu G, Chang KF, Shih IT. An exploration of the antecedents and mechanisms causing athletes' stress and twisties symptom. Heliyon 2022;8(10). e1104036276731.

81. Martorell MS, Ponseti FJ, Prats AN, et al. Competitive anxiety and performance in competing sailors. Retos 2021;39:187–91.

82. Rocha VVS, Oso rio FL. Associations between competitive anxiety, athlete characteristics and sport context: Evidence from a systematic review and meta-analysis. Rev Psiquiatr Clin 2018;45:67–74.

83. Madsen EE, Hansen T, Thomsen SD, et al. Can psychological characteristics, football experience, and player status predict state anxiety before important matches in Danish elite-level female football players? Scand J Med Sci Sports 2020;32(Suppl 1):150–60.

84. Cho S, Choi H, Youngsook K. The relationship between perceived coaching behaviors, competitive trait anxiety, and athlete burnout: a cross-sectional study. Int J Environ Res Public Health 2019;16(8):1424.

85. Pineda-Espejel HA, Alarcón E, Morquecho-Sánchez R, et al. Adaptive Social Factors and Precompetitive Anxiety in Elite Sport. Front Psychol 2021;12: 651169.

86. Kemarat S, Theanthong A, Yeemin W, et al. Personality characteristics and competitive anxiety in individual and team athletes. PLoS One 2022;17:12022, 44175-001.

87. Encel K, Mesagno C, Brown H. Facebook use and its relationship with sport anxiety. J Sports Sci 2017;35(8):756–61.

88. McDuff DR. Adjustment and anxiety disorders. In: Currie A, Owen B, editors. Sports psychiatry. Oxford, United Kingdom: Oxford University Press; 2016. p. 1–16.

89. Gouttebarge V, Bindra A, Blauwet C, et al. International Olympic Committee (IOC) Sport Mental Health Assessment Tool 1 (SMHAT-1) and Sport Mental

Health Recognition Tool 1 (SMHRT-1): towards better support of athletes' mental health. Br J Sports Med 2021;55(1):30–7.
90. Smith RE, Smoll FL, Cumming SP, et al. Measurement of multidimensional sport performance anxiety in children and adults: The Sport Anxiety Scale-2. J Sport Exerc Psychol 2006;28(4):479–501.
91. Locke AB, Kirst N, Shultz C. Diagnosis and management of generalized anxiety disorder and panic disorder in adults. Am Fam Phys 2015;91(9):617–24.
92. Fisk MZ, Steigerwald MD, Smoliga JM, et al. Asthma in swimmers: a review of the current literature. Phys Sportsmed 2010;38(4):28–34.
93. World anti-doping agency prohibited list 2023. In: World Anti-Doping Agency (WADA). Available at: https://www.wada-ama.org/sites/default/files/2022-09/2023list_en_final_9_september_2022.pdf. Accessed January 23, 2023.
94. Pickering C, Kiely J. What should we do about habitual caffeine use in athletes? Sports Med 2019;49(6):833–42.
95. Guest NS, VanDusseldorp TA, Nelson MT, et al. International society of sports nutrition position stand: caffeine and exercise performance. J Int Soc Sports Nutr 2021;18(1):1.
96. Reardon CL. Psychiatric manifestations of sport-related concussion. Curr Psychiatr 2020;19(7):22–8.
97. Champigny C, Roberts SD, Terry DP, et al. Acute Effects of Concussion in Adolescent Athletes With High Preseason Anxiety. Clin J Sport Med 2022;32(4):361–8.
98. Beidler E, Eagle S, Wallace J, et al. Anxiety-related concussion perceptions of collegiate athletes. J Sci Med Sport 2021;24(12):1224–9.
99. Thomas GA, Guty ET, Riegler KE, et al. Affective comorbidity or concussion: Can we tell the difference? Transl Issues in Psychol Sci 2022;2023:31554.
100. Wilson JJ, Wilson EM. Practical management: vocal cord dysfunction in athletes. Clin J Sport Med 2006;16(4):357–60.
101. Brun JF, Dumortier M, Fedou C, et al. Exercise hypoglycemia in nondiabetic subjects. Diabetes Metab 2001;27(2 Pt 1):92–106.
102. Luksch J, Collins PB. Thyroid disorders in athletes. Curr Sports Med Rep 2018;17(2):59–64.
103. Stillman MA, Glick ID, McDuff D, et al. Psychotherapy for mental health symptoms and disorders in elite athletes: a narrative review. Br J Sports Med 2019;53(12):767–71.
104. Vu V, Conant-Norville D. Anxiety: Recognition and Treatment Options. Psychiatr Clin North Am 2021;44(3):373–80.
105. Castaldelli-Maia JM, de Mello e Gallinaro JG, Falcao RS, et al. Mental health symptoms and disorders in elite athletes: a systematic review on cultural influences and barriers to athletes seeking treatment. Br J Sports Med 2019;53:707–21.
106. Ekelund R, Holmström S, Stenling A. Mental Health in Athletes: Where Are the Treatment Studies? Front Psychol 2022;13:781177.
107. Clark DA, Beck AT. Cognitive therapy of anxiety disorders: science and practice. New York: Guilford Press; 2010.
108. Burns L, Weissensteiner JR, Cohen M. Lifestyles and mindsets of Olympic, Paralympic and world champions: is an integrated approach the key to elite performance? Br J Sports Med 2019;53(13):818–24.
109. Hofmann SG, Gomez AF. Mindfulness-based interventions for anxiety and depression. Psychiatr Clin North Am 2017;40(4):739–49.

110. Moreton A, Wahesh E, Schmidt CD. Indirect effect of mindfulness on psychological distress via sleep hygiene in division I college student athletes. J Am Coll Health 2022;70(7):1936–40.
111. Myall K, Montero-Marin J, Gorczynski P, et al. Effect of mindfulness-based programmes on elite athlete mental health: a systematic review and meta-analysis. Br J Sports Med 2023;57(2):99–108.
112. Ramos-Sanchez CP, Schuch FB, Seedat S, et al. The anxiolytic effects of exercise for people with anxiety and related disorders: An update of the available meta-analytic evidence. Psychiatr Res 2021;302:114046.
113. Wicks C, Barton J, Orbell S, Andrews L. Psychological benefits of outdoor physical activity in natural versus urban environments: A systematic review and meta-analysis of experimental studies. Appl Psychol Health Well Being 2022; 14(3):1037–61.
114. Reardon CL, Factor RM. Sport psychiatry: a systematic review of diagnosis and medical treatment of mental illness in athletes. Sports Med 2010;40:961–80.
115. Reardon CL, Creado S. Psychiatric medication preferences of sports psychiatrists. Phys Sportsmed 2016;44(4):397–402.
116. Parise G, Bosman MJ, Boecker DR, et al. Selective serotonin reuptake inhibitors: their effect on high-intensity exercise performance. Arch Phys Med Rehabil 2001;82:867–71.
117. Meeusen R, Piacentini M, Van Den Eynde S, et al. Exercise performance is not influenced by a 5-HT reuptake inhibitor. Int J Sports Med 2001;22:329–36.
118. Marvanova M, Gramith K. Role of antidepressants in the treatment of adults with anorexia nervosa. Ment Health Clin 2018;8(3):127–37.
119. Marvin G, Sharma A, Aston W, et al. The effects of buspirone on perceived exertion and time to fatigue in man. Exp Physiol 1997;82:1057–60.
120. Johnston A, McAllister-Williams RH. Psychotropic drug prescribing. In: Currie A, Owen B, editors. Sports psychiatry. Oxford: Oxford University Press; 2016. p. 133–43.
121. Paul MA, Gray G, Kenny G, et al. Impact of melatonin, zaleplon, zopiclone, and temazepam on psychomotor performance. Aviat Space Environ Med 2003;74: 1263–70.
122. Charles RB, Kirkham AJ, Guyatt AR, et al. Psychomotor, pulmonary and exercise responses to sleep medication. Br J Clin Pharmacol 1987;24:191–7.
123. Cowan DA, abuse D, Harries M, et al. In: Oxford textbook of sports medicine. New York: Oxford University Press; 1994. p. 314–29.
124. NCAA Banned Substances. In NCAA Sport Science Institute. 2023. Available at: https://www.ncaa.org/sports/2015/6/10/ncaa-banned-substances.aspx.   Accessed 20 January 2023.
125. Ong NCH, Chua JHE. Effects of psychological interventions on competitive anxiety in sport: A meta-analysis Psychol Sport. Exerc 2021;52:101836.
126. Lachenmeier DW, Diel P. A warning against the negligent use of cannabidiol in professional and amateur athletes. Sports (Basel) 2019;7(12):251.
127. Salleh RM, Kuan G, Aziz MNA, et al. Effects of Probiotics on Anxiety, Stress, Mood and Fitness of Badminton Players, *Nutrients*, 13 (6), 2021, 1783. doi: 10.3390/nu13061783.

Depressive Disorders in Athletes

Sarah E. Beable, MBChB, FACSEP

KEYWORDS

- Depression in athletes • Athlete suicide • Depression risk factors • Life stress
- Antidepressant medication • Depression screening • SMHAT

KEY POINTS

- Depression prevalence appears to be at least as common as the general population, and possibly higher.
- Athletes have similar risk factors to the general population but also a unique set of risk factors such as injury, competition failure, performance failure, or individual sport.
- The management of depression in athletes requires an interdisciplinary team approach, often using nonpharmacological treatment such as counseling, sometimes medication, but also addressing the sporting environment and culture.
- Identifying suicidal athletes and having a mental health crisis management and action plan should be in place in all sporting organizations.
- More work is required to reduce the stigma and barriers to seeking help for those with depression.

INTRODUCTION

Depression is a significant public health issue worldwide, with approximately 18% of individuals suffering a major depressive episode in their lifetime, and rates continue to rise. The World Health Organization reports that 280 million people worldwide experience depression, now being second only to coronary artery disease as a cause of health decline.[1] Globally, depression is thought to be more common among women than men, but women are more likely to self-report symptoms of depression.[2]

The benefits of exercise and athletic participation improve self-esteem and social connectedness.[3] Furthermore, exercise in multiple forms is widely prescribed to manage depression, mental illness, and a range of other health conditions.[4] A positive correlation has been established between regular exercise and positive mental well-being.[5]

Historically, there has been an implication that only the mentally and emotionally "strong" would be competitive at the highest level and that those with significant

High Performance Sport New Zealand, Axis Sports Medicine Specialists, 15/5 Hawthorne Drive, Queenstown 9304, New Zealand
E-mail address: s.beable@axissportsmedicine.co.nz

Clin Sports Med 43 (2024) 53–70
https://doi.org/10.1016/j.csm.2023.06.011
0278-5919/24/© 2023 Elsevier Inc. All rights reserved.

mental illness would be prevented from succeeding.[6] However, athletes are not immune to what is a ubiquitous health problem worldwide. Demands of elite athlete life contribute to these athletes being as prone as their nonathletic counterparts and perhaps at an even higher risk for depressive disorders.[7–10] Unique athlete stressors such as injuries and their effects on career, pressure to perform, the physical and emotional demands of training, travel, and competition all cumulatively may negate any positive benefits of regular exercise and athletic participation.[11]

Elite athletes may not recognize, acknowledge, or seek help for depressive symptoms.[12] As Rao and Hong have suggested, there exists a need for a paradigm shift in helping identify and manage athletes who are suffering psychologically with a move toward enhanced awareness and better support systems.[13]

EPIDEMIOLOGY

Emerging studies and reviews across the globe suggest the prevalence of depression in athletes is equal to, or higher than, that of the general population. For example, a study in American collegiate athletes[9] identified 19.2% male and 25.6% female athlete demonstrated symptoms of depression. In addition, a study of German elite athletes found that approximately 15% were suffering symptoms indicative of a major depressive disorder.[10] Other studies have reported higher percentages. A study of 224 Australian athletes found 27.2% met the criteria for depression,[7] whereas in New Zealand, 21% of elite athletes were identified to have symptoms consistent with moderate depressive symptoms.[8]

In an International Olympic Committee (IOC) position statement,[11] it was noted the prevalence of depressive symptoms in athletes as high as 68%.[14] Despite this, athletes seeking the acknowledgment of, or treatment for, symptoms may not occur commonly due to the stigma surrounding mental health disorder that remains in sport.[15] A study of 13,000 elite athletes across 71 sports revealed "stigma" as the most reported factor preventing these athletes from seeking help.[16]

RISK FACTORS

Multiple factors have been proposed to account for the observed susceptibility of athletes to depression including injury,[8,10,17,18] relocating for sport,[8,19] eating disorders,[20] playing an individual sport (vs a team sport),[8,10,21,22] pain,[23] retirement[11,24–27] and the presence of high life stress.[8]

Injury

Injury can lead to difficulties coping cognitively, emotionally, and behaviorally. These can trigger degrees of psychological disturbance and potentially lead to decreased self-esteem, anger, anxiety, and depression. In addition, an injury may impact an athlete's self-identity, social structure, and concept of self-worth.[7,18,28,29] Often, the athlete has an identity intrinsically intertwined to sports participation, which is threatened in times of injury and transition from sport.[23] Depressive symptoms and life stress also have been linked to an increased susceptibility of future injury, thus addressing symptoms plays a crucial role in injury prevention.[30,31]

Relocating for Sport

Sport, particularly at more elite levels, requires extensive travel and sometimes moving. Being away from friends, family, and an established social support network is a risk factor for developing depression.[8,19]

Transitioning into and out of Sport

Transitioning into sport is high-risk period for an athlete. In the general population, individuals between the ages of 16 to 25 are considered at greater risk for depression and suicide. An elite athlete in this age group confers this same risk plus additional, as stressors associated with sport are significant. Greater training intensity, time and commitment, increased travel requirements, relocation for sport, experiencing financial struggle are just a few. Moreover, some college athletes need to balance study commitments all the while having less time for social activities.[32]

Retirement is also another high-risk time for an individual, citing loss of identity, reduction in the amount of exercise, and financial concerns as key contributors. Research has demonstrated that if the retirement is brought on suddenly and unexpectedly, this can lead to elevated feelings of vulnerability and depression.[24,32] An increased trend toward depressive symptoms was observed in a study of retired professional soccer players across six nations in which nearly 40% of the retired athletes experienced depression.[25] In New Zealand, a player survey found that one in three professional rugby players will suffer depression, anxiety, and stress upon retirement.[33] Furthermore, after retirement from high-level sport, those athletes participating in lower levels of physical activity have high reported rates of depression.[11,34]

Concussion

There are mixed reports in the literature suggesting that a history of concussion is linked with depressive disorders, with some articles suggesting a link, and others refuting this.[35–38] This is an area requiring future research.

Gender

Depression is more likely in females,[9,23,39,40] with female athletes thought to be twice more likely to report depressive symptoms than their male counterparts.[2] Male athletes tend to disclose their mental health concerns following retirement, likely skewing data collection on gender and depressive symptoms.[41]

Presence of Eating Disorders

High-performance athletes concerned with body image as well as those suffering from Relative Energy Deficiency in Sport (RED-S) are at elevated risk of depression.[42,43]

Sports in which aesthetics or leanness play a role for performance (ie, diving, gymnastics, or ballet) have higher prevalence of eating disorders and substance abuse, and risk of depression.[20,44,45]

Type of Sport

Different sports are associated with varying risks for depression. Individual sports have historically been associated with more depressive symptoms than team sports.[7,8,10,21] In addition, studies have suggested the team sport environment may even be protective of depressive symptoms.[21,22,46] As has been postulated, in an individual based sport such as track and field, there is only one winner as opposed to a team-based sport where half the competitors are winners.[23,47] In a North American study, track and field athletes had the highest rates of major depressive disorders (37.5%) compared with other college sports, with lacrosse reporting the lowest (13.5%).[23] In addition, French athletes who participated in aesthetic sports or activities requiring fine motor skills were at greater risk of experiencing depressive symptoms than those in team ball sports.[48] Higher performing elite athletes may be more at risk of depressive symptoms, with perceived competition failure thought to be associated with this.[14]

Para-athletes

There is a paucity of research in para-athletes; however, emerging studies suggest depression rates similar to non–para-athletes and the general population.[49,50]

Transgender Athletes

The transgender population, including athletes, are identified in the literature to be a psychologically vulnerable population. Although there is little research to date, this population is thought to have higher depression rates, high suicidal ideation and commit suicide at a higher rate than non-trans-gender people.[51]

Life Stress

Life events may also contribute as a risk factor. The 21st century has exposed elite athletes to multiple nonsporting factors and sports-specific stressors. There exists limited research on life stressors in elite athletes but a correlation between general life stress, sport-specific stressors, and the presence of at least moderate depressive symptoms have been reported. Major life events, including injury, are identified as increasing the risk of psychological distress and mental illness in the elite athlete.[52] It has been postulated that daily life "niggles" (ie, more frequent, and less severe stressors) perhaps have more of an impact on an individual's mood than those identified major events.[53–55] In a New Zealand study in elite athletes these daily life hassles were higher in female athletes, those who partook in an individual sport, and those who moved for their sport. There was a correlation between high levels of daily life hassles and depressive symptoms.[8]

Lower social support has also been linked with depressive symptoms. Those with a higher perceived social support were linked with fewer depressive symptoms.[56,57]

A newer, more novel factor affecting mood are the effects of the COVID-19 global pandemic.[58] A study of professional endurance athletes reported greater depressed mood despite both the increase in training and recovery. Similarly, anxiety and low motivation were noted in 40% of participants in a study of 37,000 US National Collegiate Athletic Association (NCAA) student-athletes.[55,56,59]

A summary of the risk factors of for depression is summarised in **Box 1**. This highlights some risk factors which are unique to competitive athletes.

DEFINITION OF DEPRESSION

Diagnosing an individual with a major depressive disorder requires the *presence of a depressed mood and/or little interest or pleasure from activities on most days of the week over at least a 2-week period*.[60]

As shown in **Table 1**, the formal diagnosis of depression requires at least five symptoms and a negative impact on functioning with symptoms unrelated to substance use/alcohol and not explained by an alternative diagnosis.[60]

Individuals may experience depressive symptoms without meeting full diagnostic criteria. These cases can present along a continuum ranging from "considerable detriment of wellbeing" to "minimal distress or functional impairment."

DIFFERENTIAL DIAGNOSES

Specific differential diagnoses essential to consider in the sporting setting include *low energy availability (LEA)* or *relative energy deficiency in sport (RED-S)* where energy

---

Box 1
Risk factors for depression in athletes

Female Gender

Individual Sport

Injury

Pain

Concussion

Substance or alcohol abuse

Eating disorders

Transitioning in or out of sport

Concurrent mental health diagnosis

Oher medical comorbidities

Genetic Factors

Environment factors (ie, lower social support, high life stress)

Performance factors (ie, competition failure)

Personality factors – (ie, maladaptive perfectionism)

---

expenditure exceeds energy intake, resulting in a spectrum of impaired physiologic, psychological, and performance effects. These conditions affect mood, sleep, weight, motivation, concentration, recovery, and performance. LEA and RED-s may be the result of disordered eating or a clinical eating disorder requiring further help. However, it is important to note that this energy mismatch may be inadvertent by simply under-consuming for energy expended. It is essential for the physician to distinguish between the two as care depends upon the cause.

The *overtraining spectrum* should be considered in diagnosing depression. This ranges from the short-term, supercompensation functional overreaching which is a common training loading tool. *Non-functional overreaching (NFO)* occurs with

---

Table 1
DSMV criteria for depression – as published in the IOC consensus statement[11]

At least 5 symptoms must be present for at least 2 wk (at least 1 of the symptoms must be depressed mood, or decreased interest or pleasue)	
• Depressed mood or (in children) irritable most of the day, nearly every day, as indicated by either subjective report leg (eg, feels sad or empty) or observation made by others leg (eg, appears tearful)	• Decreased interest or pleasure in most activities, most of each day
• Significant weight change or change in appetite	• Insomnia or hyersomnia
• Change in activity: psychomotor agitation or retardation	• Fatigue or loss of energy
• Feelings of worthlessness or excessive or inappropriate guit	• Diminished ability to think or concentrate, or indecisiveness
• Recurrent thought of death or suicide	

excessive training loads and insufficient recovery, leading to mood disturbances and performance deficits, but is thought to improve within 2 weeks of rest.[61,62] There is no standard diagnostic criteria for *overtraining syndrome (OTS)* but is considered more severe than NFO. This results in prolonged performance decline (greater than 2 months), and more severe psychological and/or immunologic and/or neuroendocrinological presentation.[61,63] OTS is more common in higher levels of sport and has been reported in 10% to 64% of athletes[64]

OTS should be considered when assessing and managing the depressed athlete. The "overreached" athlete will notice an improvement with a short relative rest period whereas the overtrained athlete requires prolonged rest and recovery (months and in rare cases, years). In contrast, withdrawing from exercise will often make a depressed athlete's symptoms worsen, not improve, as they lose the antidepressant effects of exercise.[11,65]

Additional depressive disorders to consider include bipolar disorder, premenstrual dysphoric disorder, seasonal affective disorder, and postpartum depression.

IMPACT OF DEPRESSION ON PERFORMANCE

Depression can considerably affect an athlete's performance, being affected by cognitive, physical, emotional, and social aspects (**Box 2**).

THE CLINICAL EVALUATION OF THE DEPRESSED ATHLETE
Screening for Depression

Following the IOC's release of their consensus statement on mental health considerations elite athletes,[11] the Sports Mental Health Assessment Tool (SMHAT-1) was introduced.[66]

The SMHAT-1 is a tool validated in athletes. It allows a range of mental health symptoms in keeping with the DSM-V of depressive disorders but also captures athletes who may benefit from intervention yet do not fully fit the criteria for the disorder. Screening for depression is just one part of the SMHAT. The tool further addresses other potential mental health disorders or risky behavior patterns such as alcohol and drug usage, sleep disturbances, and eating disorder symptoms, to name a few.[66]

The SMHAT has an initial triage component – the Athlete Psychological Strain Questionnaire (APSQ) – relating to sport-related psychological distress. The triage screening questions are assigned a certain point value. Depending on this score, further assessment of mental health symptoms may be triggered. For example, if initial screening scores return elevated for depression, this would lead to more in-depth evaluation using the Patient Health Questionnaire 9 (PHQ-9) which is validated to evaluate for depression.[66] The SMHAT guides management, monitoring, brief interventions, and when immediate action may be required.

Other standardized questionnaires used to screen for depression include the Beck Depression Inventory (BDI)[67] and the Center for Epidemiologic Studies of Depression (CESD).[68] These have been validated for depression screening in nonathletic populations[69] and widely used in research.

Although screening is useful to detect the presence and identify severity of depressive symptoms, it cannot "diagnose" depression. Diagnosis requires a clinical interview and assessment by a licensed health professional. The periodic health evaluation is an opportune time to complete screening and refer to the appropriate clinician if the athlete is identified as being at risk. These tools can additionally assist in monitoring the progression of symptoms in those receiving treatment for depression.

> **Box 2**
> **Impact of depression on performance**
>
> Cognitive impact
> - Decision-making
> - Focus and concentration
> - Reaction times
>
> Physical impact
> - Fatigue
> - Inability to recover
> - Weight loss or weight gain
> - Appetite can be decreased or increased
> - Insomnia (depression symptom and a common side effect of several commonly used antidepressant medications).
> - Low motivation can lead to difficulty engaging fully in training and competition.
>
> Emotional impact
> - Depression can lead to a heightened anxiety state, leading to performance anxiety, affecting training and competing.
> - Low self-esteem and self-confidence
> - Emotional dysregulation and poor coping strategies can be present.
>
> Social impact
> - May withdraw from social activities and group training sessions, which can enhance the feeling of loneliness and social isolation,
> - Loneliness can negatively impacting their mental state and team dynamics.
> - Communication can become challenging, amplifies the feeling of isolation, and increase the potential for interpersonal conflict.
> - Strained relationships in personal life and sporting entourage.
> - Depression can lead to an athlete exiting the sport altogether

Detailed psychological evaluation.
- *History:* A thorough mental health evaluation should be conducted to establish the diagnosis of depression, determine symptom severity, and assess for other psychological conditions. It is important to address potential comorbidities, sleep disturbances, substance and alcohol usage, and other risk-taking behaviors. This evaluation should include a detailed history of the athlete's mood, behaviors and thoughts, and ability to function. A review of past medical (including previous depression) and injury history, social history, and significant family history is also valuable. A detailed safety risk assessment must be documented.
- *Examination and investigations*: A comprehensive physical examination can assist in ruling out other medical conditions masquerading as depression, that is, thyroid dysfunction, anemia, hormonal imbalances. Laboratory tests may include blood and hormonal panels and physiologic testing.
- *Psychosocial factors:* In-depth review of risk factors and the athlete's environment, including social support network, stressors, and coping strategies may reveal important contributors. Acquiring collateral information to gain insight regarding the athlete's relationship with coaches, teammates, and family members can identify potential stressors (including daily life hassles). Understanding how they are performing academically or at work is also helpful.
- *Evaluation of training and athletic performance:* Evaluating the athlete's training load and progression, recovery practices, competition schedule, and goals is essential. This allows for determining the possibility of overreaching, overtraining, performance anxiety, and burnout.

- *Nutritional assessment*: Evaluating energy availability status and the likelihood of nutritional deficiencies is warranted as these may present similarly or contribute to depressive symptoms.

MANAGEMENT OF THE DEPRESSED ATHLETE

Early recognition is a crucial component of management. Healthcare providers should recognize that any acknowledged concern voiced about performance by the athlete or support staff may be a symptom of underlying clinical conditions such as depression or anxiety. Undiagnosed depression can affect injury and illness recovery and delay return to play. In a study of 827 sports physicians, only 80% reported "often or sometimes" asking about psychological issues relating to injury noting they found it more comfortable to ask about the injury itself rather than broaching any psychological impact from the injury.[70]

Interestingly, there seems to be a lower likelihood to diagnose depression in athletes than non-athletes[71–73] as well as a lower rate of prescribing antidepressant medication.[8] Reasons for this trend remain unclear and warrants future research.

Incorporating a "biopsychosocial model" in which biological, psychological, and social factors are examined, is advised with the use of an interdisciplinary team.[74] Each individual's needs within the sporting context are unique and thus must be tailored to when creating a management plan.

Nonpharmacological management:
1. *Psychotherapy* – "talk therapy." This involves working with a mental health professional to address thoughts, feelings, and behaviors contributing to the depression. Some evidence-based therapies include cognitive behavioral therapy (CBT), interpersonal therapy (IPT), and problem-solving therapy. 7775 In the sporting setting, for example, CBT might target identifying and addressing negative thought patterns and behaviors relating to a current injury while concurrently building more resilient and adaptive coping strategies.
2. *Lifestyle modifications* – healthy lifestyle habits should be encouraged and reinforced such as focusing on a healthy, nutrient-rich diet and avoiding alcohol.
3. Sleep hygiene education
4. *Stress management education* includes deep breathing techniques, progressive muscle relaxation, and mindfulness meditation.[76]

Pharmacologic Management

An athlete's own biology may sometimes need addressing. This can be accomplished by the addition of an antidepressant medication by a physician experienced in managing mental health in athletes with expert knowledge of the nuances between options. The prescriber must consider each unique athlete's history and be comfortable with World Anti-Doping Agency (WADA) considerations, side effect profiles, and potential effects on performance.

Serotonin Reuptake inhibitors (SSRIs): SSRIs have traditionally been the first line of treatment for depression due to their efficacy, relatively mild side effects, fewer contraindications, and permitted use in sport.[74,77,78]

- These medications function by increasing the bioavailability of serotonin-a neurotransmitter involved in mood regulation.
- Commonly prescribed SSRIs include fluoxetine, sertraline, paroxetine, citalopram, and escitalopram.
- SSRIs are not thought to negatively impact on athletic performance.[79]

- Possible side effects include gastrointestinal disturbances (especially nausea in the initial phases), sleep disturbances, and sexual dysfunction.

Selective Norepinephrine Reuptake Inhibitors (SNRIs) are less commonly used but effective antidepressants. They tend to be a second line for usage in those who have concurrent anxiety disorders and considered to be relatively energizing rather than sedating.[80]

- This class of medication increases the availability of serotonin and norepinephrine, both involved in mood regulation.
- Common SNRIs are venlafaxine and duloxetine.
- They are currently permitted in sport.
- These tend to have similar side effect profiles to SSRIs but can result in elevated pulse and blood pressure. This requires monitoring, particularly for high-intensity or endurance sports. SNRI's have not been well studied in athletic populations, thus impact on performance remains unclear.

Bupropion is an alternative to managing athletes with depression who do not have anxiety ("activating effects") nor eating disorders (increased risk of seizure).[77,81]

- This atypical antidepressant functions by inhibiting the reuptake of dopamine and norepinephrine as well as being a nicotine receptor antagonist.
- Bupropion is nonsedating and has relatively energizing properties, which may prove beneficial to those with low motivation.[77]
- Buproprion does not appear to cause weight gain, which is often appealing for the athlete.

Research suggests bupropion may be a performance enhancer by allowing athletes to push to higher heart rates and core body temperature when used in a higher, one-off dose thus improving performance. This, however, does not appear the have the same effect when taken at the lower recommended therapeutic dose.[82] At the time of writing (2023), Bupropion is currently on WADA's monitoring program given its possible effect as a stimulant. It does not currently require a therapeutic use exemption.

Tricyclic Antidepressants (TCA's) and mirtazapine should be avoided as first-line antidepressants in athletes due to the side effect profile: weight gain, sedation, and cardiac arrythmias.[62,83]

Clinics care points
- SSRIs such as fluoxetine and escitalopram are considered first-line treatment in the depressed athlete.[74,77,78]
- Bupropion is gaining popularity as an antidepressant, with possibly fewer performance impacting side effects, however as of 2023, it remains on the WADA monitoring list.
- If medication is required, it should be used in conjunction with non-pharmacological measures.

The Role of the Team Physician

The team physician has an eminent role in managing depression in athletes with the key objective being promoting wellbeing, while assisting optimizing performance. They must foster a supportive and confidential environment conducive to safe and open disclosure by athletes. If concerned, the physician must assess depression severity, collaborate as needed with other mental health professionals, and oversee the treatment plan. Once this has been established, the team physician must determine the safety and appropriateness of continued sport participation, keeping in mind that sport can confer various psychological benefits. The team physician should work to implement preventative measures, address sporting cultural concerns, and continue to advocate and educate for mental health awareness withing the sporting world. There exists a need for additional training and education for team physicians managing psychological issues in athletes.[29,70]

Sporting Culture, the Environment, and the Future

Individual sporting organizations must continue working toward reducing the stigma of mental illness. This is done by improving mental health literacy for all – with a comprehensive education program and resources directed toward depression education and mental wellbeing optimization. This education must address minority subgroups such as para-athletes, gender diverse, LGBQTI (lesbian, gay, bisexual, queer or questioning, transgender or intersex), cultural and religious sectors.

Nonaccidental injury (harassment and abuse)[84] in the sport setting can occur in physical, psychological, sexual, and emotional forms. The impact of non-accidental injury persists long after an athlete retires from a sporting programme.[84] Low self-esteem, reduced participation, anxiety, depression, self-harm, and suicide have all been identified as possible consequences of abuse in sport.[84–86] Further work needs to be done to protect all athletes. The IOC's consensus statement on harassment and abuse in sport identified a need for "no tolerance for all forms of non-accidental injury" with clear policies to safeguard athletes and a disclosure pathway outlined within a sporting organization.[84]

Widespread barriers exist which hinder athletes to seeking help for mental health issues; stigma described as the greatest obstacle.[27] Athletes remain concerned regarding how they will be perceived by support personnel, peers, and coaches if identified as needing mental health support.[87,88] Access to trained health professionals is also a significant hurdle worldwide as there exists immense social, economic, and medical disparities globally.[89]

Building athlete resilience should be a focus. In large, the aim of existing research has been in identifying the risk and predictive factors for athlete mental health issues. Dedicated high-quality research on the protective factors is indicated. Identifying common trends and learning from athletes who cope well in the face of adversity would help educate others to develop skillsets to "flourish rather than languish."[90] Potential protective factors previously identified include a feeling of autonomy, and positive relationships within the sporting setting as well as personal lives[91] needs further attention.

SUICIDE IN ATHLETES

Suicide is a significant and tragic public health concern affecting individuals across various populations and demographics, including athletes. Those experiencing a major depressive disorder are greater risk.

In general, young people are at an increased risk of suicide. As of 2019, suicide is the fourth leading cause of death in 15 to 29-year-olds.[1] This age bracket represents many athletes. Due to challenges in researching this cohort and stigma, it is possible that suicidal ideation is a larger problem than we are aware. In adolescents, sports participation is considered protective against depression and suicidal ideation, but it is possible the unique risk factors associated with mental illness in sport counteract this. Further research is required in these areas.

Some believe that athletes may actually have a lower risk for suicide compared to the general population.[92,93] This is postulated to be related to the protective mental and physical benefits of regular exercise in addition to the protective effect of sports participation – citing a sense of purpose, and social support.[93] A study investigating the rates of suicide over 9 years in American athletes found that the rate of suicide in NCAA athletes was significantly lower when comparing with age-matched nonathlete college student rate of suicide.[93]

Suicidal ideation and suicidal behavior (non-fatal, self-inflicted destructive act with the intent to die) has not been quantified in sport.[94] It is common for both suicidal ideation and attempts to peak amongst adolescents and young adults with a global lifetime prevalence between 12% and 33%.[95]

There exist additional factors identified with increased risk of suicide. Retirement, for example, is one such consideration. Approximately one in six international current and recently retired track and field athletes reported having experienced suicidal ideation in a study of 192 athletes.[94] Another includes the presence of pathologic eating patterns, thus awareness of formally diagnosed eating disorders is imperative; those suffering eating disorders in the general population have a 46% prevalence of suicidal ideation as opposed to 14% without eating disorders.[96]

Some studies have also suggested that athletes in contact sports (most citing American football) may have an increased risk of suicide.[93] This has been postulated to be due to the unclear long-term effects of repetitive traumatic brain injury and the possible development of chronic traumatic encephalopathy[97] however recent preliminary studies have not confirmed this link.[92,98] **Fig 1** summarises reported risk factors for suicide as outlined in the IOC consensus publication.[11]

Managing Suicide Risk in Athletes

Those working in the athletic environment require education and competence in psychological safety and escalating specific concerns when an individual's safety may be at risk. In addition, performance support staff, coaches, teammates, and other staff should be equipped with essential knowledge and skills on recognizing warning signs.

Early identification of warning signs is essential. For example, an athlete may exhibit changes in mood or behavior, withdraw socially or even have a considerable change in performance. In addition, they may make indirect statements or even verbalize thoughts about self-harm or suicide or cite feelings of worthlessness or hopelessness. It is thought approximately one-half of lifetime suicidal "ideators" transition to a suicide plan, and 22% of these, eventually to an attempt. Early identification and expeditious implementation a comprehensive screening program would reduce these values.[99]

Significant dedicated research has historically gone into developing emergency management plans for on-field emergencies. Similarly, developing a crisis/action plan for mental health emergencies is a necessity within all sporting organisations.[100]

The team doctor plays a critical role in assessing and managing suicide risk in athletes. **Box 3** outlines a proposed team physician approach in the setting of suicidal ideation.

Risk Factors - Suicide		
Agitation	History of childhood trauma	Interpersonal conflict
Aggression	History of suicide attempts	Physical injury/illness
Anxiety	Hopelessness	Sleep disturbance
Drug and alcohol use	Impulsivity	

Fig. 1. Risk factors for suicide. (*Adapted from* Reardon CL, Hainline B, Aron CM, et al. Mental health in elite athletes: International Olympic Committee consensus statement (2019). *Br J Sports Med*. 2019;53(11):667. https://doi.org/10.1136/bjsports-2019-100715.)

Box 3
Proposed team physician approach in the setting of suicidal ideation

The team physician should consider the following steps:

Initial risk assessment

The team doctor should ask empathetic but direct, open-ended questions in a non-judgemental fashion. Identify and document presenting concerns, and suicidal ideation, including previous attempts. They should assess the severity of the situation and any immediate safety threats to the individual or others. This step may also involve consulting with other colleagues.

Address the immediate crisis.

If the risk of suicide is imminent, immediate action is required. This could involve emergency services, informing the client's family, or coordinating with the local crisis psychiatry team on an inpatient admission.

Developing a safety plan

Work with the patient and appropriate mental health professionals to outline the steps they can take if they have suicidal thoughts or impulsive behavior. The safety plan may include recognizing triggers, avoiding drugs and alcohol, identifying supportive people to contact, and seeking professional psychological support.

Follow professional guidelines and legal obligations.

Team physicians should protect patients' right to confidentiality. It is a difficult challenge to balance their duty to protect their patient as well as the patient's right to confidentiality with imminent risk to oneself.

Documentation

Keep excellent written records of the above steps, including the assessment, actions taken, and if confidentiality was breached due to imminent safety risk. Record any consent gained from the patient. Record any consultations had with colleagues or other professionals regarding the suicide risk.

Follow-up and ongoing care

Outline and document plans for follow-up assessments and appointments, treatment recommendations, and when the plan will be revisited.

Collegial support

This is a complex issue to deal with and can take its toll. Health professionals should be encouraged to have professional supervision to debrief and be supported through complex medical challenges.

SUMMARY

Depressive disorders are a common mental health problem in the athlete. There are unique risk factors specific to the elite athlete that all of those working in the athletic environment, as well as athletes themselves, should understand.

The biopsychosocial model is a helpful model to direct interdisciplinary team approach in helping develop a management plan for a depressed individual.

Ongoing screening programs, education prevention (including mitigating risk factors, improving mental health literacy amongst all, and fostering protective factors) should be a focus. In addition, a comprehensive understanding of management options and safety risks is crucial for the team physician to have a high level of competency in.

Working toward an inclusive, safer, integrity filled environment where disclosing mental health issues and getting appropriate support is the norm, rather than the exception, should continue to be the goal.

DISCLOSURE

The author has no commercial or financial conflict of interests relating to the research described in this article. The author has no funding sources related to this article. May 2023.

REFERENCES

1. The World Health Organisation, Available at: https://www.who.int/news-room/fact-sheets/detail/depression. 2021. Accessed April 2023.
2. Gorczynski PF, Coyle M, Gibson K. Depressive symptoms in high-performance athletes and non-athletes: a comparative meta-analysis. Br J Sports Med 2017; 51(18):1348.
3. Babiss L a, Gangwisch JE. Sports participation as a protective factor against depression and suicidal ideation in adolescents as mediated by self-esteem and social support. Journal of Developmental and Behavioral Pediatrics 2009; 30(5):376–84. https://doi.org/10.1097/DBP.0b013e3181b33659.
4. Brosse AL, Sheets ES, Lett HS, et al. Exercise and the treatment of clinical depression in adults: recent findings and future directions. Sports Med 2002; 32(12):741–60.
5. Stanton R, Reaburn P. Exercise and the treatment of depression: a review of the exercise program variables. J Sci Med Sport/Sports Medicine Australia 2014; 17(2):177–82.
6. Markser VZ. Sport psychiatry and psychotherapy. Mental strains and disorders in professional sports. Challenge and answer to societal changes. Eur Arch Psychiatry Clin Neurosci 2011;261(SUPPL. 2). https://doi.org/10.1007/s00406-011-0239-x.
7. Gulliver A, Griffiths KM, Mackinnon A, et al. The mental health of Australian elite athletes. J Sci Med Sport/Sports Medicine Australia 2015;18(3):255–61.
8. Beable S, Fulcher M, Lee A. SHARP Sports mental Health Awareness Research Project. J Sci Med Sport 2017;20:1047–52.
9. Yang J, Peek-Asa C, Corlette JD, et al. Prevalence of and risk factors associated with symptoms of depression in competitive collegiate student athletes. Clin J Sport Med 2007;17(6):481–7.
10. Nixdorf I, Frank R, Hautzinger M, et al. Prevalence of depressive symptoms and correlating variables among German elite athletes. J Clin Sport Psychol 2013; 7(4):313–26.
11. Reardon CL, Hainline B, Aron CM, et al. Mental health in elite athletes: International Olympic Committee consensus statement (2019). Br J Sports Med 2019; 53(11):667.
12. Coyle M, Gorczynski P, Gibson K. "You have to be mental to jump off a board any way": Elite divers' conceptualizations and perceptions of mental health. Psychol Sport Exerc 2017;29:10–8.
13. Rao AL, Hong ES. In the mood for change: shifting the paradigm of mental health care in athletes—an AMSSM thematic issue. Br J Sports Med 2016; 50(3):133–4.
14. Hammond T, Gialloreto C, Kubas H, et al. The Prevalence of Failure-Based Depression Among Elite Athletes. Clin J Sport Med 2013;23(4):273–7.
15. Bauman NJ. The stigma of mental health in athletes: are mental toughness and mental health seen as contradictory in elite sport? Br J Sports Med 2016; 50(3):135.
16. Hainline B, Reardon CL. Breaking a taboo: why the International Olympic Committee convened experts to develop a consensus statement on mental health in elite athletes. Br J Sports Med 2019;53(11):665.
17. Appaneal RN, Levine BR, Perna FM, et al. Measuring Postinjury Depression Among Male and Female Competitive Athletes. J Sport Exerc Psychol 2009; 31:60–76.

18. Smith AM. Psychological impact of injuries in athletes. Sports Med 1996;22(6): 391–405.
19. Bruner MW, Munroe-Chandler KJ, Spink KS. Entry into Elite Sport: A Preliminary Investigation into the Transition Experiences of Rookie Athletes. J Appl Sport Psychol 2008;20(October 2014):236–52.
20. Sundgot-Borgen J, Torstveit MK. Prevalence of Eating Disorders in Elite Athletes Is Higher Than in the General Population. Clin J Sport Med 2004;14(1):25–32.
21. Nixdorf I, Frank R, Beckmann J. Comparison of Athletes' Proneness to Depressive Symptoms in Individual and Team Sports: Research on Psychological Mediators in Junior Elite Athletes. Front Psychol 2016;7.
22. Pluhar E, McCracken C, Griffith KL, et al. Team sport athletes may be less likely to suffer anxiety or depression than individual sport athletes. J Sports Sci Med 2019;18(3).
23. Wolanin A, Hong E, Marks D, et al. Prevalence of clinically elevated depressive symptoms in college athletes and differences by gender and sport. Br J Sports Med 2016;50(3):167–71.
24. Grove JR, Lavallee D, Gordon S. Coping with retirement from sport: The influence of athletic identity. J Appl Sport Psychol 1997;9(2):191–203.
25. Gouttebarge V, Frings-Dresen MHW, Sluiter JK. Mental and psychosocial health among current and former professional footballers. Occup Med (Chic III) 2015; 65(3):190–6.
26. Gouttebarge V, Castaldelli-Maia JM, Gorczynski P, et al. Occurrence of mental health symptoms and disorders in current and former elite athletes: a systematic review and meta-analysis. Br J Sports Med 2019;53(11):700.
27. Castaldelli-Maia JM, de M e Gallinaro JG, Falcão RS, et al. Mental health symptoms and disorders in elite athletes: a systematic review on cultural influencers and barriers to athletes seeking treatment. Br J Sports Med 2019;53(11):707.
28. Smith AM, Milliner EK. Injured athletes and the risk of suicide. J Athl Train 1994; 29(4):337–41.
29. Herring SA, Boyajian-O'Neill LA, Coppel DB, et al. Psychological issues related to injury in athletes and the team physician: A consensus statement. Med Sci Sports Exerc 2006;38(11):2030–4.
30. Johnson U, Ivarsson A. Psychological predictors of sport injuries among junior soccer players. Scand J Med Sci Sports 2011;21(1):129–36.
31. Williams JM, Andersen MB. Psychosocial antecedents of sport injury: Review and critique of the stress and injury model'. J Appl Sport Psychol 1998; 10(1):5–25.
32. Wippert PM, Wippert J. The Effects of Involuntary Athletic Career Termination on Psychological Distress. J Clin Sport Psychol 2010;4(2):133–49.
33. New Zealand Rugby Players Association. Retired Player Survey. 2013. Available at: https://www.yumpu.com/en/document/view/2057560/nzrpa-rw1211-dps.
34. Backmand H, Kaprio J, Kujala U. Influence of Physical Activity on Depression and Anxiety of Former Elite Athletes. Int J Sports Med 2003;24(8):609–19.
35. Guskiewicz KM, Marshall SW, Bailes J, et al. Recurrent Concussion and Risk of Depression in Retired Professional Football Players. Med Sci Sports Exerc 2007; 39(6). Available at: https://journals.lww.com/acsm-msse/Fulltext/2007/06000/Recurrent_Concussion_and_Risk_of_Depression_in.2.aspx.
36. Kerr ZY, Evenson KR, Rosamond WD, et al. Association between concussion and mental health in former collegiate athletes. Inj Epidemiol 2014;1(1):28.
37. Iverson GL, Van Patten R, Terry DP, et al. Predictors and Correlates of Depression in Retired Elite Level Rugby League Players. Front Neurol 2021;12.

38. Gouttebarge V, Kerkhoffs GMMJ. Sports career-related concussion and mental health symptoms in former elite athletes. Neurochirurgie 2021;67(3):280–2.
39. Walton CC, Rice S, Gao CX, et al. Gender differences in mental health symptoms and risk factors in Australian elite athletes. BMJ Open Sport Exerc Med 2021;7(1):e000984.
40. Prinz B, Dvořák J, Junge A. Symptoms and risk factors of depression during and after the football career of elite female players. BMJ Open Sport Exerc Med 2016;2(1):e000124.
41. Souter G, Lewis R, Serrant L. Men, Mental Health and Elite Sport: a Narrative Review. Sports Med Open 2018;4(1):57.
42. Mountjoy M, Sundgot-Borgen JK, Burke LM, et al. IOC consensus statement on relative energy deficiency in sport (RED-S): 2018 update. Br J Sports Med 2018; 52(11):687.
43. Cabre HE, Moore SR, Smith-Ryan AE, et al. Relative Energy Deficiency in Sport (RED-S): Scientific, Clinical, and Practical Implications for the Female Athlete. Dtsch Z Sportmed 2022;73(7):225–34.
44. Sundgot-Borgen J. Eating Disorders in Female Athletes. Sports Med 1994;17(3): 176–88.
45. Greenleaf C, Petrie TA, Carter J, et al. Female Collegiate Athletes: Prevalence of Eating Disorders and Disordered Eating Behaviors. J Am Coll Health 2009; 57(5):489–96.
46. Du Preez E, Graham K, Gan T, et al. Depression, Anxiety, and Alcohol Use in Elite Rugby League Players Over a Competitive Season. Clin J Sport Med 2017;27:1.
47. Chang CJ, Putukian M, Aerni G, et al. Mental Health Issues and Psychological Factors in Athletes: Detection, Management, Effect on Performance, and Prevention: American Medical Society for Sports Medicine Position Statement. Clin J Sport Med 2020;30(2):e61–87.
48. Schaal K, Tafflet M, Nassif H, et al. Psychological Balance in High Level Athletes: Gender-Based Differences and Sport-Specific Patterns. PLoS One 2011;6(5):e19007.
49. Olive LS, Rice S, Butterworth M, et al. Do Rates of Mental Health Symptoms in Currently Competing Elite Athletes in Paralympic Sports Differ from Non-Para-Athletes? Sports Med Open 2021;7(1):62.
50. Swartz L, Hunt X, Bantjes J, et al. Mental health symptoms and disorders in Paralympic athletes: a narrative review. Br J Sports Med 2019;53(12):737–40.
51. Jones BA, Arcelus J, Bouman WP, et al. Sport and Transgender People: A Systematic Review of the Literature Relating to Sport Participation and Competitive Sport Policies. Sports Med 2017;47(4):701–16.
52. Rice SM, Purcell R, De Silva S, et al. The Mental Health of Elite Athletes: A Narrative Systematic Review. Sports Med 2016;46(9):1333–53.
53. Chamberlain K, Zika S. The minor events approach to stress: Support for the use of daily hassles. Br J Psychol 1990;81(4):469–81.
54. Delongis A, Coyne JC, Dakof G, et al. Relationship of Daily Hassles, Uplifts, and Major Life Events to Health Status. Health Psychol 1982;1(2):119–36.
55. Kanner AD, Coyne JC, Schaefer C, et al. Comparison of two modes of stress measurement: daily hassles and uplifts versus major life events. J Behav Med 1981;4(1):1–39.
56. Yang J, Peek-Asa C, Lowe JB, et al. Social Support Patterns of Collegiate Athletes Before and After Injury. J Athl Train 2010;45(4):372–9.

57. Armstrong S, Oomen-Early J. Social Connectedness, Self-Esteem, and Depression Symptomatology Among Collegiate Athletes Versus Nonathletes. J Am Coll Health 2009;57(5):521–6.
58. Uroh CC, Adewunmi CM. Psychological Impact of the COVID-19 Pandemic on Athletes. Front Sports Act Living 2021;3.
59. Roche M, Sainani K, Noordsy D, et al. The Impacts of COVID-19 on Mental Health and Training in US Professional Endurance Athletes. Clin J Sport Med 2022;32(3):290–6.
60. American Psychiatric Association. Diagnostic and statistical manual of mental disorders 2013. https://doi.org/10.1176/appi.books.9780890425596.
61. Meeusen R, Duclos M, Foster C, et al. Prevention, diagnosis and treatment of the overtraining syndrome: Joint consensus statement of the European College of Sport Science (ECSS) and the American College of Sports Medicine (ACSM). Eur J Sport Sci 2013;13(1):1–24.
62. Weakley J, Halson SL, Mujika I. Overtraining Syndrome Symptoms and Diagnosis in Athletes: Where Is the Research? A Systematic Review. Int J Sports Physiol Perform 2022;17(5):675–81.
63. Kreher JB, Schwartz JB. Overtraining Syndrome. Sports Health: A Multidisciplinary Approach 2012;4(2):128–38.
64. Chang C, Putukian M, Aerni G, et al. Mental health issues and psychological factors in athletes: detection, management, effect on performance and prevention: American Medical Society for Sports Medicine Position Statement—Executive Summary. Br J Sports Med 2020;54(4):216.
65. Reardon CL, Factor RM. Sport psychiatry a systematic review of diagnosis and medical treatment of mental illness in athletes. Sports Med 2010;40(11):961–80.
66. Gouttebarge V, Bindra A, Blauwet C, et al. International Olympic Committee (IOC) Sport Mental Health Assessment Tool 1 (SMHAT-1) and Sport Mental Health Recognition Tool 1 (SMHRT-1): towards better support of athletes' mental health. Br J Sports Med 2021;55(1):30.
67. Upton J. Beck Depression Inventory (BDI). In: Gellman MD, editor. Encyclopedia of Behavioral Medicine. Cham: Springer; 2020. https://doi.org/10.1007/978-3-030-39903-0_441.
68. Eaton WW, Muntaner C, Smith C, et al. Center for Epidemiologic Studies Depression Scale: Review and Revision (CESD and CESDR). In: The Use of Psychological Testing for Treatment Planning and Outcomes Assessment. Vol 3: Instruments for Adults. Vol III; 2004:363-378. Available at: http://www.amazon.com/Use-Psych-Test-Set-Psychological-Instruments/dp/0805843310. Accessed August 2015.
69. Smarr KL, Keefer AL. Measures of depression and depressive symptoms: Beck Depression Inventory-II (BDI-II), Center for Epidemiologic Studies Depression Scale (CES-D), Geriatric Depression Scale (GDS), Hospital Anxiety and Depression Scale (HADS), and Patient Health Questionna. Arthritis Care Res 2011; 63(S11):S454–66.
70. Mann BJ, Grana WA, Indelicato P a, et al. A survey of sports medicine physicians regarding psychological issues in patient-athletes. Am J Sports Med 2007;35(12):2140–7.
71. Hirschfeld RM, Keller MB, Panico S, et al. The National Depressive and Manic-Depressive Association consensus statement on the undertreatment of depression. JAMA 1997;277(4):333–40.
72. Schwenk TL. The stigmatisation and denial of mental illness in athletes. Br J Sports Med 2000;34(1):4–5.

73. Guillemin M, Barnard E, George LE. The Biopsychosocial Model and the Construction of Medical Practice. In: Collyer F, editor. The Palgrave Handbook of social theory in health, illness and medicine. Palgrave Macmillan UK; 2015. p. 236–50. https://doi.org/10.1057/9781137355621_15.

74. Glick ID, Horsfall JL. Diagnosis and psychiatric treatment of athletes. Clin Sports Med 2005;24(4 SPEC. ISS):771–81.

75. Stillman MA, Glick ID, McDuff D, et al. Psychotherapy for mental health symptoms and disorders in elite athletes: a narrative review. Br J Sports Med 2019; 53(12):767–71.

76. Myall K, Montero-Marin J, Gorczynski P, et al. Effect of mindfulness-based programmes on elite athlete mental health: a systematic review and meta-analysis. Br J Sports Med 2023;57(2):99.

77. Reardon CL, Creado S. Psychiatric medication preferences of sports psychiatrists. Phys Sportsmed 2016;44(4):397–402.

78. Ciocca M, Stafford H, Laney R. The Athlete's Pharmacy. Clin Sports Med 2011; 30(3):629–39.

79. Meeusen R, Piacentini M, Van Den Eynde S, et al. Exercise Performance is not Influenced by a 5-HT Reuptake Inhibitor. Int J Sports Med 2001;22(05):329–36.

80. Roelands B, Goekint M, Heyman E, et al. Acute norepinephrine reuptake inhibition decreases performance in normal and high ambient temperature. J Appl Physiol 2008;105(1):206–12.

81. Davidson J. Seizures and bupropion: a review. J Clin Psychiatry 1989;50(7): 256–61.

82. Roelands B, Hasegawa H, Watson P, et al. Performance and thermoregulatory effects of chronic bupropion administration in the heat. Eur J Appl Physiol 2009;105(3):493–8.

83. Fowler NO, McCall D, Chou TC, et al. Electrocardiographic changes and cardiac arrhythmias in patients receiving psychotropic drugs. Am J Cardiol 1976; 37(2):223–30.

84. Mountjoy M, Brackenridge C, Arrington M, et al. International Olympic Committee consensus statement: harassment and abuse (non-accidental violence) in sport. Br J Sports Med 2016;50(17):1019–29.

85. Hodge K, Lonsdale C. Prosocial and Antisocial Behavior in Sport: The Role of Coaching Style, Autonomous vs. Controlled Motivation, and Moral Disengagement. J Sport Exerc Psychol 2011;33(4):527–47.

86. Gervis M, Dunn N. The emotional abuse of elite child athletes by their coaches. Child Abuse Rev 2004;13(3):215–23.

87. Ong NCH, Harwood C. Attitudes toward sport psychology consulting in athletes: Understanding the role of culture and personality. Sport Exerc Perform Psychol 2018;7(1):46–59.

88. Barnard JD. Student-Athletes' Perceptions of Mental Illness and Attitudes Toward Help-Seeking. J College Stud Psychother 2016;30(3):161–75.

89. Thornicroft G, Chatterji S, Evans-Lacko S, et al. Undertreatment of people with major depressive disorder in 21 countries. Br J Psychiatry 2017;210(2):119–24.

90. Kuettel A, Pedersen AK, Larsen CH. To Flourish or Languish, that is the question: Exploring the mental health profiles of Danish elite athletes. Psychol Sport Exerc 2021;52:101837.

91. Kuettel A, Larsen CH. Risk and protective factors for mental health in elite athletes: a scoping review. Int Rev Sport Exerc Psychol 2020;13(1):231–65.

92. Pichler E, Ewers S, Ajdacic-Gross V, et al. Athletes are not at greater risk for death by suicide: A review. Scand J Med Sci Sports 2023;33(5):569–85.

93. Rao AL, Asif IM, Drezner JA, et al. Suicide in National Collegiate Athletic Association (NCAA) Athletes. Sports Health: A Multidisciplinary Approach 2015;7(5): 452–7.
94. Timpka T, Spreco A, Dahlstrom O, et al. Suicidal thoughts (ideation) among elite athletics (track and field) athletes: associations with sports participation, psychological resourcefulness and having been a victim of sexual and/or physical abuse. Br J Sports Med 2021;55(4):198–205.
95. Turecki G, Brent DA. Suicide and suicidal behaviour. Lancet 2016;387(10024): 1227–39.
96. Patel RS, Machado T, Tankersley WE. Eating Disorders and Suicidal Behaviors in Adolescents with Major Depression: Insights from the US Hospitals. Behav Sci 2021;11(5). https://doi.org/10.3390/bs11050078.
97. Omalu BI, Bailes J, Hammers JL, et al. Chronic Traumatic Encephalopathy, Suicides and Parasuicides in Professional American Athletes: The Role of the Forensic Pathologist. Am J Forensic Med Pathol 2010;31(2). https://journals.lww.com/amjforensicmedicine/Fulltext/2010/06000/Chronic_Traumatic_Encephalopathy,_Suicides_and.7.aspx.
98. Morales JS, Castillo-García A, Valenzuela PL, et al. Mortality from mental disorders and suicide in male professional American football and soccer players: A meta-analysis. Scand J Med Sci Sports 2021;31(12):2241–8.
99. Mortier P, Cuijpers P, Kiekens G, et al. The prevalence of suicidal thoughts and behaviours among college students: a meta-analysis. Psychol Med 2018;48(4): 554–65.
100. Currie A, McDuff D, Johnston A, et al. Management of mental health emergencies in elite athletes: a narrative review. Br J Sports Med 2019;53(12):772.

Mental Health and Disordered Eating in Athletes

Andrea Kussman, MD[a],*, Hyunwoo June Choo, MD, MPH[b]

KEYWORDS

- Eating disorder • Disordered eating • Athlete • Mental health • Anorexia nervosa
- Bulimia nervosa • Binge eating disorder

KEY POINTS

- Athletes are at an increased risk for eating disorders (EDs) or disordered eating (DE) when compared with nonathletes.
- Female athletes and athletes in lean sports are at an increased risk for developing ED or DE.
- EDs are associated with wide-ranging and severe medical complications and impaired performance in athletes.
- Early identification and treatment improve outcomes, so physicians should screen for DE/ED annually at the preparticipation physical evaluation, and whenever athletes present with potentially related complaints, such as fatigue.
- Treatment of DE/EDs requires a multidisciplinary care team consisting of (at minimum) a physician, a dietitian, and a mental health provider. Partial or full restriction from sport may be required in some cases.

INTRODUCTION

Eating disorders (EDs) are devastating health conditions that can have severe effects on an athlete's well-being and performance. Clinical outcomes are improved by early identification and treatment, so it is crucial that sports medicine providers are familiar with the screening, diagnosis, workup, and treatment of DE/EDs. Athletes with DE/EDs face many unique considerations, including the delicate balance between dysfunctional exercise and the high levels of training required for athletic participation. In addition, athletes must balance adequate fueling with the demands of their training. These unique constraints make the sports medicine provider a key resource for athletes with DE/EDs.

[a] Department of Family Medicine, University of Washington; [b] Division of Physical Medicine and Rehabilitation, Stanford University Department of Orthopaedics, 450 Broadway, MC 6342, Redwood City, CA 94063, USA
* Corresponding author. 3800 Montlake Boulevard NE, Box 354060, Seattle, WA 98195.
E-mail address: akussman@uw.edu

Clin Sports Med 43 (2024) 71–91
https://doi.org/10.1016/j.csm.2023.07.001
0278-5919/24/© 2023 Elsevier Inc. All rights reserved.

DEFINITIONS

EDs include several conditions, as defined by the Diagnostic and Statistical Manual V (DSM-V). These include anorexia nervosa (AN), bulimia nervosa (BN), binge eating disorder (BED), avoidant/restrictive food intake disorder (ARFID), other specified feeding and eating disorder (OSFED), and unspecified feeding and eating disorder (UFED).[1] Please refer to **Table 1** for details on diagnostic criteria for each of these disorders. Athletes may also present with rumination disorder, which is characterized by repeated effortless regurgitation of recently ingested food, which may be rechewed, reswallowed, or spit out. This behavior must be ongoing for at least 1 month and may not be associated with a general medical condition such as gastroesophageal reflex disease. Furthermore, regurgitation may not occur solely during the course of AN, BN, BED, or ARFID.[1] Although diagnoses of ARFID and Rumination Disorder are less common, it is important to avoid confusing them with other ED diagnoses.

In addition, many athletes will present with complicated relationships with food and body image, which do not meet criteria for an ED. These occur on a spectrum of disordered eating (DE), which range from mildly dysfunctional to bordering on meeting full criteria for an ED. Athletes can move along this spectrum over time. It is more common for athletes to present with DE than with ED.[2]

Signs and symptoms of DE may include but are not limited to the following:

- Frequent dieting
- Skipping meals
- Anxiety associated with specific foods or types of foods
- Chronic weight fluctuations
- Rigid rituals and routines surrounding food and exercise
- Feelings of guilt and shame associated with eating
- Preoccupation with food, weight, and body image that negatively influences quality of life
- Making eating contingent on exercise (eg, skipping meals if they have not completed a workout)

Orthorexia is not an official diagnosis per the DSM-V but it is commonly used in the athletic community to refer to an obsession with healthy eating.[3] Orthorexia is typically used when the obsessive focus on healthy eating is associated with compulsive behaviors or mental preoccupation with following specific dietary practices for optimal health, when violating the self-prescribed dietary practices results in fear of negative outcomes or guilt and shame, and when these dietary practices escalate over time to become more restrictive or incorporate more foods.[4] Ultimately, these behaviors may result in malnutrition or weight loss, intrapersonal distress, impaired psychosocial functioning, and negative influences on body image or assessment of self-worth.[4] For the purposes of this article, orthorexia can be understood as part of the DE spectrum.

PREVALENCE

In the general population, the lifetime prevalence estimates of AN are 0.9% in women and 0.3% in men, estimates of BN are 1.5% in women and 0.5% in men, and estimates of BED are 3.5% in women and 2.0% in men.[5] This study relied on the narrower DSM-IV diagnoses of AN, BN, and BED, so current lifetime prevalence rates are likely higher. In addition, a survival analysis based on retrospective age-of-onset cohorts suggests that the risk of BN and BED may be increasing with successive birth cohorts.[5]

Table 1
Sport categories that are at increased risk for disordered eating/eating disorders - these include sports where having a lean body habitus could be perceived as a benefit

Condition	Definition	Specifications
AN	1. Restriction of energy intake relative to requirements, leading to significantly low body weight in the context of age, sex, developmental trajectory, and physical health. Significantly low weight is defined as a weight that is less than minimally normal or, for children and adolescents, less than minimally expected 2. Intense fear of gaining weight or of becoming fat, or persistent behavior that interferes with weight gain, even though at a significantly low weight 3. Disturbance in the way in which one's body weight or shape is experienced, undue influence of body weight or shape on self-evaluation, or persistent lack of recognition of the seriousness of the current low body weight	• Restricting type: During the last 3 mo, the individual has not engaged in recurrent episodes of binge eating or purging behavior. This subtype describes presentations in which weight loss is accomplished primarily by dieting, fasting, and/or excessive exercise • Binge eating/purging type: During the last 3 mo, the individual has engaged in recurrent episodes of binge eating or purging behavior • In partial remission: Full criteria for anorexia were previously met but currently the first criteria (low body weight) is not met; however, the second and third criteria are still met

BN	1. Recurrent episodes of binge eating, which are characterized by both of the following:
	   a. Eating, in a discrete period of time, an amount of food that is definitely larger than what most people would eat during a similar period of time and under similar circumstances
	   b. A sense of lack of control over eating during the episode
	2. Recurrent inappropriate compensatory behavior to prevent weight gain, such self-induced vomiting; misuse of laxatives, diuretics, enemas, or other medications; fasting; or excessive exercise
	3. The binge eating and inappropriate compensatory behaviors both occur on average at least once per week for 3 mo
	4. Self-evaluation is unduly influenced by body shape and weight
	5. The disturbance does not occur exclusively during episodes of AN	

(continued on next page)

Table 1
(continued)

Condition	Definition	Specifications

BED	1. Recurrent episodes of binge eating, which are characterized by both of the following:
	  a. Eating, in a discrete period of time, an amount of food that is definitely larger than what most people would eat during a similar period of time and under similar circumstances
	  b. A sense of lack of control over eating during the episode
	2. Binge eating episodes are marked by at least 3 of the following:
	  a. Eating more rapidly than normal
	  b. Eating until feeling uncomfortably full
	  c. Eating large amounts of food when not feeling physically hungry
	  d. Eating alone because of embarrassment about the amount of food consumed
	3. Feeling disgusted with oneself, depressed, or guilty after overeating
	4. Episodes occur, on average, at least once per week for 3 mo
	5. No regular use of inappropriate compensatory behaviors, as seen in AN and BN
	6. Binge eating does not occur solely during the course of AN or BN	

ARFID	1. Avoiding or restricting food intake, based on one or more of the following:
	  a. Lack of interest in food or low appetite.
	  b. Aversion or disgust to sensory characteristics of certain foods or food types
	  c. A conditioned negative response (such as anxiety or disgust) associated with food intake following an aversive experience (such as choking, vomiting, or abdominal pain)
	2. Restriction in the types of foods eaten leads to a persistent failure to meet nutritional and/or energy needs, manifested by at least one of the following:	

(continued on next page)

Table 1 (continued)		
Condition	**Definition**	**Specifications**
	a. Clinically significant weight loss, or in children, poor growth or failure to achieve expected weight gain b. Nutritional deficiency c. Supplementary enteral feeding or oral nutrition supplements are required to provide adequate intake d. Impaired psychosocial functioning 3. The eating or feeding disturbance is not due to lack of available food or associated with a culturally sanctioned practice 4. The disturbance does not occur solely during the course of AN or BN, and body weight and shape are not distorted 5. The disturbance is not due to a general medical condition (such as gastrointestinal disease or food allergies) or another psychiatric disorder	
OSFED	OSFED applies to patients with symptoms that cause significant distress or impair psychosocial functioning but who do not meet full criteria for a specified feeding or eating disorder. Clinicians record the diagnosis "Other Specified Feeding and Eating Disorder" followed by the reason the condition does not meet full criteria for an eating disorder	Examples: • Atypical AN—all criteria for AN are met, except BMI is $\geq$ 18.5 kg/m^2 • BN of low frequency and/or limited duration—all criteria for BN are met except episodes of binge eating and inappropriate compensatory behaviors occur less than once per week or for <3 mo
UFED	Unspecified Feeding or Eating Disorder is used when the symptoms of a feeding or eating disorder cause significant distress or impair psychosocial functioning but do not meet full criteria for a specific eating disorder	When possible, it is preferred to use OSFED and specify the reason why the patient does not meet criteria

From: Association., A.P., *Diagnostic and Statistical Manual of Mental Disorders, Fifth Edition (DSM-5)*. American Psychiatric Association. 2013.

Athletes have higher rates of ED than the general population, and female athletes are at an increased risk compared with male athletes. In a Norwegian study, female athletes were more likely to have ED than female nonathletes (20% vs 9%), and male athletes were more likely to have ED than male nonathletes (8% vs 0.5%).[6] Rates of ED in athletes may also increase longitudinally during an athletic career. In a 2-year study of Norwegian female adolescent elite athletes, ED diagnoses increased from 15.3% to 20.8%.[7] In another study, the percentage of collegiate female athletes with subclinical ED diagnoses increased from 18.7% during competition days to 26.7% 6 years later at the time of their retirement from sport.[8]

The rates of DE behaviors that do not meet full criteria for an ED are likely much higher, and athletes are more likely to present with DE than with an ED.[9] In one study, 40% of female artistic swimmers and divers were actively attempting to lose weight during their World Championships,[10] and a high percentage of athletes in weight class sports start using extreme weight loss methods early in their career.[11] Concerning rates of DE have also been noted in the para-athlete community.[12]

Unfortunately, rates of DE/EDs have been increasing. From 2007 to 2017, the years lost to disability rates remained constant or slightly decreased for all causes, noncommunicable diseases, and mental disorders overall; however, they increased by 6% for AN and 10% for BN.[13] Furthermore, a recent study demonstrated a surge in DE among current and former athletes because of the SARS-CoV-2 (COVID-19) pandemic response.[14] It is important to keep these changing trends in mind because many sports medicine providers may see a significant increase in the number of athletes presenting with DE/EDs.

RISK FACTORS

There are multiple risk factors that can increase an athlete's individual risk of developing DE/EDs. First, women are at an increased risk relative to men. Second, although athletes in any sport can develop an eating disorder, athletes who participate in sports in which there is a perceived benefit to maintaining a lean body habitus are at an increased risk (**Table 2**).[6,15–17] Third, environmental factors such as coaching staff and personality traits of individual athletes can influence their risk level. Athletes have reported their coach is one of the most influential people in determining their dieting patterns, weight loss, and body image.[18,19] In one qualitative analysis among endurance athletes, there were 2 larger themes associated with the development of DE: conflating physical appearance and sporting ability (particularly with social comparisons and expectations about what an "athletic body" looks like), and the lifestyle of an athlete, which requires discipline, sacrifice, and balance.[20] A study of female collegiate distance runners similarly found that expectations about "sport body ideals" influenced body image and DE.[19] Thus, societal expectations and sport-specific pressures may both contribute to the development of DE in the athletic population.

Table 2	
Sport categories that are at increased risk for disordered eating/eating disorders—these include sports where having a lean body habitus is perceived as a benefit	
Category of Sport	**Examples**
Esthetic sports	• Gymnastics • Artistic swimming • Diving • Figure skating
Endurance sports	• Long-distance running • Cycling • Rowing
Weight class sports	• Wrestling • Lightweight rowing
Aerial sports	• Gymnastics • Ski jumping

COMMON COMORBIDITIES AND COMPLICATIONS

Athletes with DE/EDs frequently have other mental health conditions, such as depression, anxiety, bipolar disorder, substance use, suicidality, and posttraumatic stress disorder. Even after controlling for factors such as age and sex, patients who were diagnosed with an ED were likely to have other core psychiatric diagnoses—this applied to 94.5% of patients with BN, 78.9% of patients with BED, and 56.2% of patients with AN.[5]

There are several medical conditions that are more common among patients with ED, including diabetes mellitus Type 1, gastroesophageal reflux disease, celiac disease, delayed gastric emptying, and lactose intolerance.[21–24] It is challenging to ascertain whether these medical conditions predispose an athlete to develop an ED, or whether these medical conditions are sequelae/complications of the ED itself.

In addition, EDs cause severe impairments in nearly every organ system of the body.[25] Due to the extensive medical complications that can develop, as well as associations with suicidality, EDs have one of the highest morbidity rates of all mental health conditions, with approximately 3.3 million healthy life years lost to ED-related disability.[26] Among the types of ED, the standardized mortality ratio is highest for AN, at 5.9.[27] One out of every 5 patients who dies with AN, dies by suicide.[27]

Those patients with EDs who also engage in dysfunctional exercise are more likely to experience poor physical and psychosocial outcomes.[25] Dysfunctional exercise can be defined as a pathologic relationship with exercise, which results in negative physical or psychological impairment, and includes compulsive exercise, exercise addiction, obligatory exercise, and exercise dependence.[25] Many athletes with EDs have features of dysfunctional exercise, given their relationship to their sport. This remains an important area for future research, and a challenging area to treat.

One of the most common complications of DE is the Female or Male Athlete Triad (Triad), or Relative Energy Deficiency in Sport (RED-S). In the Female Athlete Triad, low energy availability (EA) leads to functional hypothalamic amenorrhea and impaired bone health (**Fig. 1**).[28] This may manifest as oligomenorrhea or amenorrhea, infertility, increased risk of bone stress injuries (BSI), and osteoporosis. Similarly, the Male Athlete Triad describes the interrelated conditions of low EA, hypogonadotropic hypogonadism, and impaired bone health in the male athlete (**Fig. 2**).[29] This could manifest with increased fatigue, decreased libido, absence of morning erections, decrease in facial hair growth, infertility, increased risk of BSI, and osteoporosis.[29] The RED-S model was proposed by the International Olympic Committee as a unifying term, which includes both male and female athletes. It describes how relative energy deficiency can lead to a range of medical and performance-related complications (**Figs. 3 and 4**).[30,31]

It is important to note that low EA may be intentional (such as from an ED), or may be unintentional, as is frequently seen in athletes who increase their training intensity or volume without also increasing their fueling practices. Furthermore, not all athletes with DE will have low EA, and not all athletes with low EA will have DE. However, in many cases, athletes with DE/EDs may initially present for medical attention with one of the components of the Triad or one of the sequelae of RED-S. The most common example is an athlete who presents with a history of multiple BSI and is subsequently found to have low EA. Detailed evaluations are necessary when athletes present with one of the potential sequelae of the Triad or RED-S, in order to identify occult energy deficiency and whether this may be associated with DE/EDs.

In addition to the well-established link between DE/EDs and BSI, research shows that both male and female athletes with DE/EDs are at increased risk of other types of injury as well.[32]

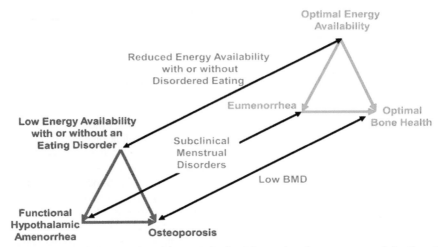

Fig. 1. Spectra of the Female Athlete Triad. The 3 interrelated components of the Female Athlete Triad are EA, menstrual status, and bone health. EA directly affects menstrual status, and in turn, EA and menstrual status directly influence bone health. Optimal health is indicated by optimal EA, eumenorrhoea, and optimal bone health, whereas, at the other end of the spectrum, the most severe presentation of the Female Athlete Triad is characterized by low EA with or without an eating disorder, functional hypothalamic amenorrhoea, and osteoporosis. An athlete's condition moves along each spectrum at different rates depending on her diet and exercise behaviors. BMD, bone mineral density. (*From*: Adapted with permission from Lippincott Williams and Wilkins/Wolters Kluwer Health: Medicine and Science in Sport and Exercise. De Souza MJ, Nattiv A, Joy E, et al. 2014 Female Athlete Triad Coalition Consensus Statement on Treatment and Return to Play of the Female Athlete Triad: 1st International Conference held in San Francisco, California, May 2012 and 2nd International Conference held in Indianapolis, Indiana, May 2013. Br J Sports Med. 2014 Feb;48(4):289. doi:10.1136/bjsports-2013 to 093218.

SCREENING

Early identification of EDs leads to better clinical outcomes, thus sports medicine providers should regularly screen athletes for EDs.[33] Athletes should be screened at the time of their preparticipation physical evaluation (PPE) from an early age. The PPE monograph includes several screening questions about DE/EDs, summarized in **Table 3**.[34] Additionally, including menstruation questions in the assessment of female athletes can be helpful in identifying functional hypothalamic amenorrhea, which is associated with low EA.[28]

There are also signs of EDs, which may be appreciated on physical examination at the time of the PPE. Some examples of physical examination findings that may indicate an ED include[35] the following:

- Fluctuations in weight
- Failure to gain expected weight in children
- Dental erosions
- Oral trauma or lacerations
- Parotid enlargement
- Hypotension
- Bradycardia
- Cardiac arrhythmias
- Lanugo
- Russell's sign (calluses/abrasions on the dorsum of hand from inducing emesis)

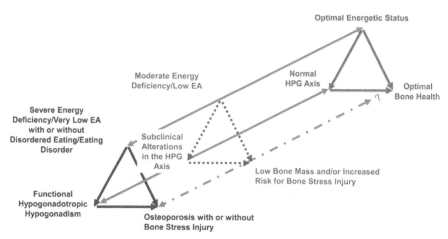

Fig. 2. Model of the Male Athlete Triad. The unidirectional arrows from energetic status/EA toward bone health and the hypothalamic-pituitary-gonadal (HPG) axis indicate the causal role of EA on both bone health and HPG axis function. Similarly, the unidirectional arrow from HPG toward bone health indicates the causal effect of reproductive hormones on bone health. Furthermore, the bidirectional arrows along each continuum of severity represent the "reversibility" of the condition such that an individual can improve or worsen over time. The line showing reversal of bone health outcomes is dashed with a question mark because the reversal of BMD is less known, and more research is needed. Notably, with the Male Athlete Triad, the subclinical and clinical sequelae present at lower EA levels than what is often required for the development of health consequences in exercising women. (*From*: Nattiv A, De Souza MJ, Koltun KJ, et al. The Male Athlete Triad-A Consensus Statement From the Female and Male Athlete Triad Coalition Part 1: Definition and Scientific Basis. Clin J Sport Med. 2021 Jul 1;31(4):345–353. doi: 10.1097/JSM.0000000000000946.)

The National Collegiate Athletic Association (NCAA) has recommended that mental health screening questionnaires be considered part of the PPE.[36] There are multiple screening measures for ED or low EA. When determining which screening measure is ideal, it is important to consider factors such as the population where the tool has been validated (athletes vs nonathletes, men vs women, and so forth), and the feasibility of administering the screening measure.

It is also important to screen athletes for DE/EDs anytime they present with signs or symptoms that could be attributed to an ED or low EA. Due to the secrecy and shame which often surround EDs, patients may be more likely to present with related complaints, such as BSI, fatigue, or decreased performance. In one study, less than half of participants with BN or BED had ever sought or received medical treatment of their EDs.[5]

MAKING THE DIAGNOSIS

The history is the most crucial part of the evaluation for suspected DE/EDs. Please refer to **Fig. 5** for some questions that may help guide a more detailed exploration of an athlete's relationship to their nutrition.[35] A nonexhaustive list of important areas to assess during the medical history is suggested in **Table 4**.

Concerning physical examination findings, as noted above, increase a physician's suspicion for ED. If there is concern for DE/EDs after performing a history and physical examination, additional workup is recommended. For a suggested list of diagnostic studies, please refer to **Fig. 6**.[35] The clinician should exercise their clinical judgment and tailor their workup to their patient's individual presentation. It is particularly

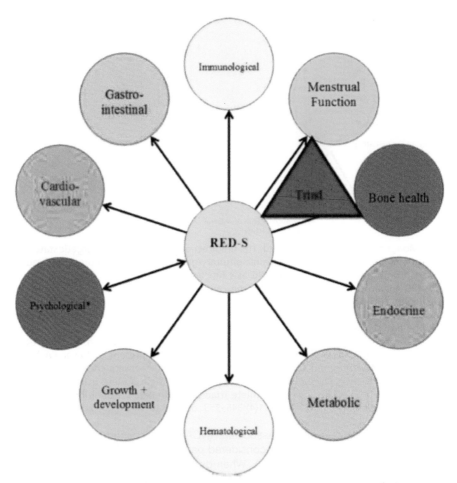

Fig. 3. Health Consequences of Relative Energy Deficiency in Sport (RED-S) showing an expanded concept of the Female Athlete Triad to acknowledge a wider range of outcomes and the application to male athletes (*Psychological consequences can either precede RED-S or be the result of RED-S). Adapted from Constantini. (Mountjoy M, Sundgot-Borgen J, Burke L, et alThe IOC consensus statement: beyond the Female Athlete Triad—Relative Energy Deficiency in Sport (RED-S)British Journal of Sports Medicine 2014;48:491-497.)

important to assess hormonal profiles and investigate any menstrual irregularities. Although functional hypothalamic amenorrhea is a common cause of amenorrhea in active women, there are other potential causes of amenorrhea that must also be ruled out, such as pregnancy or polycystic ovarian syndrome. In many athletes, bone mineral density (BMD) will be a concern. This is crucial to evaluate in adolescents with DE/EDs, who will be at a critical time to achieve peak bone accrual.[2] Even among older athletes, it is important to monitor BMD to prevent excessive bone loss.

DIAGNOSING EATING DISORDERS IN MALE ATHLETES

Male athletes present with EDs less frequently than female athletes. Although many athletes perceive there to be stigma associated with an ED diagnosis, male athletes

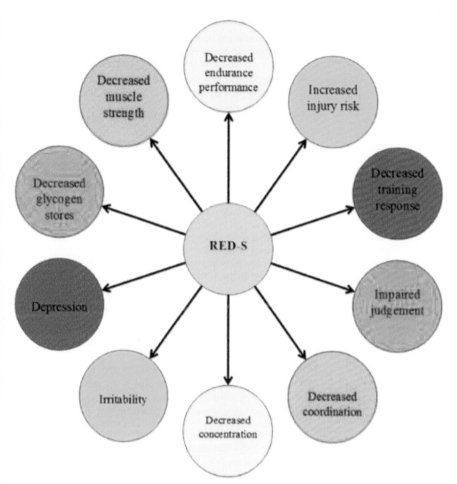

Fig. 4. Potential Performance Effects of Relative Energy Deficiency in Sport (*Aerobic and anaerobic performance). (Mountjoy M, Sundgot-Borgen J, Burke L, et alThe IOC consensus statement: beyond the Female Athlete Triad—Relative Energy Deficiency in Sport (RED-S) British Journal of Sports Medicine 2014;48:491-497.)

Table 3
Screening questions related to disordered eating/eating disorders on the preparticipation physical evaluation form

Medical Questions	Menstrual Questions
1. Do you worry about your weight?	1. Have you ever had a menstrual period?
2. Are you trying to or has anyone recommended that you gain or lose weight?	2. How old were you when you had your first menstrual period?
3. Are you on a special diet, or do you avoid certain types of foods or food groups?	3. When was your most recent menstrual period?
4. Have you ever had an eating disorder?	4. How many periods have you had in the past 12 mo?

From: American Academy of Pediatrics, A.A.o.F.P., American College of Sports Medicine, American Medical Society for Sports Medicine, American Medical Society for Sports Medicine, American Orthopedic Society for Sports Medicine, and American Osteopathic Academy of Sports Medicine. , *Preparticipation Physical Evaluation Monograph, 5th Edition.* 2019: American Academy of Pediatrics.

Topic	Questions
Questions to start the conversation	▶ How have you been feeling in general? How do you feel about yourself? ▶ Do you mind if we talk about your eating habits?
Initial critical questions	▶ Are there foods or food groups that you avoid eating? How do you feel about dieting in general? ▶ How do you feel about your body size? ▶ In what ways does your weight affect the way you think about yourself? ▶ What percentage of your waking hours do you spend thinking about weight, food and body image?
Diet and dieting	▶ Do you worry that you have lost control of how much you eat? ▶ Are you happy with your eating behaviour? ▶ Do you eat in secret? ▶ What did you have for breakfast today/yesterday? Lunch? Dinner? Snacks? ▶ Do you count your calories? Watch fat grams? Avoid certain foods? ▶ Do you ever eat a lot in one sitting—enough that you feel sick afterward? ▶ Are you worried because sometimes you can't stop eating?
Vomiting/purging	▶ Do you make yourself throw-up because you feel uncomfortably full? ▶ Do you use diuretics, laxatives or diet pills?
Weight and self-perception	▶ When you look in the mirror, what do you see? ▶ What do you think you should weigh? What are you doing to reach or maintain that weight? ▶ Have you recently lost or gained a lot of weight in a short period of time? ▶ What was your lowest weight in the last year? Your highest weight?
Exercise and training	▶ Do you exercise above and beyond what is required for your sport? ▶ Do you feel anxious if you miss a workout?
Family and support	▶ Does your family have any history of obesity, eating disorders, depression, mental illness or substance abuse (parents or other family members)? ▶ Who are your primary sources of emotional support? How do they support you?
Health	▶ Female patients: When did you have your first period? Are your periods regular? When was your last period? ▶ Do you have constipation? Diarrhoea? ▶ Are you ever dizzy? Weak? Tired? Have you ever fainted? ▶ Do you get cold easily? ▶ Have you lost any hair? Grown new hair? Do you have dry skin? ▶ Do you ever feel bloated? Have abdominal pain? ▶ Do you have muscle cramps, bone pain?

Fig. 5. Sample questions to evaluate for DE/ED behaviors. (*From*: Joy E, Kussman A, and Nattiv A. 2016 update on eating disorders in athletes: A comprehensive narrative review with a focus on clinical assessment and management. Br J Sports Med, 2016. 50(3): p. 154–62. Reprinted with permission.)

Table 4
Suggested Elements of the medical history in athletes with suspected disordered eating/eating disorder

Areas to Consider	Example Questions
Eating/nutrition related behaviors	• Whether any specific diets are followed (eg, vegetarian) • Average daily food/beverage intake, including timing and number of meals and snacks • Presence of binge episodes • Use of compensatory behaviors • Rigidity around food choices • Amount of time spent thinking about food or body image • Whether the patient is trying to lose or gain weight • Food security • Social patterns around eating, for example, eating alone
Training related factors	• Current phase of training • Recent changes to sport participation, including increases in intensity or changes to starting line-up • Recent athletic performance • Whether there are sport specific weight requirements
Injury history	• Pattern of overuse injuries, with particular attention to BSI
Medical history	• Endocrine disorders • Menstrual pattern (including age of menarche and number of periods within the past 12 mo) • Symptoms which might suggest hypogonadotropic hypogonadism in male athletes, such as a decrease in libido, or a decrease in the need to shave facial hair • Use of medications, such as COCs
Psychiatric history	• Previous mental health diagnoses • Current mental health symptoms, including screening for depression and anxiety • Assessment for suicidality
Family history	• Particularly of eating disorders, mental health conditions, or osteoporosis
Social history	• Drug or alcohol use • Pressure from coaches, peers, or parents to maintain a certain physique or weight • Level of social function

may perceive increased stigma due to misperceptions that this is predominantly a "female" problem. In addition, male athletes do not have menstrual cycle, which can serve as a helpful clinical indicator of low EA. These factors may combine to cause male athletes to present later with EDs than their female peers.[37] Furthermore, the body dysmorphia experienced by male athletes may take the form of "muscle dysmorphia," which refers to a desire to have a more muscular physique.[37] Thus, male athletes may present more with preoccupations about muscularity and lean muscle mass, rather than preoccupations with weight.

TREATMENT
Level of Care

The initial step when establishing a treatment plan is to determine the necessary level of care—inpatient, intensive outpatient, or outpatient. Indications that an athlete may need a higher level of care include severe electrolyte abnormalities, cardiac

Lab/test	When to use
Basic blood chemistry: serum electrolytes; renal function (BUN, Cr); calcium; liver function tests; thyroid stimulating hormone (TSH); complete blood count (CBC), differential and platelets; urinalysis	All patients with suspected eating disorders
Additional blood chemistry: iron studies; vitamin D; vitamin B12; magnesium; phosphorous	Malnourished and severely symptomatic patients
Additional blood chemistry: serum luteinizing hormone; follicle stimulating hormone; prolactin; estradiol; thyroid stimulating hormone (TSH)—if not previously obtained; urine pregnancy test	▸ Patients with delayed menarche—no menses by age 15 ▸ Absence/delay of secondary sexual characteristics by age 13; ▸ Secondary amenorrhea (no menses for three consecutive months)
Toxicology screen	Patients with suspected substance use
Radiological imaging: dual energy X-ray absorptiometry (DXA), radiographs, advanced imaging	▸ DXA for patients with amenorrhoea for 6 mo or more of prolonged oligomenorrhoea (<6 periods in 24 mo); ▸ Radiographs to evaluate for stress fractures, or more advanced imaging if needed
ECG	▸ Patients with syncope, recurrent near syncope, palpitations, resting supine heart rate <50 bpm ▸ Rapid weight loss; weight <80% of ideal body weight ▸ Hypophophatemia

Fig. 6. Suggested workup for patients with suspected DE/EDs. (*From*: Joy E, Kussman A, and Nattiv A. 2016 update on eating disorders in athletes: A comprehensive narrative review with a focus on clinical assessment and management. Br J Sports Med, 2016. 50(3): p. 154–62. Reprinted with permission.)

arrhythmias, syncope, rapid weight loss, or suicidal ideation. Most athletes can be treated in the outpatient setting, and the goal is to identify patients with EDs before they reach a severe condition, which requires hospitalization.[35]

The Multidisciplinary Care Team

When proceeding with outpatient treatment, it is crucial to establish a multidisciplinary treatment team. This has been associated with positive influences on treatment outcomes in patients with oligomenorrhea or amenorrhea and low EA.[38] At a minimum, this team should consist of a physician, a dietitian, and a mental health professional (**Fig. 7**).[2,35] Providing counseling regarding nutritional recommendations will not be successful unless the patient also engages with the underlying cognitive processes that fuel their DE behaviors. Similarly, athletes require guidance about how to gradually increase their energy intake. A focus on "optimizing fueling" can be more helpful than emphasizing "increasing calories." Although many patients will require an increase in their caloric intake, others would benefit from changing the timing or content of their meals, or from reducing inappropriate compensatory behaviors instead. Although some providers raise concerns that increasing dietary intake while undergoing psychological counseling could exacerbate negative eating behaviors, a recent randomized controlled trial found that modest increases in dietary intake (guided by a dietitian and a psychologist) led to increases in body and

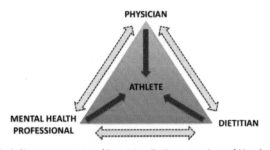

Fig. 7. The multidisciplinary care team. (*From*: Joy E, Kussman A, and Nattiv A. 2016 update on eating disorders in athletes: A comprehensive narrative review with a focus on clinical assessment and management. Br J Sports Med, 2016. 50(3): p. 154–62. Reprinted with permission.)

fat mass without increasing DE-related attitudes, stress, or depressive symptoms.[38] Thus, it is most helpful to approach ED treatment from multiple angles at once — providing guidance on gradually increasing nutrient intake, processing challenging relationships with body image or nutrition, and providing medical support for potential complications.

Frequent communication between team members is essential to avoid misunderstandings and to closely monitor the patient's clinical stability. In some cases, the treatment team may include consultants, athletic trainers, coaches, or parents. Frequency of medical appointments with members of the care team will vary considerably, depending on the acuity of the case and where the patient is in their recovery. When the severity of EDs is concerning, patients may require weekly physician visits. These may be spaced out as the patient recovers. Anyone can refer a patient who is at risk for DE/EDs to the multidisciplinary treatment team. This team is also responsible for liaising with sports and support staff.[2]

The Physician's Role in Eating Disorder Treatment

A suggested agenda for a physician visit is as follows. This agenda should be personalized to the individual patient.

1. Assess mood symptoms and inquire about mental health. Screen for suicidality if relevant.
2. Assess current ED symptoms, including frequency of bingeing, recent nutritional intake levels, and current volume of exercise.
3. Discuss the patient's function in different domains, including academic, interpersonal, or sport-related.
4. Review physical symptoms, such as palpitations, lightheadedness, or menstrual pattern. Menstrual irregularities should not be interpreted as the "normal" outcome of intense training.
5. Vital signs should be measured, including a blind weight, a resting heart rate, and a blood pressure. It is important to closely monitor the patient's weight trajectory to ensure they are not continuing to lose weight. However, a stable weight does not necessarily mean adequate nutritional intake is occurring because the patient may have a decreased resting metabolic rate (RMR) due to their low EA.
6. A relevant physical examination should be performed, as guided by the patient's level of illness and their symptoms.
7. Repeat laboratory or diagnostic studies may be indicated, depending on the patient's presentation and prior workup.
8. A plan of care should be established in collaboration with the patient. This may include medical prescriptions or additional referrals as indicated. It should also explicitly include clearance status for sports participation (full participation, limited participation, or restriction from training) and the timing of the next follow-up visit.

Pharmacologic Treatment

The majority of treatment for DE/EDs should be nonpharmacological and should consist of psychological support, nutrition education, and increasing EA. If this proves insufficient, then medications may be considered. Although there are psychiatric medications, which may be used in the treatment of mental health conditions that are frequently associated with EDs, such as depression or anxiety, it is worth noting that many patients experience improvement in their depressive and anxious symptoms as their EDs are treated and their EA is optimized.[39]

Multiple medications have been tested as a treatment of AN, and none has proven successful.[39] However, multiple medications (most notably antidepressants) have shown efficacy in treating BN. The most well-studied treatment of BN is high-dose fluoxetine (60 mg/day).[39] This should be initiated in lower doses, and gradually uptitrated as needed. BED has responded well to numerous psychiatric medications including fluoxetine, sertraline, citalopram, escitalopram, duloxetine, bupropion, lamotrigine, and topiramate; however, most of these cause a reduction in binge eating episodes without weight loss (which is a goal for some patients but is not indicated in all cases of BED).[39] Most recently, lisdexamfetamine has been approved by the Federal Drug Administration for the treatment of BED and has resulted in decreased binge episodes and modest weight loss.[39]

If amenorrhea or oligomenorrhea are present, combined oral contraceptives (COCs) should not be considered an appropriate treatment method (unless the patient also desires this for the prevention of pregnancy or management of other symptoms such as acne). Prescribing COCs to patients with DE/EDs does not address the underlying problem which is causing the irregular menses (low EA) and also does not improve BMD.[2,28] If a patient continues to have low BMD despite greater than 1 year of nonpharmacologic treatment, then they could consider transdermal estrogen with cyclic progesterone.[2,28] However, it is worth noting that this pattern of hormonal medication does not provide contraception.

Athletes with ED should be tested for electrolyte disturbances or nutrient deficiencies and treated accordingly. Whenever possible, athletes should obtain important micronutrients such as calcium, vitamin D, iron, and potassium from their diet; however, in some cases, supplementation may be necessary.[40]

Clearance Decisions

Decisions regarding clearance for sport in athletes with EDs are challenging and require an individualized assessment. If DE/EDs are diagnosed, an athlete may be allowed to continue full participation while engaging in treatment, or they may be partially or fully restricted from participation until further improvement is noted. The Female and Male Athlete Triad Coalition have a Cumulative Risk Assessment Tool and the RED-S model provides a Clinical Assessment Tool; these can assist the team physician in determining clearance status for an athlete with low EA.[28,29,31] However, these assessment tools should always be applied with the physician's clinical judgment, and should acknowledge individual aspects of an athlete's presentation.

Severe manifestations of ED should warrant removal from participation until further recovery is noted. These include a severely low body mass index (BMI) less than 16 kg/m^2, a significant percentage of weight loss, or frequent purging episodes occurring more than 4 times per wk.[35] Additionally, there may be red flags identified in the athlete's ED workup, which would warrant restriction from participation, such as cardiac arrhythmias or severe electrolyte disturbances.

For some higher risk athletes, it may be helpful to use a treatment contract. This specifies the treatment plan and clarifies the criteria for ongoing sports participation or for return-to-sport. It is signed by both the physician and the athlete and helps to prevent miscommunications between members of the treatment team. A sample treatment contract can be found in the 2014 Female Athlete Triad Consensus Statement.[28]

Prevention

Given the prevalence of DE/EDs in the athletic community, increasing rates of DE/EDs, and the devastating effects that EDs can have, preventative efforts are crucial. These should focus on education for athletes, coaches, parents, and other sports support staff.

There is evidence to support educational programs for athletes. A 1-year school-based intervention designed to prevent the development of new cases of EDs reduced the total prevalence of EDs among elite female athletes by 90%.[7] Bodies in Motion is a program developed based on cognitive dissonance and mindful self-compassion principles, and participants in this program had decreased "thin ideal internalization" when compared with controls during 4 months.[41] The Female Athlete Body (FAB) project is another educational intervention, which includes an 80-minute session once per week for 3 weeks. Data show significant reductions in dietary restraint, binge episodes, and thin-ideal internalization at 18-months of follow-up for participants in the FAB project when compared with controls.[42] In addition, a recent study found that the Male Athlete Body project (adapted from the FAB project) resulted in decreased body dissatisfaction, muscle dysmorphia, and body-ideal internalization in male athletes.[43]

Education would also be helpful to coaches. Several studies have found that coaches are not more likely to correctly identify an ED when compared with community members, and in one study, interviews showed that coaches tended to minimize the issue of ED in athletes.[44,45] By empowering our coaches to recognize the warning signs of DE/EDs in their athletes, and educating them about the potential negative health and performance outcomes of DE/EDs, coaches could be a valuable ally and could promote early identification and treatment.

Similarly, providing education for parents or athletic trainers could help to facilitate earlier identification and treatment of athletes. Being mindful of word choice and language surrounding appearances, nutrition, and performance can be helpful in reducing some of the pressures which contribute to DE/EDs. Whenever possible, staff should emphasize outcomes or results (such as personal records or amount of weight bench pressed) rather than commenting on physical appearance. Staff should also avoid labeling certain foods as "good" or "bad." There should be an overarching emphasis on health and well-being, rather than on athlete weight.[2] When body composition testing (such as the use of dual energy x-ray absorptiometry [DXAs] or regular weigh-ins) are used, there should be a clear rationale for performing the assessment, these should be done with athlete consent, and they should be managed by a sports dietitian, rather than the coach.[2]

Future Research

Given the increasing rates of DE/EDs in the wake of the COVID-19 pandemic, it will be important to continue to monitor these trends over time so that institutions and providers can appropriately allocate resources. In particular, more information is needed regarding the prevalence of DE/EDs in athlete subpopulations, such as para-athletes. Efforts to improve early identification of patients with DE/EDs will be helpful, as well as more knowledge about the presentation and treatment of ED in male athletes, or in individuals with compulsory exercise. Furthermore, research into programming, which can help prevent DE/EDs, would play a valuable role in reducing the influence these severe health conditions have on the athletics community.

SUMMARY

DE/EDs can have wide-ranging and devastating consequences on athlete health and performance. It is important that sports medicine providers are familiar with diagnostic criteria for EDs and comfortable screening for DE/EDs in the sports medicine clinic.

When DE/EDs are diagnosed, the team physician plays a crucial role as a member of the multidisciplinary treatment team and is responsible for making complex decisions regarding clearance status for sport participation. Educational programs can be effective in reducing DE behaviors or cognitions. Whenever possible, the sports medicine community should seek to prevent DE/EDs, destigmatize treatment, and promote healthy relationships with nutrition, which support the well-being and goals of our athletes.

CLINICS CARE POINTS

- Athletes can have a stable weight while still having an ED or being in a state of low EA due to adjustments in the body's RMR.
- All athletes who are suspected of having a DE/ED should undergo laboratory workup. Additionally, some athletes may need other studies such as an electrocardiogram (ECG) or DXA, depending on their presentation.
- In some cases, it may be necessary to partially or fully restrict an athlete with ED from participation until further recovery is noted. Treatment contracts may be used with high-risk athletes.
- Use neutral language such as "optimizing fueling" when recommending nutritional changes to athletes. This process of improving fueling may include increasing caloric intake but can also include changes to the timing or content of meals and snacks.

DISCLOSURE

None of the authors has any disclosures.

REFERENCES

1. Association AP. Diagnostic and Statistical Manual of Mental Disorders, Fifth Edition (DSM-5). American Psychiatric Association; 2013.
2. Wells KR, Jeacocke NA, Appaneal R, et al. The Australian Institute of Sport (AIS) and National Eating Disorders Collaboration (NEDC) position statement on disordered eating in high performance sport. Br J Sports Med 2020;54(21): 1247–58.
3. Koven N, Abry A. The clinical basis of orthorexia nervosa: emerging perspectives. Neuropsychiatric Dis Treat 2015;385.
4. Dunn TM, Bratman S. On orthorexia nervosa: a review of the literature and proposed diagnostic criteria. Eat Behav 2016;21:11–7.
5. Hudson JI, Hiripi E, Pope HG, et al. The prevalence and correlates of eating disorders in the National Comorbidity Survey Replication. Biol Psychiatry 2007;61(3): 348–58.
6. Sundgot-Borgen J, Torstveit MK. Prevalence of eating disorders in elite athletes is higher than in the general population. Clin J Sport Med 2004;14(1):25–32.
7. Martinsen M, Bahr R, Borresen R, et al. Preventing Eating Disorders among Young Elite Athletes: A Randomized Controlled Trial. Med Sci Sports Exerc 2014;46(3):435–47.
8. Thompson A, Petrie T, Tackett B, et al. Eating disorder diagnosis and the female athlete: A longitudinal analysis from college sport to retirement. J Sci Med Sport 2021;24(6):531–5.

9. Bonci CM, Bonci LJ, Granger LR, et al. National athletic trainers' association position statement: preventing, detecting, and managing disordered eating in athletes. J Athl Train 2008;43(1):80–108.

10. Mountjoy M, Junge A, Magnusson C, et al. Beneath the Surface: Mental Health and Harassment and Abuse of Athletes Participating in the FINA (Aquatics) World Championships, 2019. Clin J Sport Med 2022;32(2):95–102.

11. Sundgot-Borgen J, Torstveit MK. Aspects of disordered eating continuum in elite high-intensity sports. Scand J Med Sci Sports 2010;20(Suppl 2):112–21.

12. Brook EM, Tenforde AS, Broad EM, et al. Low energy availability, menstrual dysfunction, and impaired bone health: A survey of elite para athletes. Scand J Med Sci Sports 2019;29(5):678–85.

13. Disease, G.B.D., I. Injury, and C. Prevalence. Global, regional, and national incidence, prevalence, and years lived with disability for 354 diseases and injuries for 195 countries and territories, 1990-2017: a systematic analysis for the Global Burden of Disease Study 2017. Lancet 2018;392(10159):1789–858.

14. Buckley GL, Hall LE, Lassemillante AM, et al. Disordered eating & body image of current and former athletes in a pandemic; a convergent mixed methods study - What can we learn from COVID-19 to support athletes through transitions? J Eat Disord 2021;9(1):73.

15. Gorrell S, Nagata JM, Hill KB, et al. Eating behavior and reasons for exercise among competitive collegiate male athletes. Eat Weight Disord 2021;26(1):75–83.

16. Thiemann P, Legenbauer T, Vocks S, et al. Eating disorders and their putative risk factors among female German professional athletes. Eur Eat Disord Rev 2015;23(4):269–76.

17. Reinking MF, Alexander LE. Prevalence of disordered-eating behaviors in undergraduate female collegiate athletes and nonathletes. J Athl Train 2005;40(1):47–51.

18. Pensgaard AM, Roberts GC. Elite athletes' experiences of the motivational climate: the coach matters. Scand J Med Sci Sports 2002;12(1):54–9.

19. Carson TL, Tournat T, Sonneville K, et al. Cultural and environmental associations with body image, diet and well-being in NCAA DI female distance runners: a qualitative analysis. Br J Sports Med 2021;55(8):433–7.

20. Stoyel H, Delderfield R, Shanmuganathan-Felton V, et al. A qualitative exploration of sport and social pressures on elite athletes in relation to disordered eating. Front Psychol 2021;12:633490.

21. Mehler PS, Brown C. Anorexia nervosa - medical complications. J Eat Disord 2015;3:11.

22. Mehler PS, O'Melia A, Brown C, et al. Medical complications of bulimia nervosa. Br J Hosp Med 2017;78(12):672–7.

23. Rosen DS, A.A.o.P.C.o. Adolescence. Identification and management of eating disorders in children and adolescents. Pediatrics 2010;126(6):1240–53.

24. Baechle C, Castillo K, Strassburger K, et al. Is disordered eating behavior more prevalent in adolescents with early-onset type 1 diabetes than in their representative peers? Int J Eat Disord 2014;47(4):342–52.

25. Quesnel DA, Cooper M, Fernandez-Del-Valle M, et al. Medical and physiological complications of exercise for individuals with an eating disorder: A narrative review. J Eat Disord 2023;11(1):3.

26. van Hoeken D, Hoek HW. Review of the burden of eating disorders: mortality, disability, costs, quality of life, and family burden. Curr Opin Psychiatry 2020;33(6):521–7.

27. Arcelus J, Mitchell AJ, Wales J, et al. Mortality rates in patients with anorexia nervosa and other eating disorders. A meta-analysis of 36 studies. Arch Gen Psychiatry 2011;68(7):724–31.

28. De Souza MJ, Nattiv A, Joy E, et al. Female Athlete Triad Coalition Consensus Statement on Treatment and Return to Play of the Female Athlete Triad: 1st International Conference held in San Francisco, California, May 2012 and 2nd International Conference held in Indianapolis, Indiana, May 2013. Br J Sports Med 2014; 48(4):289.

29. Fredericson M, Kussman A, Misra M, et al. The Male Athlete Triad-A Consensus Statement From the Female and Male Athlete Triad Coalition Part II: Diagnosis, Treatment, and Return-To-Play. Clin J Sport Med 2021;31(4):349–66.

30. Mountjoy M, Sundgot-Borgen J, Burke L, et al. The IOC consensus statement: beyond the Female Athlete Triad–Relative Energy Deficiency in Sport (RED-S). Br J Sports Med 2014;48(7):491–7.

31. Mountjoy M, Sundgot-Borgen J, Burke L, et al. International Olympic Committee (IOC) Consensus Statement on Relative Energy Deficiency in Sport (RED-S): 2018 Update. Int J Sport Nutr Exerc Metab 2018;28(4):316–31.

32. Eichstadt M, Luzier J, Cho D, et al. Eating Disorders in Male Athletes. Sports Health 2020;12(4):327–33.

33. Chang P, Delgadillo J, Waller G. Early response to psychological treatment for eating disorders: A systematic review and meta-analysis. Clin Psychol Rev 2021;86:102032.

34. American Academy of Pediatrics, A.A.o.F.P., American College of Sports Medicine, American Medical Society for Sports Medicine, American Medical Society for Sports Medicine, American Orthopaedic Society for Sports Medicine, and American Osteopathic Academy of Sports Medicine. In: Preparticipation physical evaluation monograph. 5th edition. American Academy of Pediatrics; 2019.

35. Joy E, Kussman A, Nattiv A. Update on eating disorders in athletes: A comprehensive narrative review with a focus on clinical assessment and management. Br J Sports Med 2016;50(3):154–62.

36. Association, N.C.A. Mental Health Best Practices. 2016 (cited 2023 May 25); Available at: https://www.ncaa.org/sports/2016/5/2/mental-health-best-practices.aspx.

37. Gaudiani JL. Sick enough : a guide to the medical complications of eating disorders. New York, NY: Routledge; 2019.

38. Strock NCA, De Souza MJ, Mallinson RJ, et al. 12-months of increased dietary intake does not exacerbate disordered eating-related attitudes, stress, or depressive symptoms in women with exercise-associated menstrual disturbances: The REFUEL randomized controlled trial. Psychoneuroendocrinology 2023;152: 106079.

39. Crow SJ. Pharmacologic Treatment of Eating Disorders. Psychiatr Clin North Am 2019;42(2):253–62.

40. Ross AC, Manson JE, Abrams SA, et al. The 2011 report on dietary reference intakes for calcium and vitamin D from the Institute of Medicine: what clinicians need to know. J Clin Endocrinol Metab 2011;96(1):53–8.

41. Voelker DK, Petrie TA, Huang Q, et al. Bodies in Motion: An empirical evaluation of a program to support positive body image in female collegiate athletes. Body Image 2019;28:149–58.

42. Stewart TM, Pollard T, Hildebrandt T, et al. The Female Athlete Body project study: 18-month outcomes in eating disorder symptoms and risk factors. Int J Eat Disord 2019;52(11):1291–300.

43. Perelman H, Schwartz N, Yeoward-Dodson J, et al. Reducing eating disorder risk among male athletes: A randomized controlled trial investigating the male athlete body project. Int J Eat Disord 2022;55(2):193–206.
44. Macpherson MC, Harrison R, Marie D, et al. Investigating coaches' recognition of symptoms of eating disorders in track athletes. BMJ Open Sport Exerc Med 2022;8(3):e001333.
45. Nowicka P EK, Ng J, Apitzsch E, et al. Moving from knowledge to action; a qualitative study of elite coaches' capacity for early intervention in cases of eating disorders. Int J Sports Sci 2013;(8):343–55.

Sleep in the Athlete

Carly Day, MD[a],*, Naoya Nishino, MD[b], Yuka Tsukahara, MD, PhD[c]

KEYWORDS

- Sleep • Athlete • Mental health • Performance • Jet lag • Insomnia

KEY POINTS

- Sleep disorders are prevalent in both the general population and athletes, but there are unique factors that athletes face due to the high-stress competitive environment.
- Sleep is crucial for general health, cognitive function, lowering injury risk, and maintaining athletic performance.
- Taking a sleep history, evaluating sleep objectively, and addressing other related factors such as mental health and substance abuse are essential in diagnosing and understanding sleep disorders.
- Treatment options for sleep disorders include sleep hygiene, cognitive behavioral therapy, medication, and addressing contributing factors.
- Sleep is also affected by factors such as travel fatigue and jet lag, which should be taken into consideration for athletes.

DEFINITIONS

Sleep disorders refer to a group of conditions that affect a person's ability to get adequate sleep. Some common examples include insomnia, sleep apnea, restless leg syndrome (RLS), and narcolepsy. These conditions can have a significant impact on a person's overall health and well-being, leading to fatigue, irritability, and an increased risk of health problems.[1-3]

Insomnia

Insomnia is a sleep disorder characterized by difficulty falling or staying asleep, despite having adequate opportunity and circumstances, and must be associated with negative impact of daily activities or mood-related symptoms.[4,5] People with insomnia may also experience difficulty concentrating, irritability, mood swings, and

[a] Department of Health and Kinesiology, Purdue University, 900 John R Wooden Drive, West Lafayette, IN 47907, USA; [b] Sleep and Circadian Neurobiology Laboratory, Department of Psychiatry and Behavioral Sciences, Stanford University School of Medicine, 3155 Porter Drive, Palo Alto, CA 94304, USA; [c] Department of Sports Medicine, Tokyo Women's College of Physical Education, 3-40-1 Fujimidai, Kunitachi, Tokyo 1868668, Japan
* Corresponding author. 900 John R Wooden Drive, West Lafayette, IN 47907.
E-mail address: carlykreps@gmail.com
Twitter: @CarlyDayMD (C.D.)

Clin Sports Med 43 (2024) 93–106
https://doi.org/10.1016/j.csm.2023.06.007
0278-5919/24/© 2023 Elsevier Inc. All rights reserved.

sportsmed.theclinics.com

a decrease in overall quality of life. Insomnia can be caused by a variety of factors including stress, anxiety, depression, poor sleep hygiene, medications, and medical conditions.[6] A diagnosis of insomnia is established when the patient expresses dissatisfaction with sleep on at least 3 nights per week over a period of more than 3 months, along with accompanying symptoms such as daytime drowsiness, reduced attention span, and mood changes. A polysomnogram (PSG) may also be conducted to rule out other sleep disorders and to evaluate the patient's sleep patterns.

Sleep Apnea

Sleep apnea is a disorder characterized by repeated episodes of interrupted breathing during sleep. The symptoms of sleep apnea include loud snoring, pauses in breathing during sleep, choking or gasping during sleep, and difficulty staying asleep.[7] It can also lead to daytime sleepiness, morning headache, dry mouth, and difficulty concentrating. Sleep apnea can lead to serious health problems if left untreated, such as high blood pressure, heart attack, stroke, diabetes, and depression.[8] It is also important to note that sleep apnea can occur in people of all ages and is not limited to older adults or overweight individuals. Sleep apnea is caused by a partial or complete blockage of the airway during sleep. This blockage can be caused by a variety of factors, including obesity, a large tongue or tonsils, and is associated with family history of sleep apnea. It is typically diagnosed based on a patient's reported symptoms and a PSG.[7]

Restless Leg Syndrome

RLS is a neurologic disorder characterized by an irresistible urge to move the legs, often accompanied by unpleasant sensations such as tingling, creeping, crawling, or aching. The symptoms typically occur at night and can disrupt sleep, leading to daytime fatigue and impaired quality of life. The exact cause of RLS is unknown, but it is believed to be related to a deficiency of dopamine, a neurotransmitter that plays a role in movement and sensation. Other factors that may contribute to the development of RLS include iron deficiency, peripheral neuropathy, kidney failure, pregnancy, and certain medications.[9] The diagnosis of RLS is made through a clinical history and is often accompanied by periodic limb movements in sleep (PLMS). PLMS is present in 80% to 90% of RLS patients and can be confirmed with a PSG if necessary. Owing to the absence of a reliable biological diagnostic marker for RLS, the clinical assessment, especially the acquisition of the patient's medical history, plays a vital role in accurately diagnosing this condition.[9]

Narcolepsy

Narcolepsy is a disorder characterized by excessive daytime sleepiness along with other symptoms such as cataplexy (sudden loss of muscle tone), sleep paralysis, and vivid hallucinations during sleep onset or wakefulness. The primary cause of narcolepsy is a deficiency in the neurotransmitter hypocretin (also known as orexin), which regulates wakefulness and rapid eye movement (REM) sleep.[10] The diagnosis of narcolepsy is typically made by a sleep specialist through a combination of patient history, physical examination, and sleep studies such as PSG and multiple sleep latency test.[5]

NATURE OF THE PROBLEM
Sleep Disorders in the General Population

Sleep disorders are common among the general population, with a significant number of people experiencing difficulty sleeping. According to data from the National Center for Health Statistics, approximately 50 to 70 million adults in the United States have a sleep disorder.[11] Insomnia is the most common sleep disorder, with an estimated 30% of adults experiencing symptoms of insomnia at some point in a given year and roughly 10% of the adult population meeting the criteria for insomnia disorder. Sleep apnea affects an estimated 25 million people in the United States, with 80% of moderate to severe cases remaining undiagnosed and higher rates observed in men and older adults[12] RLS affects around 2% to 10% of adults, whereas narcolepsy is estimated to affect one in 2000 people in the United States.[12] However, the prevalence of sleep disorders can vary widely depending on the population studied and the diagnostic criteria used. It is also not uncommon for people to experience multiple sleep disorders at the same time.

Sleep Disorders in Athletes

The prevalence of sleep disorders in athletes has received increased attention in recent years, with research suggesting that athletes may be at higher risk for certain sleep disorders due to factors such as training schedules, travel, and competition stress. Although research in the field is still limited, studies have suggested that athletes have higher rates of insomnia symptoms compared with the general population.[13] This may be caused by the physical and mental exertion aspects of sports training. In addition, certain athletes (especially those in contact sports such as rugby and American football) may have physical attributes such as a higher body mass index or larger neck circumference and the altered upper airway dynamics that come with it, which may lead to a higher risk of obstructive sleep apnea (OSA).[14]

Another aspect that may be common for athletes to face is the sleep disorders that can be caused by the psychological stress of competition and the pressure to perform. Athletes may experience insomnia, anxiety, and depression that can affect their sleep patterns.[15]

Gender Differences

There are some differences in sleep patterns and disorders between men and women, which may be influenced by a variety of factors including hormonal, physiologic, and lifestyle differences. Women are 1.4 times more likely to experience insomnia than men.[16] Women are also more likely to experience sleep-related movement disorders, such as RLS.[17] On the other hand, sleep-disordered breathing, such as OSA, is more prevalent in men than women.[18]

Although sleep disorder disparities between men and women are apparent in the general population, research on elite athletes has produced conflicting results. Studies have shown that women had a higher prevalence of sleep disorders, specifically difficulty initiating and maintaining sleep, and male athletes had longer total sleep times than female athletes.[19,20] However, other research found that men who competed at an elite level had more sleep complaints than women.[21]

CLINICAL RELEVANCE

Sleep is essential for maintaining physical and mental health and well-being. Adequate sleep is important for the proper functioning of the body's systems and plays a crucial role in the healing and repair of the heart and blood vessels, muscles, and other tissues.[22]

General Health Benefits

Maintaining a healthy immune system that can defend against infections and illnesses requires sufficient sleep.[23] The regulation of the body's metabolism is another essential function of sleep, which is important for maintaining a healthy weight and preventing chronic diseases such as obesity, diabetes, and heart disease.[24]

Cognition

Sleep plays a critical role in cognitive function and brain health. Some of the cognitive benefits of sleep include.

Memory consolidation: Sleep helps to consolidate and solidify memories, allowing them to be stored and retrieved more easily. Sleep plays a crucial role in the consolidation of both declarative and procedural memories.[25]

Learning and cognitive flexibility: Adequate sleep is essential for learning new information and skills and for being able to adapt to new situations. Sleep-deprived individuals have difficulty adapting to new information and learning new tasks.[26]

Improved attention, reaction time, and decision-making: Sleep deprivation can lead to decreased attention and reaction time, impaired judgment, and increased accident risk.[27]

Problem-solving and creativity: Sleep is essential for the brain to be able to process information and find new solutions to problems. Sleep-deprived individuals have difficulty solving problems and coming up with new ideas.[28]

Emotional regulation: Sleep also plays a role in regulating emotions, which can affect cognitive processes such as decision-making, problem-solving, and attention.[29]

Injury Reduction

Insufficient sleep can lead to slower reaction times, decreased attention, and impaired judgment, all of which can lead to greater risk of sports and musculoskeletal injuries.[30] Less than 8 hours of sleep per night was associated with higher injury risk in high school athletes.[31] Most evidence points to chronic sleep deprivation having a larger impact than acute sleep issues.[30] It has been suggested that there is a link between sleep extension and enhancement of muscle injury recovery via the boosting of Insulin-like Growth Factor 1 (IGF-1) levels and potential regulation of localized inflammation.[32]

Athletic Performance

Sleep is critical for not only physical and mental health but for optimal athletic performance. Some of the demonstrated effects of sleep on performance include:[33,34]

Endurance: Sleep deprivation is associated with an increase in perceived exertion and decreased time to exhaustion.

Anaerobic power: Sleep deprivation leads to decreased mean and peak power output during the Wingate test (a cycle ergometer test that measures anaerobic capacity and power output).

Accuracy: Sleep extension improved basketball free throw and three-point field goal percentage. Sleep restriction decreased tennis serve and dart-throwing accuracy.

Mental Health and Sleep

The relationship between mental health and sleep is bidirectional and complex. The interconnected nature of the two can pose a challenge to the physician, but it is important to assess both and take steps to treat any problems identified. The stress of performance and competition can impact sleep in athletes. Some theories suggest a hormonal mechanism. Salivary cortisol levels and perceived stress are higher following competition compared with training and rest days and this was accompanied by reduced sleep quantity and quality.[35]

Anxiety and depression: Some data suggest that order of onset can vary based on the type of mental health disorder. In young adults, anxiety was more likely to precede insomnia, whereas depression more commonly had a later onset than insomnia.[36] Treating anxiety and depression with cognitive behavioral therapy can improve insomnia severity.[37]

Suicidal ideation: Suicidal thoughts are more prevalent in athletes with sleep disorders, such as onset insomnia and insufficient sleep (not getting enough sleep to feel rested).[38]

Eating disorders: The prevalence of sleep disturbance in patients with eating disorders is greater than 50%, and patients with a higher binge frequency were more likely to have sleep difficulties.[39]

Attention-deficit hyperactivity disorder: Adolescents with attention-deficit hyperactivity disorder have a longer sleep onset and shorter sleep duration than age-matched controls.[40]

APPROACH

Taking a detailed sleep history allows physicians to best determine diagnosis and treatment of sleep disorders.

Basic Sleep History Questions

To better understand the sleep habits of an athlete, the following issues should be addressed when evaluating an athlete according to the National Collegiate Athletic Association (NCAA) Interassociation Task Force on Sleep and Wellness:[41]

- Bedtime
- Wake time
- How long it takes to fall asleep
- Nap frequency, timing, and duration
- Sleep quality
  - Number of nightly awakenings and reason
  - Issues with sleep onset or sleep maintenance
  - Waking feeling rested
  - Daytime sleepiness
- Sleep disorders
  - Hallucinations, sleep paralysis, or cataplexy
  - Nighttime leg discomfort relieved by movement
  - Sleep walking or night terrors
  - Snoring, witnessed apnea, choking, gasping, or shortness of breath
- Medication and drug use
  - Stimulants (prescription medications, caffeine)
  - Sedative hypnotics
  - Drug and alcohol use
- Mental health status
- Environmental conditions
  - Exposure to light
  - Electronic device use

Athlete-Specific Questions

High-level athletes experience unique circumstances that may affect their sleep. Inquiring about these topics will help the physician understand potential barriers to adequate sleep. Examples include.

- What time of day do you typically train?
- Do you have any current injuries or pain that affect your sleep?
- Is fear of reinjury or reliving a traumatic event on your mind often?
- Does worrying about playing time or performance affect your ability to sleep?
- How often do you travel for games/training?
- Is your sleep worse when you are away from home?
- Do you travel to other time zones?
- Does your sleep vary in relation to being in-season versus out-of-season?

Advanced Questions

Although the above sleep history suggestions will address the majority of sleep difficulties, a physician may need to consider less common causes if the source of sleep difficulty cannot be determined.

Diet: Meals high in protein may improve sleep quality, and diets high in fat may shorten the duration of sleep.[42,43] Hidden sources of caffeine may also be uncovered as some sports drinks now contain caffeine.

Eating disorders: Although female athletes and those in esthetic and endurance sports are at higher risk of developing disordered eating/eating disorders, any athlete can have an eating disorder or low energy availability.[44] Malnutrition increases orexin, a hormone that promotes wakefulness.

Food insecurity: Greater odds of depression, anxiety, and suicidal ideation as well trouble falling asleep and staying asleep are seen in people who deal with food insecurity.[45] This could be easily missed as athletes may not be forthright about difficulty affording adequate nutrition.

Menstrual cycles: Premenstrual and menstrual periods are associated with insomnia and poor sleep quality.[46] Premenstrual syndrome is associated with symptoms such as headaches and mood disturbances which may impact sleep. The luteal phase is associated with poor sleep quality and daytime sleepiness, possibly due to changes in melatonin and body temperature.[47]

Mental health: Although screening for anxiety and depression is common in athletes, attention should also be paid to disorders such as schizophrenia, bipolar disorder, or post-traumatic stress disorder (PTSD). PTSD can occur in athletes after musculoskeletal injuries but asking about recent concussions can also be helpful.[48]

Overtraining syndrome: Athletes with fatigue, muscle soreness, reduced performance, sleep disturbance, and mood changes may be dealing with overtraining syndrome.[49] Asking about training volume and recovery strategies may help uncover this diagnosis.

Medical conditions: Asthma and gastroesophageal reflux disease are common medical conditions that can have an impact on sleep, especially when they are not adequately treated.[50]

EVALUATION

If a sleep disorder is suspected, the physician must decide the best way to evaluate the athlete to provide a diagnosis or determine the factors contributing to their problem.

Polysomnography

Considered the gold standard for diagnosing sleep problems, PSG is used to capture physiologic characteristics such as brain activity, muscle activity, eye movement, and heart activity during sleep. It also provides information on sleep onset latency, wake after sleep onset, sleep efficiency, frequency of sleep awakenings, and sleep fragmentation. In addition, both REM sleep and non-REM sleep can be evaluated. Some less desirable aspects of PSG include high cost, needing specialized equipment and a laboratory environment with a trained technician, and sleeping in a foreign location that may not accurately mimic the home sleep environment, thus skewing outcomes.

Actigraphy

Actigraphy is a method for determining sleep and wake patterns based on movement data collected by a device that may be worn on the wrist or ankle and is less expensive and easier to wear than PSG. It is possible to evaluate total sleep time, sleep-onset latency, waking after sleep onset, and sleep efficiency. It is recommended that the device is worn for at least 5 days, and measurements are usually taken every minute.[51] Actigraph data can be incorrect if the device is worn inconsistently as lack of motion when not attached to the person can be interpreted as sleep. It also tends to overestimate total sleep time because it is hard to detect brief awakenings.

Sheet Sensors

Sheet sensors were first used in nursing homes or by the elderly living alone. A device is placed under the sheet to detect sleep/wake patterns, heart rate, body movement, and respiration patterns. However, because it can only be used while an individual is sleeping in the bed, this option may miss naps taken in locations other than the bed or nights where the person sleeps away from their home.[52] It is inexpensive, inconspicuous, and longitudinal data can be obtained.

Smartphone Applications

Owing to the increase in smartphone usage, there are numerous sleep measurement applications.[53] Most are required to be placed on the bed and measure the subject's movement using the smartphone's integrated sensors or some can record sounds to evaluate sleep. However, evidence is scant and additional research is required, particularly to confirm the application's quality compared with PSG or other well-studied techniques.

Sleep Diaries

Sleep diaries are cost-effective and should normally be kept for at least 1 week. Athletes should record their bedtime and waking time, daytime napping, assessments of drowsiness and alertness, caffeine and alcohol use, and use of light-emitting devices before going to bed. However, they may be subjective and, because they are generally based on memory, are not always accurate.

Questionnaires

Questionnaires may be subjective, but they are frequently used to evaluate the sleep habits and disorders of athletes due to being cost-effective. They can be the best option for mass screening of large athlete populations. Commonly used questionnaires include:

Athlete Sleep Behavior Questionnaire: The Athlete Sleep Behavior Questionnaire (ASBQ) is also for athletes and consists of 18 questions that examine sleep behavior using a five-point scale. Three main categories included are routine/environmental factors (naps, consistent bedtimes, travel), behavioral factors (medications, alcohol, and late-night technology use), and sport-related factors (late night training, pain, and worrying about performance). A higher global score suggests a larger risk of poorer sleep-related behaviors; the investigators of the ASBQ advise that a global score $\leq$ 36 corresponds to "excellent" sleep behavior, 37 to 41 corresponds to "moderate" sleep behavior, and ≥ 42 corresponds to "bad" sleep behavior. The ASBQ has demonstrated low-to-moderate correlations with other sleep questionnaires and high test–retest consistency.[54]

Athlete Sleep Screening Questionnaire: The Athlete Sleep Screening Questionnaire is a survey that is designed to assess athletes for clinical sleep disorders and suggest if further workup is needed using 16 questions. A "Sleep Difficulty Score" (SDS) is calculated using five questions based on total sleep time, satisfaction with sleep, use of medicine to help sleep, and the presence of insomnia symptoms. The SDS is paired with several additional questions assessing chronotype and sleep-disordered breathing.[55] The SDS was incorporated into the International Olympic Committee's (IOC) Sport Mental Health Assessment Tool 1 to screen for mental health symptoms and disorders.[56]

Epworth Sleepiness Scale: The Epworth Sleepiness Scale is a questionnaire used to assess daytime sleepiness. Questions evaluate the likelihood of falling asleep in various situations such as reading, watching TV, or riding in a car.[57] This is not specific to athletes.

Insomnia Severity Index: Insomnia Severity Index consists of seven questions investigating difficulty falling asleep, staying asleep, and waking early as the impact of sleep on quality of life over a 2-week period.[58] This is not specific to athletes.

Pittsburgh Sleep Quality Index: This is used to evaluate sleep length, habitual sleep efficiency, sleep latency, sleep disruption, daytime dysfunction, sleep medication use, and subjective sleep quality. Participants are asked to rate the frequency of each item over the preceding month. The questions are not athlete-specific but have been validated in many languages.[59]

TREATMENT

Addressing sleep difficulties in athletes involves targeting deficiencies and treating co-morbid conditions.

Sleep Hygiene

Educating athletes on proper sleep hygiene is almost always the first step of addressing sleep disorders. This can be done via handouts to large groups or one-on-one sessions if time and resources allow. The NCAA Interassociation Task Force on Sleep and Wellness recommend following these sleep hygiene guidelines:[41]

- Maintain a regular sleep schedule
- Seek bright light during the day and avoid bright light at night
- Keep the sleep environment cool, dark, and comfortable
- Avoid caffeine at least 6 hours before bedtime
- Avoid excessive food and liquids at night
- Avoid obsessive clock watching
- Consider avoiding naps, although some people may function better with naps so this recommendation may vary on an individual basis
- Use beds for sleep only

Cognitive Behavioral Therapy

Cognitive behavioral therapies are beneficial and are extensively used for insomnia.[60] Cognitive behavioral therapy for insomnia (CBTI) is a structured program that identifies and replaces sleep-disrupting thoughts and actions with sleep-promoting routines. The patient can learn how to support and naturalize the body's sleep process, resulting in long-term improvements. CBTI consists of sleep restriction, stimulus control, cognitive therapy, sleep hygiene training, and relaxation training. CBTI is a safe and highly effective treatment for insomnia, but it may be underused due to a shortage of skilled CBTI practitioners and because athletes' busy schedules may make it difficult for them to attend therapy sessions. Thus, physicians and medical practitioners can play a role in educating athletes about the significance and benefit of CBTI.[61]

Medications and Anti-Doping Considerations

Both the NCAA and the IOC recommend CBTI over medication when treating sleep disorders in athletes.[41,62] With that said, some athletes use medication despite a lack of high-level research on efficacy in their population. Over-the-counter melatonin is a common treatment, often acquired by athletes without seeing a physician. Melatonin receptor agonists and benzodiazepine receptor agonists (BZRAs) are used for sleep-onset disorders, whereas dual orexin receptor antagonists, low-dose doxepin, and BZRAs are used for sleep-maintenance insomnia.[63] Some off-label prescription medications are used such as sedating antidepressants and gabapentin, although these are probably most effective when being used to also address concomitant mental health or pain conditions.[63] Owing to the sedating nature of many of these medications, the athlete should monitor for side effects that may carry over to the next day and impact training.[64] Stimulants, sometimes prescribed to treat daytime drowsiness, are prohibited by World Anti-Doping Agency (WADA) and steps need to be taken to assure that compliance with all WADA documentation occurs.

Lifestyle Changes

Sleep disorders including sleep apnea and RLS can be treated with lifestyle changes. For sleep apnea, this may include weight loss, exercise, and avoiding alcohol and sedatives. In patients with RLS, regular exercise and avoiding caffeine and alcohol as well as medications such as dopaminergic drugs, iron supplements, and anticonvulsants are recommended.[65]

Continuous Positive Airway Pressure

The treatment of sleep apnea typically involves a combination of lifestyle changes and medical devices. Continuous positive airway pressure (CPAP) machines deliver air pressure through a mask and oral appliances reposition the jaw to help keep the airway open. Surgery, which may help to remove or shrink excess tissue in the airway that may be causing the blockage, may also be an option for some individuals with sleep apnea if CPAP and lifestyle changes do not work.[66]

CONSIDERATIONS
Travel Fatigue

Travel fatigue is a combination of physical, physiologic, and psychological issues leading to exhaustion and tiredness and can occur from various modes of travel (bus, train, and airplane). Some proposed contributors to travel fatigue include restricted movement, impaired nutritional intake, concerns about travel logistics, disruption of daily routine, and noise stress. The four key factors of travel fatigue severity are total distance traveled, time of travel, frequency of travel, and time available for recovery.[67] Travel fatigue can occur without crossing time zones and is a separate entity than jet lag (explained below). Symptoms of travel fatigue include persistent fatigue, recurrent illness, behavior and mood changes, and loss of motivation. Management of travel fatigue is multifactorial. Pretravel athletes should be as well rested as possible and plan their nutrition and hydration in advance. During travel, it is important to move frequently and stretch when possible, consider noise-cancelling headphones, and follow illness prevention strategies such as hand washing.[67]

Jet Lag

Jet lag is a "temporary impairment of sleep and wakefulness, as well as other biological functions, associated with rapid eastward or westward travel across 3 or more time-zones."[67] This is due to a circadian desynchronization between the athlete's internal clock and the external cues of the new time zone. The severity of jet lag is affected by number of time zones traveled and travel direction (eastward vs westward). Ideal performance likely occurs during daytime of the time zone the athlete came from and evaluation of professional athletes suggests that traveling westward for an evening competition gives the greatest disadvantage.[68] Symptoms of jet lag include daytime sleepiness, sleep disruption, and lack of concentration.[67] One validated tool that can be used to assess the effect of trans-meridian travel on athletes is the Liverpool Jet Lag Questionnaire.

Jet lag can be explained in part by two markers of circadian rhythm. First, core body temperature (CBT) in the human body has daily fluctuations. Sleep can be initiated most easily when CBT is low or falling. Conversely, when CBT is high or rising it is difficult to sleep.[67] Second, melatonin is a hormone that aids with sleep and is typically secreted approximately 2 hours before habitual bedtime (often referred to as dim light melatonin onset).[67] Traveling across times zones creates a mismatch in timing of CBT and melatonin which can impact ability to fall asleep and stay asleep.

Two commonly proposed solutions to jet leg are light exposure and melatonin.[69] Although some assume that bright light in the morning and melatonin before bedtime will help manage jet leg, timing of these interventions is complex and depends on eastward versus westward travel.[67] Light exposure and exogenous melatonin recommendations can be found in sleep publications, although evidence behind these recommendations is low quality.[67,69,70] Other suggestions for assisting with phase shifting or combating symptoms of jet leg include exercise, caffeine, strategic napping, and following good general sleep hygiene practices.[67,69]

CLINICS CARE POINTS

- Evaluation of an athlete's sleep involves taking a thorough sleep history but ruling out contributions from medical conditions such as sleep apnea, asthma, and gastroesophageal reflux disease.

- When screening large groups of athletes for sleep disorders, consider the Athlete Sleep Screening Questionnaire or Athlete Sleep Behavior Questionnaire, athlete-specific questionnaires.

- Cognitive behavioral therapy for insomnia is recommended as a first-line treatment for insomnia over medications by prominent sporting organizations including both the National Collegiate Athletic Association and International Olympic Committee.

- Understanding the effects of jet lag and travel fatigue, and creating plans in advance for athletes who travel frequently, will optimize health and performance.

DISCLOSURE

The authors have nothing to disclose.

REFERENCES

1. Ford DE, Cooper-Patrick L. Sleep disturbances and mood disorders: an epidemiologic perspective. Depress Anxiety 2001;14(1):3–6.
2. Lockley SW, Barger LK, Ayas NT, et al. Effects of health care provider work hours and sleep deprivation on safety and performance. Jt Comm J Qual Patient Saf 2007;33(11 Suppl):7–18.
3. Finan PH, Goodin BR, Smith MT. The association of sleep and pain: an update and a path forward. J Pain 2013;14(12):1539–52.
4. American Psychiatric Association D, Association AP. Diagnostic and statistical manual of mental disorders: DSM-5. Washington, DC: American psychiatric association; 2013.
5. Sateia MJ. International classification of sleep disorders. Chest 2014;146(5): 1387–94.
6. Morin CM, Drake CL, Harvey AG, et al. Insomnia disorder. Nat Rev Dis Prim 2015; 1(1):1–18.
7. Gottlieb DJ, Punjabi NM. Diagnosis and management of obstructive sleep apnea: a review. JAMA 2020;323(14):1389–400.
8. Maeder MT, Schoch OD, Rickli H. A clinical approach to obstructive sleep apnea as a risk factor for cardiovascular disease. Vasc Health Risk Manag 2016;12: 85–103.
9. Manconi M, Garcia-Borreguero D, Schormair B, et al. Restless legs syndrome. Nat Rev Dis Prim 2021;7(1):80.
10. Mignot E, Lammers GJ, Ripley B, et al. The role of cerebrospinal fluid hypocretin measurement in the diagnosis of narcolepsy and other hypersomnias. Arch Neurol 2002;59(10):1553–62.
11. Harvey R, Colten B, Altevogt M, Institute of Medicine (US) Committee on Sleep Medicine and Research. Sleep disorders and sleep deprivation. Washington, DC, USA: National Academies Press (US); 2006.
12. Ohayon MM. Epidemiological overview of sleep disorders in the general population. Sleep Medicine Research 2011;2(1):1–9.
13. Gupta L, Morgan K, Gilchrist S. Does elite sport degrade sleep quality? A systematic review. Sports Med 2017;47:1317–33.
14. Swinbourne R, Gill N, Vaile J, et al. Prevalence of poor sleep quality, sleepiness and obstructive sleep apnoea risk factors in athletes. Eur J Sport Sci 2016;16(7): 850–8.
15. Grandner MA, Hall C, Jaszewski A, et al. Mental health in student athletes: associations with sleep duration, sleep quality, insomnia, fatigue, and sleep apnea symptoms. Athl Train Sports Health Care 2021;13(4):e159–67.
16. Nowakowski S, Meers J, Heimbach E. Sleep and women's health. Sleep medicine research 2013;4(1):1.
17. Wesström J, Nilsson S, Sundström-Poromaa I, et al. Restless legs syndrome among women: prevalence, co-morbidity and possible relationship to menopause. Climacteric 2008;11(5):422–8.
18. Senaratna CV, Perret JL, Lodge CJ, et al. Prevalence of obstructive sleep apnea in the general population: a systematic review. Sleep Med Rev 2017;34:70–81.
19. Schaal K, Tafflet M, Nassif H, et al. Psychological balance in high level athletes: gender-based differences and sport-specific patterns. PLoS One 2011;6(5): e19007.
20. Leeder J, Glaister M, Pizzoferro K, et al. Sleep duration and quality in elite athletes measured using wristwatch actigraphy. J Sports Sci 2012;30(6):541–5.

21. Silva A, Narciso FV, Rosa JP, et al. Gender differences in sleep patterns and sleep complaints of elite athletes. Sleep Science 2019;12(4):242.
22. Everson CA, Henchen CJ, Szabo A, et al. Cell injury and repair resulting from sleep loss and sleep recovery in laboratory rats. Sleep 2014;37(12):1929–40.
23. Besedovsky L, Lange T, Born J. Sleep and immune function. Pflügers Archiv-European Journal of Physiology 2012;463(1):121–37.
24. Cappuccio FP, Miller MA. Sleep and cardio-metabolic disease. Curr Cardiol Rep 2017;19:1–9.
25. Stickgold R. Sleep-dependent memory consolidation. Nature 2005;437(7063):1272–8.
26. Walker MP, Stickgold R. Sleep-dependent learning and memory consolidation. Neuron 2004;44(1):121–33.
27. Goel N, Rao H, Durmer J, et al. Sleep deprivation and clinical performance. Sleep 2002;34(3):387–91.
28. Wagner U, Gais S, Haider H, et al. Sleep inspires insight. Nature 2004;427(6972):352–5.
29. Ten Brink M, Dietch JR, Tutek J, et al. Sleep and affect: A conceptual review. Sleep Med Rev 2022;65:101670.
30. Gao B, Dwivedi S, Milewski MD, et al. Lack of sleep and sports injuries in adolescents: a systematic review and meta-analysis. J Pediatr Orthop 2019;39(5):e324–33.
31. Milewski MD, Skaggs DL, Bishop GA, et al. Chronic lack of sleep is associated with increased sports injuries in adolescent athletes. J Pediatr Orthop 2014;34(2):129–33.
32. Chennaoui M, Vanneau T, Trignol A, et al. How does sleep help recovery from exercise-induced muscle injuries? J Sci Med Sport 2021;24(10):982–7.
33. Mah CD, Mah KE, Kezirian EJ, et al. The effects of sleep extension on the athletic performance of collegiate basketball players. Sleep 2011;34(7):943–50.
34. Watson AM. Sleep and athletic performance. Curr Sports Med Rep 2017;16(6):413–8.
35. O'Donnell S, Bird S, Jacobson G, et al. Sleep and stress hormone responses to training and competition in elite female athletes. Eur J Sport Sci 2018;18(5):611–8.
36. Johnson EO, Roth T, Breslau N. The association of insomnia with anxiety disorders and depression: exploration of the direction of risk. J Psychiatr Res 2006;40(8):700–8.
37. Mason EC, Harvey AG. Insomnia before and after treatment for anxiety and depression. J Affect Disord 2014;168:415–21.
38. Khader WS, Tubbs AS, Haghighi A, et al. Onset insomnia and insufficient sleep duration are associated with suicide ideation in university students and athletes. J Affect Disord 2020;274:1161–4.
39. Kim KR, Jung Y-C, Shin M-Y, et al. Sleep disturbance in women with eating disorder: prevalence and clinical characteristics. Psychiatr Res 2010;176(1):88–90.
40. Hvolby A, Jørgensen J, Bilenberg N. Actigraphic and parental reports of sleep difficulties in children with attention-deficit/hyperactivity disorder. Arch Pediatr Adolesc Med 2008;162(4):323–9.
41. Kroshus E, Wagner J, Wyrick D, et al. Wake up call for collegiate athlete sleep: narrative review and consensus recommendations from the NCAA Interassociation Task Force on Sleep and Wellness. Br J Sports Med 2019;53(12):731–6.
42. Doherty R, Madigan S, Warrington G, et al. Sleep and nutrition interactions: implications for athletes. Nutrients 2019;11(4):822.

43. Halson SL. Sleep in elite athletes and nutritional interventions to enhance sleep. Sports Med 2014;44(Suppl 1):13–23.
44. Sundgot-Borgen J, Larsen S. Pathogenic weight-control methods and self-reported eating disorders in female elite athletes and controls. Scand J Med Sci Sports 1993;3(3):150–5.
45. Nagata JM, Palar K, Gooding HC, et al. Food insecurity is associated with poorer mental health and sleep outcomes in young adults. J Adolesc Health 2019;65(6):805–11.
46. Baker FC, Driver HS. Self-reported sleep across the menstrual cycle in young, healthy women. J Psychosom Res 2004;56(2):239–43.
47. Shibui K, Uchiyama M, Okawa M, et al. Diurnal fluctuation of sleep propensity and hormonal secretion across the menstrual cycle. Biol Psychiatr 2000;48(11):1062–8.
48. Brassil HE, Salvatore AP. The frequency of post-traumatic stress disorder symptoms in athletes with and without sports related concussion. Clin Transl Med 2018;7:1–9.
49. Meeusen R, Duclos M, Foster C, et al. Prevention, diagnosis and treatment of the overtraining syndrome: Joint consensus statement of the European College of Sport Science (ECSS) and the American College of Sports Medicine (ACSM). Eur J Sport Sci 2013;13(1):1–24.
50. Shibli F, Skeans J, Yamasaki T, et al. Nocturnal gastroesophageal reflux disease (GERD) and sleep: an important relationship that is commonly overlooked. J Clin Gastroenterol 2020;54(8):663–74.
51. Fekedulegn D, Andrew ME, Shi M, et al. Actigraphy-Based Assessment of Sleep Parameters. Ann Work Expo Health 2020;64(4):350–67.
52. Uchida S, Endo T, Suenaga K, et al. Sleep evaluation by a newly developed PVDF sensor non-contact sheet: a comparison with standard polysomnography and wrist actigraphy. Sleep Biol Rhythm 2011;9:178–87.
53. Choi YK, Demiris G, Lin S-Y, et al. Smartphone applications to support sleep self-management: review and evaluation. J Clin Sleep Med 2018;14(10):1783–90.
54. Driller MW, Mah CD, Halson SL. Development of the athlete sleep behavior questionnaire: a tool for identifying maladaptive sleep practices in elite athletes. Sleep Science 2018;11(1):37.
55. Bender AM, Lawson D, Werthner P, et al. The Clinical Validation of the Athlete Sleep Screening Questionnaire: an Instrument to Identify Athletes that Need Further Sleep Assessment. Sports Medicine - Open 2018;4(1):23.
56. Gouttebarge V, Bindra A, Blauwet C, et al. International Olympic Committee (IOC) sport mental health assessment tool 1 (SMHAT-1) and sport mental health recognition tool 1 (SMHRT-1): towards better support of athletes' mental health. Br J Sports Med 2021;55(1):30–7.
57. Johns MW. A new method for measuring daytime sleepiness: the Epworth sleepiness scale. sleep 1991;14(6):540–5.
58. Bastien CH, Vallières A, Morin CM. Validation of the Insomnia Severity Index as an outcome measure for insomnia research. Sleep Med 2001;2(4):297–307.
59. Buysse DJ, Reynolds CF III, Monk TH, et al. The Pittsburgh Sleep Quality Index: a new instrument for psychiatric practice and research. Psychiatr Res 1989;28(2):193–213.
60. Espie CA, MacMahon KM, Kelly H-L, et al. Randomized clinical effectiveness trial of nurse-administered small-group cognitive behavior therapy for persistent insomnia in general practice. Sleep 2007;30(5):574–84.

61. Rossman J. Cognitive-Behavioral Therapy for Insomnia: An Effective and Underutilized Treatment for Insomnia. Am J Lifestyle Med 2019;13(6):544–7.
62. Reardon CL, Hainline B, Aron CM, et al. Mental health in elite athletes: International Olympic Committee consensus statement (2019). Br J Sports Med 2019; 53(11):667–99.
63. Winkelman JW, Benca R, Eichler A. Overview of the treatment of insomnia in adults. Waltham, MA, USA: UpToDate; 2020.
64. Taylor L, Chrismas BC, Dascombe B, et al. Sleep Medication and Athletic Performance-The Evidence for Practitioners and Future Research Directions. Front Physiol 2016;7:83.
65. Gossard TR, Trotti LM, Videnovic A, et al. Restless legs syndrome: contemporary diagnosis and treatment. Neurotherapeutics 2021;18(1):140–55.
66. Certal V, Nishino N, Camacho M, et al. Reviewing the systematic reviews in OSA surgery. Otolaryngology-Head Neck Surg (Tokyo) 2013;149(6):817–29.
67. Janse van Rensburg DC, Jansen van Rensburg A, Fowler PM, et al. Managing travel fatigue and jet lag in athletes: a review and consensus statement. Sports Med 2021;51(10):2029–50.
68. Walsh NP, Halson SL, Sargent C, et al. Sleep and the athlete: narrative review and 2021 expert consensus recommendations. Br J Sports Med 2020;bjsports(2020): 102025.
69. Roach GD, Sargent C. Interventions to minimize jet lag after westward and eastward flight. Front Physiol 2019;10:927.
70. Van Rensburg DCCJ, Van Rensburg AJ, Fowler P, et al. How to manage travel fatigue and jet lag in athletes? A systematic review of interventions. Br J Sports Med 2020;54(16):960–8.

Mental Health in the Youth Athlete

Mary M. Daley, MD^{a,*}, Claudia L. Reardon, MD^b

KEYWORDS

- Youth sports • Mental health • Sports medicine • Sports psychiatry
- Sports psychology

KEY POINTS

- Overtraining can result in depressed mood, fatigue, and physiologic and hormonal changes that perpetuate declines in performance, all of which can lead to burnout or withdrawal from sports.
- Perfectionism is a common trait in athletes and has been associated with depression, anxiety, and eating disorders.
- Injured athletes should be closely monitored for signs of depression, anxiety, post-traumatic stress disorder, disordered eating, and substance misuse.
- Future directions should emphasize the advancement of mental health literacy, decreasing stigma, and implementation of effective screen practices to optimize recognition and management of mental health concerns in young athletes.

INTRODUCTION AND HISTORICAL CONTEXT

As trends and transformations in the landscape of youth sports exert tremendous influence on the mental health of young athletes, it may be helpful to understand this landscape's origins and how it has evolved to the multi-billion-dollar industry it is today. Although children have presumably always engaged in play, the development of organized adult-directed structured play activities and sport programs in the United States began in the late nineteenth century in an effort not only to socialize children, but also as a vehicle to instill morals and values.[1] While the early programs were largely led by religious institutions, by the 1920s organized sports were increasingly funded by private organizations, often drawing criticism for overemphasis on winning, commercialization, injury risk due to overtraining, and even over-specialization.[1]

In addition to religious institutions and private organizations taking an interest in the utility of youth sports, the government directed its attention to the health and fitness of

^{a} Department of Orthopaedic Surgery, Division of Sports Medicine, Children's Hospital of Philadelphia, Perelman School of Medicine at the University of Pennsylvania, 3401 Civic Center Boulevard, Philadelphia, PA 19104, USA; ^{b} Department of Psychiatry, University of Wisconsin School of Medicine and Public Health, 6001 Research Park Boulevard, Madison, WI 53719, USA
* Corresponding author.
E-mail address: daleym2@chop.edu

Clin Sports Med 43 (2024) 107–126
https://doi.org/10.1016/j.csm.2023.06.003
0278-5919/24/© 2023 Elsevier Inc. All rights reserved.

the youth of the nation as well. One of the first examples of this was the establishment of the President's Council on Youth Fitness in 1956 under Dwight Eisenhower, thought to possibly reflect the emphasis on military preparedness during the Cold War era.[1] Throughout the first century of the existence of organized youth sports, the opportunity to participate was one that was afforded exclusively to white males. It was not until after the Civil Rights Movement of the 1960s that African American youth were allowed to compete against and alongside their white peers, and it was later still that Title IX was passed, with subsequent drastic increases in opportunities for females to participate in organized sports as well.[1,2]

The evolution of the nature of parental involvement in youth sports is also worth considering in the context of the parent-child dyad. In the 1950s and 1960s, sports presented an opportunity for bonding between parents (usually fathers) and children. Youth were more likely to participate in sports if their parents were interested in sports and fitness and encouraged their participation. The emphasis on scheduling activities for children became more prominent in the 1980s, resulting in a shift away from free and spontaneous play toward more organized achievement-driven engagement in sports.[3] It was during this time that researchers began characterizing parental involvement in sport based on the multidimensional construct of pressure and support, and sought to explore the impact of this dichotomy on enjoyment, burnout, and self-esteem.[4] They found that supportive parenting practices such as offering praise, positive feedback, and unconditional love were associated with higher levels of self-perceived competence in sport, enjoyment, self-esteem, and coping skills in young athletes. In contrast, those who felt pressured by parents with unrealistic expectations, harsh criticisms, and an over-emphasis on winning or achievement tended to report decreased enjoyment, greater anxiety around competition, lower motivation, and feeling less competent in their sport.[3] Further research has shed light on factors that influence parental behaviors, including their own past experiences and knowledge of sports, investment of time and finances, challenges with sharing authority over their child with coaches to varying degrees, and the social implications of identity formation as a sport parent within the unique culture of each sport.[3,5] In recognizing the implications of parental involvement, models have emerged for workshops and other educational endeavors to support and empower parents in ways that seek to foster healthy experiences for youth athletes at all levels.[5–7]

TRENDS IN YOUTH SPORT PARTICIPATION

Current trends in youth sport participation are multifaceted, and are subject to a variety of economic, social, and cultural factors. According to the Aspen Institute, youth sport participation peaked in 2008, at which time 45% of children ages 6 to 12 years participated in team sports on a regular basis. That number has continually declined to a low of 37% in 2021, the most recent year for which data was available at the time of this publication.[8] Similar patterns in participation rates in this age group were seen across racial and ethnic groups, with the most significant declines seen in those of lower socioeconomic status.[8] These trends are thought to be due to a multitude of factors, including the economic recession, rising costs of participation, early sport specialization, the relative lack of high-quality recreational opportunities, and the declining birth rate in the United States.[8] The last decade has seen a shift from school- and community-based sports to private, club, or travel sports, contributing to the rising costs of participation and resultant disparities for youth from low-income households. A 2016 survey found that 63% of parents reported spending $1200 to $6000 per year for sports participation, with 19% of parents spending $1000 or more per child per month.[9] In addition to participation fees and equipment and travel costs, transportation can present a further challenge to lower income families. Considering all of these barriers, in 2021 only 24% of children ages 6 to 12 years and 28% of adolescents ages 13 to 17 years from households with an annual income of less than $25,000 played sports on a regular basis, compared with 40% and 48% of those with an annual income greater than $100,000, respectively.[8]

SPORT SPECIALIZATION

While rates of participation may be declining, the average number of hours per week seems to be increasing in youth who do engage in sports. A 2022 survey study of youth ages 5 to 18 years in the United States found that parents reported their child engaged in their primary sport (including practice, competitions, free play, and training outside of practice) an average of 18 hours per week.[10] This is likely reflective of the trend toward early sport specialization, an increasingly common practice defined by the year-round participation in a single sport (greater than 8 months per year), often to the exclusion of other sports, with prevalence estimates ranging from 17% to 41%.[11] Multiple medical organizations including the American Academy of Pediatrics (AAP), American Medical Society of Sports Medicine (AMSSM), and American Orthopedic Society of Sports Medicine (AOSSM) have published position statements addressing the potential for early specialization to lead to increased risk of injury, psychological burnout, depression, and anxiety.[11–15]

Due in part to the significant variations across sports, current guidelines on sport specialization admittedly lack specificity, but share an overarching goal of optimizing the benefits of youth sport participation while limiting risks.[16] Though more evidence is needed to better inform the formulation of sport-specific guidelines regarding training load, **Box 1** outlines current recommendations for youth athletes.

ATHLETIC IDENTITY

Central to understanding the psychology of sports is the construct of athletic identity, which has been defined as the degree and exclusivity to which a person identifies with the athlete role or the degree to which one devotes special attention to sport relative to other engagements or activities in life.[17,18] In other words, athletic identity refers to the extent to which one's sense of self is constructed around their role as an athlete. Athletic identity is subject to several cognitive, emotional, and social factors–both internal and external–and can fluctuate over the course of one's lifetime and even over the course of the season, including in response to performance-related success or failures.[18,19] The Athlete Identity Measurement Scale (AIMS) is a validated psychometric

---

Box 1
Sport specialization recommendations

- Sport specialization should be delayed until late adolescence for most sports[88]
- Athletes should have at least 1 to 2 rest days per week[89]
- Limit hours per week of sport-specific training to the equivalent of child's age in years, or to no more than 16 hours per week[15,88,90]
- Limit sport-specific training to no more than 8 months per year[12,89]
- Youth who specialize in a single sport should plan periods of isolated and focused integrated neuromuscular training to enhance diverse motor skill development and reduce injury risk[14]
- Youth athletes should be monitored for signs of burnout[15,91]

instrument that has been reliably applied to athletes of all levels and to non-athletes as well.[18] The most recent iteration of this questionnaire consists of 7 questions with responses based on a 7-point Likert scale. Responses range from "strongly disagree" to "strongly agree", with higher scores reflecting higher degrees to which one identifies as an athlete. This instrument is based on the conceptualization of athletic identity as a multidimensional construct, with questions designed to assess social identity (the extent to which one views oneself as an athlete), exclusivity (the extent to which one's self worth is determined solely by their performance or achievements as an athlete), and negative affectivity (the extent to which one experiences negative affect in response to undesirable outcomes or perceived failures in sport).[18]

Multiple studies have found that higher levels of athletic identity are associated with improved athletic performance, enhanced commitment to training, and higher level of enjoyment of sports.[18,20–22] These benefits, however, are not without cost, as other studies have demonstrated associations with overtraining, playing while injured, difficulty coping with temporary or permanent discontinuation of sport due to injury and/or retirement, and high-risk behaviors such as disordered eating and use of performance-enhancing substances.[23–25] Therefore despite the well-recognized psychological benefits of physical activity and participation in organized sports, athletes are certainly not exempt from mental illness.[26–28]

DEPRESSION
Prevalence

According to 2019 data from Mental Health America, 15% of youth ages 0 to 17 years reported having had at least one major depressive episode in the past year, a number which had nearly doubled from 5 years prior.[29,30] More alarming still is that existing literature is strongly suggestive that the prevalence of depression and suicidality in children and adolescents has significantly increased even more since 2019 in the setting of the Covid-19 pandemic, prompting the American Academy of Pediatrics (AAP), American Academy of Child and Adolescent Psychiatry (AACAP) and the Children's Hospital Association (CHA) to declare a national state of emergency in children's mental health in October 2021.[31] As of 2021, suicide was the second leading cause of death in youth ages 10 to 14 years, and the third leading cause of death in those age 15 to 19 years.[32] The drastic rise in mental illness seen during this time has been attributed not only to fear and anxiety related to the pandemic itself, but perhaps even more so to the widespread restrictions resulting in isolation from peers, loneliness, academic burnout, lack of autonomy, and being stripped of the opportunity to celebrate or participate in important milestones, with immeasurable long-term implications.[33]

Though there is a relative paucity of evidence specifically examining mental health in child and adolescent athletes involved in organized sports, a 2016 systematic review found that the prevalence of depression and anxiety in elite athletes is comparable to non-athletes, while a 2020 systematic review and meta-analysis suggests slightly lower rates of depression and anxiety in adolescent athletes compared with their non-athlete peers.[34–36] Nonetheless, a comprehensive exploration of the potential risk factors for and clinical manifestations of mental illness in this population is essential to the mission of fostering well-being and promoting healthy outcomes both within and outside of sports.

Depression in Athletes During the COVID-19 Pandemic

One study specifically examined the mental health of adolescent athletes approximately 2 months after school closures and other restrictions were implemented in the United States, and found increased depression and anxiety, lower levels of physical activity, and decreased quality of life scores, with findings most pronounced in females, athletes in grade 12, team sport athletes, and those of lower socioeconomic status.[37] The disproportionate impacts on the mental health of females compared with males and those of lower compared with higher socioeconomic status are consistent with patterns seen in other settings, with these regarded as more vulnerable populations. However, this study also demonstrated that team sport athletes had worsening depression, anxiety, and quality of life compared with individual sport athletes, in contrast to prior studies that have shown a greater likelihood of depression and anxiety in individual sport athletes.[26,37] This discrepancy can likely be understood in the context of pandemic restrictions, wherein the cancellation of organized sports and enforcement of social distancing disproportionately affected team sport athletes, while individual sport athletes such as runners or even tennis players could more easily continue to engage in their sport to some degree.

The other unique finding in this study was that physical health, mental wellbeing, and quality of life were all negatively correlated with grade in school, whereas prior investigations yielded mixed results based on grade level. Pre-pandemic studies had suggested that the prevalence of depression in females peaked at age 15 and then declined, while the prevalence of depression in males peaked at age 17, and that quality of life remained relatively constant throughout the high school years.[38,39] The finding that athletes in higher grade levels fared worse during the pandemic than their younger peers might be explained by several factors. For some, there were implications for college recruitment and scholarships, and many others had unexpectedly lost their final opportunity to compete in the sport they loved. Although this study did not directly compare athletes with non-athletes, it does highlight some of the nuance involved when seeking to understand the factors contributing to mental health that are specific to the athletic population.

Clinical Presentation

Recognizing signs of clinical depression is especially important when considering that the current culture often encourages young athletes to exhibit mental toughness and avoid the appearance of weakness, thereby potentially deterring help-seeking behavior.

Similar to adults, adolescents often experience what are considered melancholic symptoms of depression, including withdrawal, psychomotor slowing, lack of motivation, loss of weight or appetite, and inability to take pleasure in activities they previously enjoyed. Younger children, however, are less likely to exhibit these symptoms classically associated with depression.[40] They might instead present with more externalizing symptoms such as frustration, refusal to participate in their normal activities, or even aggression. This discrepancy may be due in part to cognitive and emotional development, as younger children may struggle to conceptualize, much less articulate, their experience, resulting in outward expressions of frustration. This inability to integrate the internal experience may also explain the association of depression with somatic manifestations such as stomach aches or migraines, which are perhaps more common in but certainly not unique to younger children with depression. Somatic symptoms are also frequently seen in those with anxiety, trauma, or other causes of emotional disturbance—a reminder of the inextricable link between our psychological and physiologic state.

Among children and adolescents with depression, the most common comorbidity is anxiety, with estimates ranging from 15% to 75%.[41] Depression has also been found to be strongly correlated with social phobia, competitive anxiety, and perfectionistic concerns in elite athletes.[42]

OVERTRAINING AND BURNOUT
Definitions

Depression in athletes can also be seen in the setting of overtraining and burnout. Excessive training in sport can be characterized on a spectrum from overreaching to overtraining syndrome, with symptoms that can overlap to varying degrees with clinical depression and/or anxiety. Overreaching may be functional or non-functional, the latter of which leads to longer periods of declines in performance (weeks to months as opposed to days to weeks) and is more likely to be associated with psychological symptoms.[13,43] Functional overreaching can be understood in the context of periodization, in which a period of high effort, high-intensity training is followed by a period of rest to allow recovery and adaptation. Depending in part on its implementation, this is a practice that should be used judiciously in young athletes, as risks may outweigh the potential gains.[44] Overtraining syndrome represents the extremes of nonfunctional overreaching, with declines in performance lasting more than 2 months, psychological symptoms including depressed mood and withdrawal, and physiologic and hormonal changes that perpetuate the detrimental impacts on performance.[13] In addition to declining athletic performance, increased risk of injury, and potential withdrawal from sport, the stress of overtraining can lead to decreased sleep and appetite, unexplained weight loss, and impaired immune function, each of which begets myriad physiologic consequences.[13,43] Burnout refers to the potential culmination of overtraining in which the athlete lacks motivation to participate in their sport and may withdraw from sports altogether.[45] See **Table 1** for a comparison of terms.

Prevalence and Risk Factors

Prevalence estimates of overtraining and burnout are limited, due in part to the lack of consistent terminology and clear diagnostic criteria. A study of more than 300 young English athletes ages 11 to 18 years with the representation of 19 different sports at all levels of play found that 20% self-reported having experienced nonfunctional

Table 1 Overreaching, overtraining, and burnout		
	Definition	**Recovery Time**
Functional Overreaching	Short term period of accumulated training above the normal level of intensity and/or duration followed by a recovery period, thought to result in super-compensation effect	Days to weeks
Non-functional Overreaching	Short to medium-term period of training above the normal level of intensity and/or duration followed by performance decrement	Weeks to months
Overtraining	Extreme non-functional overreaching resulting in declining performance, fatigue, depressed mood, and physiologic and hormonal changes	≥ 2 mo
Burnout	Lack of motivation to participate and potential withdrawal from sport	Not applicable

overreaching or overtraining syndrome at some point in their athletic career, with 3.5% reporting experiencing those symptoms at the time of the survey.[43]

Factors that contribute to the development of overtraining syndrome and burnout include low self-esteem, perfectionism, decreased locus of control, heightened anxiety, and lack of confidence in performance capabilities relative to the perception of excessive demands or expectations.[13] As such, efforts to foster confidence while ensuring that expectations placed on young athletes are appropriate for their age, developmental stage, and athletic capabilities are essential, and may help to mitigate the propensity toward burnout. Additional preventative measures include ensuring training volume is developmentally appropriate and limiting the frequency and intensity of competition, while focusing instead on skill development and enjoyment.

Clinical Presentation

It is important to distinguish overtraining syndrome from clinical depression, particularly in light of the overlap in clinical presentation, including depressed mood, changes in sleep and appetite, loss of interest in activities, fatigue, and feelings of worthlessness.[46] One key distinction is that overtraining syndrome results in functional impairment within the context of sport, whereas depression is more likely to impact other aspects of life including academic performance and relationships with family and friends. The other feature that differentiates the two conditions is response to treatment. Symptoms of overtraining syndrome should improve with rest from sport, as this is the cornerstone of treatment for this condition. In contrast, for a young athlete struggling with depression, participation in sport may serve as a protective factor, and removal from sport might therefore lead to *worsening* symptoms.

ANXIETY
Prevalence and Clinical Presentation

Anxiety disorders represent the most common mental health diagnoses in children and adolescents, likely affecting 15% to 20% of this population, with some estimates as high as 30%.[47–49] Anxiety is a reflexive response to danger, designed to protect the individual from perceived threats, which can become maladaptive if it becomes frequent, severe, or persistent enough to disrupt normal function.[49] It is important to consider the developmental age of the child in distinguishing appropriate emotional responses from pathology, and further to recognize that the clinical presentation of anxiety disorders in youth may differ from that of adults. Examples of fears that are considered to be developmentally appropriate include separation anxiety in infants and toddlers, and specific phobias (eg, monsters, germs, natural disasters) in school-age children.[49] In terms of normative anxiety more relevant to young athletes, school and performance anxiety in school-age children and fear of rejection in adolescents may be developmentally appropriate; both of which may fall under the umbrella of social anxiety and/or generalized anxiety disorders should they progress to the extent of significant distress and/or functional impairment.[49] Anxiety in school-age children may present with sleep disturbances, behavioral outbursts, or extreme shyness, whereas adolescents are more likely to exhibit withdrawal, avoidance, and perfectionist tendencies in an effort to evade negative evaluation.[49]

Anxiety in Athletes

One of the key contributing factors to anxiety is the uncertainty of outcome. This, along with the tendency toward self-critical comparisons typical of adolescents and the vulnerability to judgment or criticism from peers, coaches, and other spectators renders athletic competition a potentially threating endeavor. Performance or competitive anxiety is associated with decreased enjoyment, poor performance, increased injury risk, and discontinuation of sport.[50–54] Existing literature often differentiates between somatic and cognitive anxiety. Somatic anxiety refers to the physiologic response, including increased levels of cortisol, elevated heart rate, and muscle tension. Cognitive anxiety consists of two components: worry about the situation and potential outcomes, and disruptions in focus or concentration.[50,55,56] A study of athletes ages 9 to 14 years utilizing this three-factor model found higher levels of worry and total anxiety in 12 to 14 year olds compared with the younger cohort.[50] The authors suggested this may be explained by a combination of the normative increase in anxiety symptoms in early adolescence and higher levels of competitive pressure in the older age group.[50] They also found that female athletes exhibited greater worry, whereas males reported more concentration disruption.[50]

When evaluating a broader age range to include young adults, older and more experienced athletes tend to have lower levels of anxiety, which has been attributed to a higher level of mastery, more experience with adversity in competition, enhanced cognitive and coping skills, and better emotional regulation.[55,57–60] Higher levels of competitive anxiety are seen in individual compared with team sport athletes, which is likely due to the sole responsibility of success or failure resting with the individual as opposed to being shared among team members.[60] Additional risk factors for performance anxiety in athletes include playing away from the home setting and having had a prior poor performance or negative experience such as a loss.[60]

It is also important to note that anxiety disorders are associated with increased risk of subsequent development of depressive and/or substance use disorders, and therefore represent a significant predictive factor in terms of mental health outcomes.[49]

PERFECTIONISM
Origins of Perfectionist Tendencies

As previously alluded to in the context of burnout, the discrepancy between a child's self-perceived competency in sport and their ability to meet external demands and expectations can result in psychological distress, perhaps best understood at least in part as the construct of shame. Shame refers to a negative evaluation of one's inherent value, and is distinct from guilt, which refers to a negative assessment of a particular action or behavior.[61] Perfectionism can be understood as the manifestation of a predisposition to neuroticism, which may lend itself to achievement-oriented successes, corrupted by the development of maladaptive striving and a tendency toward harsh self-criticism.[62,63] Some suggest that perfectionism invariably emerges from a sense of shame, whether conscious or otherwise, and further that a reciprocal relationship very likely exists between the two.[64]

Perfectionism in Athletes

Regardless of its origins, it is not uncommon for athletes to identify as perfectionists. This can be understood as a potential strength in terms of having exceedingly high personal standards (ie, perfectionistic striving), and/or a vulnerability insofar as the obsessive preoccupation with fear of failure or inability to meet those standards (ie, perfectionistic concerns) can be detrimental to overall wellbeing and potentially performance.[62] Some evidence suggests that compared with young adult athletes, adolescent athletes are more likely to experience perfectionistic *concerns,* which represent the maladaptive dimension of perfectionism.[42] The motivational factors that drive perfectionistic tendencies are an important consideration. Athletes who are internally motivated by mastery and performance goals may have higher levels of enjoyment, perceived athletic ability, and self-esteem, but are not immune to the heightened anxiety associated with perfectionism. Those who are influenced more by external factors (eg, pressure from parents or coaches or comparison to peers) and by fear of failure experience greater degrees of self-criticism, depressive symptoms, and anxiety, and tend to have lower self-esteem.[62]

Accordingly, there is some evidence to suggest that athletes characterized as self-oriented or intrinsically motivated perfectionists may be at lower risk than those for whom perfectionism is driven by external forces or expectations.[65,66] This may be explained by the notion that a self-motivated athlete presumably has a greater sense of ownership over their performance capabilities, and therefore may be less susceptible to feelings of helplessness and the emotional fatigue or amotivation that can lead to burnout. In either case, self-worth of the perfectionist is inextricably linked to one's ability to meet expectations that are often unrealistic and/or unattainable, and perfectionism may therefore best be viewed as a potential risk factor for young athletes in terms of mental health and wellbeing. Existing literature supports associations of perfectionism with depression and anxiety in athletes, particularly when the preoccupation with fear of failure is dominant.[62] Perfectionism is also intrinsically linked to eating disorders, wherein one continually strives toward an intangible goal, seeking a sense of pride in their ability to control and resist a human drive as powerful as hunger, in an effort to temporarily suppress the shame that inevitably dominates the entire cycle.[64]

MUSCULOSKELETAL INJURY
Implications of Athletic Identity

Though widely accepted as one of the risks of participation, injuries necessitating time away from sports can be devastating to an athlete. In the immediate aftermath of an injury and the early stages of recovery, those with higher levels of athletic identity may experience a greater degree of emotional disturbance.[67] In these athletes for whom the sense of self is constructed around their role as an athlete, the loss of involvement with their sport and the loss of the physical ability to participate, even when temporary, can be extremely difficult. However, existing literature also suggests that a stronger athletic identity may be beneficial over the broader course of recovery, as these patients demonstrate greater adherence to rehabilitation exercises, presumably reflective of a strong desire to return to sports.[68]

Depression

One of the most common responses to injury is depressed mood, which in some cases may progress to clinical depression, characterized by feelings of helplessness or hopelessness, irritability or anger, sleep disturbance, decreased energy, changes in weight or appetite, apathy, and/or withdrawal or isolative behaviors.[46,69] Depression and other negative emotions such as confusion, anger, and frustration may fluctuate over the course of recovery, but in general negative emotions tend to dissipate over time.[70] While those with pre-existing mental health conditions are likely at increased risk, it is important to recognize that any athlete may suffer the psychological consequences of injury, with some estimates of post-injury depression in young athletes as high as 40%.[71]

Anxiety, Fear, and Post-Traumatic Stress

Anxiety, fear of re-injury, and post-traumatic stress disorder (PTSD) can also emerge in the aftermath of injury in sport. Anxiety is often heightened when there is uncertainty of outcome, so efforts to ensure the athlete has an age-appropriate understanding of the nature and extent of the injury and realistic expectations for the rehabilitative process may prove useful. It is also important to note that anxiety can be correlated with pain, as demonstrated by a study examining patients who had undergone anterior cruciate ligament (ACL) reconstruction, which found that anxiety was the sole predictor of pain at 24 hours postoperatively, over and above gender, postoperative medication consumption, or depression.[72] Fear of reinjury is associated with the decreased likelihood of returning to pre-injury level of sport participation and significantly increased risk of re-injury among those who do return to sports, when compared with athletes with lower levels of self-reported fear.[73-76]

PTSD is characterized by avoidance, hyperarousal, intrusive symptoms, and alterations in mood or cognition in the aftermath of a traumatic experience. A study of 24 athletes aged 21 years or younger who had sustained ACL rupture evaluated PTSD symptoms at the medical visit following the initial diagnosis. They found that more than 75% experienced symptoms of avoidance (eg, feelings of numbness, avoiding thinking about the injury), intrusive symptoms (eg, strong waves of emotion or strong physical reactions brought about by thinking about the injury), and/or symptoms of hyperarousal (eg, feeling on guard, startling easily, sleep disturbance).[77] Female sex, age 15 years or greater, and high athletic identity were associated with greater severity of symptoms, although the latter was not statistically significant.[77]

Maladaptive Responses to Injury

Behavioral responses to injury may include various efforts to cope, including rigorous engagement in the rehabilitative process, avoidance or distraction, and self-destructive behaviors including substance use/misuse or disordered eating.[69,70] Careful attention and monitoring is particularly important for adolescents, as this age group is already at increased risk for engaging in these potentially lethal behaviors. In terms of substance use, providers aim to strike a balance between using caution when prescribing opioid pain medications, while avoiding *under*treating pain, which could create an opportunity for young people to seek out illicit substances in an effort to achieve adequate relief. Recent years have seen a shift toward a multimodal approach to post-operative pain management after ACL reconstruction to include nerve blocks, intra-articular or periarticular injections of local anesthotics, and non-opiate analgesics.[78] Disordered eating or clinical eating disorders can also emerge in the aftermath of injury, often in response to a fear of gaining weight in the setting of abrupt discontinuation of physical activity, and can be associated with feelings of unworthiness, depression, and/or a sense of loss of control over one's circumstances.[69,79]

CONCUSSION
Mental Health Implications

Concussion represents a unique form of injury, as the injury itself results in a conglomeration of physical, cognitive, and emotional sequelae, the latter of which include depression, anxiety, irritability, and emotional lability. This is all further complicated by the nature of concussion, often considered an "invisible injury", as associated impairments are generally not readily observable to others in the way that other injuries might require the use of crutches or casts. This can lead to feelings of isolation and a sense of not being seen or understood, which can lead to worsening depression and irritability. Compounding this already potentially isolating experience is that in addition to not being able to compete, athletes with concussion may not be able to tolerate the stimulating environment of school, social events, or practices during recovery, so the option of observing from the sideline while injured may not be available to them.

The indeterminate timeline for concussion recovery can contribute to anxiety as well, so efforts to mitigate this by acknowledging the uncertainty and discussing general expectations may be helpful. Providers are also well-positioned not only to empower athletes by arming them with rehabilitative tools such as vestibular exercises, academic accommodations, and sleep hygiene counseling to optimize recovery, but also to encourage conversations about the emotional aspects of concussion, and thereby increase the likelihood that any mental health concerns are identified and appropriately addressed.

Impact of Cognitive, Somatic, and Sleep-Related Symptoms

Cognitive, somatic, and sleep-related difficulties associated with concussion can have tremendous impact on the psychological and emotional experience as well. For example, athletes often have difficulty falling asleep and changes in sleep duration and quality after concussion. Inadequate sleep is known to be associated with depression, inattentiveness, and impairments in behavioral and emotional regulation.[80] In addition to headaches, fatigue, and difficulty tolerating screen time, cognitive deficits such as difficulty with concentration and memory can further impede an athlete's efforts to keep up with school work. As a result, it is very common for athletes to fall behind and to see significant declines in academic performance, all of which further contribute to heightened anxiety. This in turn can lead to increased frustration, depressed mood, and misguided efforts to continually push beyond their capacity, further worsening symptoms and likely prolonging recovery. It is incumbent upon providers, parents, teachers, and school administrators to support recovery by advocating for the student and ensuring appropriate accommodations to minimize any detrimental academic consequences.

RECOGNITION AND TREATMENT
Mental Health Literacy

The ability to recognize and treat the mental health needs of athletes begins with awareness, education, and continually fostering conversations among youth, parents, coaches, and providers across disciplines and specialties. Mental health literacy refers to one's knowledge, beliefs and perceptions of mental health, and can influence the ability to recognize warning signs, support those experiencing mental health concerns, and identify available resources.[81] A 2020 study by Vella, and colleagues demonstrated improvements in mental health literacy and resilience among adolescent male athletes as well as their parents and coaches by implementing a combination of in person workshops and online modules.[81] Further interventions would ideally include efforts directed not only to athletes, parents and coaches, but also to club or league administrators and sport governing bodies. Widespread implementation of this type of program could potentially have far reaching impacts on protecting the mental wellbeing of young athletes.

Screening

Despite the tremendous gains that have been made toward decreasing stigma around mental health in recent years, many athletes operate in an environment in which mental toughness is celebrated, and they may hesitate to disclose struggles due to fears of being perceived as weak. This may be particularly true for elite athletes, as evidenced by a 2019 survey administered by the International Olympic Committee Mental Health Working Group (IOC MHWG), which found that nearly two-thirds of respondents agreed that talking about mental health was taboo in elite sports and that there was no recognition of mental health symptoms in their sport, while 90% were in favor of routine screening.[82] In response, the IOC MHWG developed the Sport Mental Health Assessment Tool (SMHAT-1) and Sport Mental Health Recognition Tool (SMHRT-1) to aide in the identification and management of mental health concerns in elite athletes.[82] The SMHAT-1 utilizes a triage model, starting with the administration of the Athlete Psychological Strain Questionnaire (APSQ): a 10-item questionnaire with responses based on a 5-point Likert scale to assess the risk of psychological stress specific to the context of sport. Athletes who score ≥ 17 points (of a total range of 10–50 points) are then administered a series of six disorder-specific questionnaires to screen for symptoms of depression, anxiety, sleep disturbance, alcohol or other substance misuse, and eating disorders. Those results are used to determine whether to proceed with further clinical assessment, brief interventions, or referrals to mental health providers. The companion tool (SMHRT-1) was designed to be used by peers, coaches, parents, or others close to the athlete to promote the early detection of mental health concerns.[82]

Though designed specifically for elite athletes aged 16 years and older, the recommendations of the IOC MHWG have applications for athletes at all levels. For example, the triage model for screening starting with the routine administration of a single brief self-assessment questionnaire is a practical approach that can be utilized in most settings and can help providers determine whether any further evaluation is indicated. As recommended by the IOC MHWG, this process can be implemented not only with routine pre-season medical evaluations, but also in times of increased risk such as in the setting of injury or performance concerns.[82] The APSQ was designed for elite athletes with questions geared specifically toward psychological stress in the context of sports. For younger patient populations, providers might consider using an alternative triage tool in its place to assess more broadly for psychological distress in all domains (whether within or outside of sports), taking care to ensure an appropriate degree of validation in and/or applicability to the population in question. Though further study and expert consensus would be needed to determine the most appropriate assessment tool to use in place of the APQS, screening instruments often deployed in the primary care setting include the Pediatric Symptom Checklist (PSC) and the Strengths and Difficulties Questionnaire (SDQ).[00] While screening questionnaires are not diagnostic tools, they serve an integral role in the identification and management of youth with mental health concerns. See **Table 2** for examples of screening instruments that could be used for young athletes.

Referrals and Evaluation

Given the significant limitations in mental health resources, in the event that referral is indicated, expertise in caring for children and adolescents should be prioritized over expertise in sports, although a provider who specializes in caring for young athletes would be ideal. It is crucial for diagnosis and management to be approached with attention to the athlete's developmental stage, and that this be incorporated into a comprehensive biopsychosocial formulation. Successful treatment of mental health concerns in the youth athlete requires an understanding of their role within the family unit, the team, and the community, and the exploration of their relationships within each of those systems.[84]

Treatment

Perhaps the most substantial distinction between psychological treatment of children and adolescents compared with adults is that it generally necessitates parental or family involvement, both during the diagnostic process and throughout the course of

Table 2
Screening instruments that could be used for young athletes

Screening Instrument	Format	Goal	Age
Pediatric Symptom Checklist (PSC)[92]	35-item self- and/or parent report; 3-point Likert scale (Also validated in a 17-item format)	Identify behavioral and emotional changes in children	6–17 y (parent-report) 11–17 y (self-report)
Strengths and Difficulties Questionnaire (SDQ)[93]	25-item self- and/or parent report; 3-point Likert scale	Identify behavioral, emotional, or social concerns	2–17 y
Athlete Psychological Strain Questionnaire (APSQ)[82,94]	10-item self-report; 5-point Likert scale	Assess psychological stress specific to athletic domain	≥ 16 y
Patient Health Questionnaire (PHQ)-9[95]	9-item self-report; 4-point Likert scale	Screen for depressive symptoms and suicidality	≥ 12 y
Patient Reported Outcomes Measurement Information System (PROMIS) Anxiety[96]	13-item self-report or 10-item parent-report; 5-point Likert scale	Screen for anxiety symptoms	6–17 y (parent-report) 11–17 y (self-report)
PROMIS Depression[97]	14-item self-report or 11-item parent-report; 5-point Likert scale	Screen for depressive symptoms	6–17 y (parent-report) 11–17 y (self-report)
General Anxiety Disorder (GAD)-7[98]	7-item self-report; 4-point Likert scale	Screen for anxiety symptoms	≥ 13 y
Athlete Sleep Screening Questionnaire (ASSQ)[99]	15-item self-report	Identify maladaptive sleep behaviors in athletes	≥ 18 y
Childhood and Adolescent Sleep Evaluation Questionnaire (CASEQ)[100]	36-item self- and/or parent-report; Yes/No	Screen for sleep disorders	2–18 y
Brief Eating Disorder in Athletes Questionnaire (BEDA-Q)[101]	9-item self-report; 6-point Likert scale, Yes/No	Identify eating disorders in adolescent female elite athletes	≥ 15 y
Cutting Down, Annoyance by Criticism, Guilty Feeling, and Eye-openers Adapted to Include Drugs (CAGE-AID)[102]	4-item self- and/or parent-report; 3-point Likert scale	Screen for substance use disorders in adolescents	12–18 y

treatment. The nature and extent of family involvement depend in part on the diagnosis, the developmental stage of the athlete, and family dynamics. As one of the primary objectives of treatment is to restore the healthy functioning of the athlete within their home and social settings, a collaborative effort is required. Specific psychotherapeutic treatment modalities for mental health concerns including depression or anxiety include cognitive behavioral therapy (CBT), acceptance and commitment therapy, and mindfulness-based interventions, all of which can be provided by licensed mental health professionals.[85,86] In terms of pharmacologic treatment, many commonly used psychotropic agents carry the risk of side effects that could be particularly problematic for athletes, including sedation, weight gain, tremor, tachycardia, or orthostatic hypotension, necessitating appropriate counseling and symptom monitoring. If and when psychopharmacological treatment is indicated, providers should give careful consideration to any potential impacts on health, safety, and performance, and, especially for athletes performing at high levels of competition, should be knowledgeable on regulations regarding medication use and prohibited substances specific to the relevant sport governing body.[87]

SUMMARY

Recent decades have seen several changes in the landscape of youth sports, with declining rates of participation, increased early sport specialization, and disparities emerging in the face of rising costs of participation and a trend toward private and club-based organizations. There are important considerations that are unique to the athletic population, including but not limited to depression in the context of overtraining and burnout, performance anxiety, perfectionism and disordered eating, mental health implications of musculoskeletal injuries, and psychological sequalae of concussion. Effective management of mental health concerns in the athletic population requires continued efforts to improve mental health literacy, decrease stigma, promote help-seeking behaviors, and encourage the routine implementation of effective screening practices.

CLINICS CARE POINTS

- Although more research is needed, most organizations recommend delaying sport specialization until late adolescence, ensuring training load is developmentally appropriate, and monitoring youth athletes for signs of burnout.
- Clinical presentation of depression and anxiety can vary with age, as young children are more likely to exhibit externalizing symptoms, behavior changes, and somatic complaints, while adolescents are more likely to present with withdrawal, lack of motivation, and avoidance.
- Overtraining can result in depressed mood, fatigue, and physiologic and hormonal changes that perpetuate declines in performance, all of which can lead to burnout or withdrawal from sports.
- Perfectionism is a common trait in athletes, and has been associated with depression, anxiety, and eating disorders.
- Injured athletes should be closely monitored for signs of depression, anxiety, post-traumatic stress disorder, disordered eating, or substance misuse.
- Psychological sequelae of concussion are complex and multifactorial, and often require a multidisciplinary approach to treatment.
- Efforts to optimize mental health literacy and implement routine screening are essential steps toward improving the recognition and management of mental health concerns in young athletes.

DISCLOSURE

The authors have nothing to disclose.

REFERENCES

1. Wiggins DK. A Worthwhile Effort? History of Organized Youth Sport in the United States. Kinesiol Rev 2016;2(1):65–75.
2. Acosta R, Carpenter L. Women in Intercollegiate Sport: A Longitudinal, National Study. Thirty Three Year Update, 1977-2010. 2010.
3. Dorsch TE, Wright E, Eckardt VC, et al. A History of Parent Involvement in Organized Youth Sport: A Scoping Review. Sport Exerc Perform Psychol 2021;10(4): 536–57.
4. Leff SS, Hoyle RH. Young athletes' perceptions of parental support and pressure. J Youth Adolesc 1995;24(2):187–203.
5. Knight CJ, Berrow SR, Harwood CG. Parenting in sport. Curr Opin Psychol 2017;16:93–7.
6. Lafferty ME, Triggs C. The working with parents in sport model (WWPS-Model): A practical guide for practitioners working with parents of elite young performers. J Sport Psychol Action 2014;5(2):117–28.
7. Vincent AP, Christensen DA. Conversations With Parents: A Collaborative Sport Psychology Program for Parents in Youth Sport. J Sport Psychol Action 2015; 6(2):73–85.
8. State of Play 2022: Our Annual Report on Trends in Youth Sports and Project Play's Contributions to the Field.; 2022.
9. TD Ameritade. Investor Survey: Parent Perspectives on the Cost of Competitive Youth Sports.; 2016. Available at: file:///Users/marydaley/Downloads/TDAmeritrade_SportsParentsSurveyReport_2016 (1).pdf.
10. Dorsch TE, Blazo JA. Youth Sports Parents Surveys, 2021 and 2022.; 2022.
11. Jayanthi NA, Post EG, Laury TC, et al. Health consequences of youth sport specialization. J Athl Train 2019;54(10):1040–9.
12. Brenner JS, LaBella CR, Brooks MA, et al. Sports specialization and intensive training in young athletes. Pediatrics 2016;138(3). https://doi.org/10.1542/peds.2016-2148.
13. Difiori JP, Benjamin HJ, Brenner JS, et al. Overuse injuries and burnout in youth sports: A position statement from the American Medical Society for Sports Medicine. Br J Sports Med 2014;48(4):287–8.
14. LaPrade RF, Agel J, Baker J, et al. AOSSM Early Sport Specialization Consensus Statement. Orthop J Sport Med 2016. https://doi.org/10.1177/2325967116644241.
15. Herman DC, Nelson VR, Montalvo AM, et al. Systematic Review of Health Organization Guidelines Following the AMSSM 2019 Youth Early Sport Specialization Summit. Sports Health 2022;14(1):127–34.
16. Kliethermes SA, Marshall SW, LaBella CR, et al. Defining a Research Agenda for Youth Sport Specialization in the United States: The AMSSM Youth Early Sport Specialization Summit. Clin J Sport Med 2021;31(2):103–12.
17. Brewer BW, Van Raalte JL, Linder DE. Construct validity of the Athletic Identity Measurement Scale. In: In Proceedings of the North American Society for the psychology of sport and physical activity annual Conference. Monterey, CA; 1991:13-16.
18. Edison BR, Christino MA, Rizzone KH. Athletic identity in youth athletes: A systematic review of the literature. Int J Environ Res Public Health 2021;18(14). https://doi.org/10.3390/ijerph18147331.
19. Brewer BW, Selby CL, Under DE, et al. Distancing oneself from a poor season: Divestment of athletic identity. J Pers Interpers Loss 1999;4:149–62.

20. Brewer B, Boin P, Petitpas A, et al. Dimensions of Athletic Identity. In: Proceedings of the North American Society for the psychology of sport and physical activity annual Conference. Toronto, ON: Canada; 1993. p. 19–22.
21. Babic V, Sarac J, Missoni S, et al. Athletic engagement and athletic identity in top Croatian sprint runners. Coll Anthr 2015;39:521–8.
22. Horton RS, Mack DE. Athletic Identity in Marathon Runners. J Sport Behav 2000; 23(2):101–19.
23. Coker-Cranney A, Watson JC, Berstein M, et al. How far is too far? Understanding identity and overconformity in collegiate wrestlers. Qual Res Sport Exerc Heal 2018;10:92–116.
24. Lavallee D, Robinson HK. In pursuit of an identity: A qualitative exploration of retirement from women's artistic gymnastics. Psychol Sport Exerc 2007;8(1): 119–41.
25. Manuel JC, Shilt JS, Curl WW, et al. Coping with sports injuries: An examination of the adolescent athlete. J Adolesc Heal 2002;31(5):391–3.
26. Pluhar E, McCracken C, Griffith KL, et al. Team sport athletes may be less likely to suffer anxiety or depression than individual sport athletes. J Sport Sci Med 2019;18(3):490–6.
27. SA V, CA M, et al. Associations between sports participation and psychological difficulties during childhood: a two-year follow up. J Sci Med Sport 2015;18(3): 304–9. Available at: https://pubmed.ncbi.nlm.nih.gov/24908361/.
28. Vella SA, Swann C, Allen MS, et al. Bidirectional associations between sport involvement and mental health in adolescence. Med Sci Sports Exerc 2017; 49(4):687–94.
29. Reinert M, Fritze D, Nguyen T. The State of Mental Health in America 2022. Alexandria, VA; 2021.
30. Nguyen T. Parity or Disparity: The State of Mental Health in America 2015.; 2015.
31. American Academy of Pediatrics. A declaration from the American Academy of Pediatrics. United States: American Academy of Child and Adolescent Psychiatry and Children's Hospital Association; 2021.
32. Centers for Disease Control and Provention, National Center for Health Statistics. National Vital Statistics System, Mortality 2018-2021 on CDC WONDER Online Database, released in 2021. http://wonder.cdc.gov/ucd-icd10-expanded. html. Accessed February 26, 2023.
33. Branje S, Morris AS. The Impact of the COVID-19 Pandemic on Adolescent Emotional, Social, and Academic Adjustment. J Res Adolesc 2021;31(3): 486–99.
34. Rice SM, Purcell R, De Silva S, et al. The Mental Health of Elite Athletes: A Narrative Systematic Review. Sport Med 2016;46(9):1333–53.
35. Weber S, Puta C, Lesinski M, et al. Symptoms of anxiety and depression in young athletes using the hospital anxiety and depression scale. Front Physiol 2018;9(MAR):1–12.
36. Panza MJ, Graupensperger S, Agans JP, et al. Adolescent Sport Participation and Symptoms of Anxiety and Depression: A Systematic Review and Meta-Analysis. J Sport Exerc Psychol 2020;42(3):201–18.
37. McGuine TA, Biese KM, Petrovska L, et al. Mental health, physical activity, and quality of life of us adolescent athletes during COVID-19-related school closures and sport cancellations: A study of 13 000 athletes. J Athl Train 2021;56(1):11–9.
38. Breslau J, Gilman S, Stein B, et al. Sex differences in recent first-onset depression in an epidemiological sample of adolescents. Transl Psychiatry 2017;7(5).

39. Lam KC, Snyder Valier AR, Bay RC, et al. A unique patient population? Health-related quality of life in adolescent athletes versus general, healthy adolescent individuals. J Athl Train 2013;48(2):233–41.
40. Birmaher B, Williamson DE, Dahl RE, et al. Clinical presentation and course of depression in youth: Does onset in childhood differ from onset in adolescence? J Am Acad Child Adolesc Psychiatry 2004;43(1):63–70.
41. Cummings CM, Caporino NE, Kendall PC. Comorbidity of anxiety and depression in children and adolescents: 20 years after. Psychol Bull 2014;140(3):816–45.
42. Jensen SN, Ivarsson A, Fallby J, et al. Depression in Danish and Swedish elite football players and its relation to perfectionism and anxiety. Psychol Sport Exerc 2018;36(June 2017):147–55.
43. Matos NF, Winsley RJ, Williams CA. Prevalence of nonfunctional overreaching/overtraining in young english athletes. Med Sci Sports Exerc 2011;43(7):1287–94.
44. Pass J, Nelson L, Doncaster G. Real world complexities of periodization in a youth soccer academy: An explanatory sequential mixed methods approach. J Sports Sci 2022;40(11):1290–8.
45. Gustafsson H, Kenttä G, Hassmén P, et al. Prevalence of burnout in competitive adolescent athletes. Sport Psychol 2007;21(1):21–37.
46. Americam Psychiatric Association. Diagnostic and Statistical Manual of Mental Disorders. 5th edition Washington, DC; 2013.
47. Xanthopoulos MS, Benton T, Lewis J, et al. Mental Health in the Young Athlete. Curr Psychiatry Rep 2020;22(11):1–15.
48. Lebrun-Harris LA, Ghandour RM, Kogan MD, et al. Five-Year Trends in US Children's Health and Well-being, 2016-2020. JAMA Pediatr 2022;176(7):2016–20.
49. Beesdo K, Knappe S, Pine DS. Anxiety and Anxiety Disorders in Children and Adolescents: Developmental Issues and Implications for DSM-V. Psychiatr Clin North Am 2009;32(3):483–524.
50. Grossbard JR, Smith RE, Smoll FL, et al. Competitive anxiety in young athletes: Differentiating somatic anxiety, worry, and concentration disruption. Hist Philos Logic 2009;22(2):153–66.
51. Scanlan T, Babkes M, Scanlan L. Participation in sport: A developmental glimpse at emotion. In: Mahoney J, Larson R, Eccles J, editors. Organized activities as contexts of development: extracurricular activities, after-school and community programs. Mahwah, NJ: Lawrence Erlbaum; 2005.
52. Smith R, Smoll FL. Behavioral research and intervention in youth sports. Behav Ther 1991;22:329–44.
53. Williams J, Scherzer C. Injury risk and rehabilitation: Psychological considerations. In: Williams J, editor. Applied sport psychology: personal growth to peak performance. Boston, MA: McGraw-Hill; 2006.
54. Smith R, Ptacek J, Patterson E. Moderator effects of cognitive and somatic trait anxiety on the relation between life stress and physical injuries. Hist Philos Logic 2000;13(3):269–88.
55. González-Hernández J, Gomariz-Gea M, Valero-Valenzuela A, et al. Resilient resources in youth athletes and their relationship with anxiety in different team sports. Int J Environ Res Public Health 2020;17(15):1–11.
56. Smith R, Smoll FL. Anxiety and coping in sport: Theoretical models and approaches to anxiety reduction. In: Morris T, Summer J, editors. Sports psychology: theories, applications, and issues. 2nd edition. Sydney, Australia: Wiley; 2004. p. 294–321.

57. Hanton S, Neil R, Mellalieu S, et al. Competitive experience and performance status: An investigation into multidimensional anxiety and coping. Eur J Sport Sci 2008;8:143–52.

58. Almeida P, Luciano R, Lameiras J, et al. Perceived benefits of sports injuries: A qualitative study in professional and semi-professional footballers. J Sport Psychol 2014;23:457–64.

59. Mellalieu S, Hanton D, O'Brien M. Intensity and direction of competitve anxiety as a function of sport type and experience. Scand J Med Sci Sport 2004;14: 326–34.

60. Rocha VVS, Osório F de L. Associations between competitive anxiety, athlete characteristics and sport context: Evidence from a systematic review and meta-analysis. Rev Psiquiatr Clin 2018;45(3):67–74.

61. Brown B. Shame resilience theory: A grounded theory study on women and shame. Fam Soc 2006;87(1):43–52.

62. Hill AP, Mallinson-Howard SH, Jowett GE. Multidimensional perfectionism in sport: A meta-analytical review. Sport Exerc Perform Psychol 2018;7(3):235–70.

63. Smith MM, Sherry SB, Vidovic V, et al. Perfectionism and the Five-Factor Model of Personality: A Meta-Analytic Review. Personal Soc Psychol Rev 2019;23(4): 367–90.

64. Howard TLM, Williams MO, Woodward D, et al. The relationship between shame, perfectionism and Anorexia Nervosa: A grounded theory study. Psychol Psychother Theory, Res Pract 2022;(August 2022):40–55. https://doi.org/10. 1111/papt.12425.

65. Appleton PR, Hill AP. Perfectionism and athlete burnout in junior elite athletes: The mediating role of motivation regulations. J Clin Sport Psychol 2012;6(2): 129–45.

66. Appleton PR, Hall H, Hill A. Relations between multidimensional perfectionism and burnout in junior-elite male athletes. Psychol Sport Exerc 2009;10:457–65.

67. Brewer BW, Cornelius AE, Sklar JH, et al. Pain and negative mood during rehabilitation after anterior cruciate ligament reconstruction: A daily process analysis. Scand J Med Sci Sport 2007;17(5):520–9.

68. Brewer BW, Cornelius AE, Van Raalte JL, et al. Age-Related Differences in Predictors of Adherence to Rehabilitation After Anterior Cruciate Ligament Reconstruction. J Athl Train 2003;38(2):158–62.

69. Daley MM, Griffith K, Milewski MD, et al. The Mental Side of the Injured Athlete. J Am Acad Orthop Surg 2021;29(12):499–506.

70. Brewer BW. Psychological responses to sport injury. Oxford University Press; 2020. Available at;. https://oxfordre.com/psychology/psychology/psychology/view/10.1093/acrefore/9780190236557.001.0001/acrefore-9780190236557-e-172.

71. Garcia GH, Wu HH, Park MJ, et al. Depression Symptomatology and Anterior Cruciate Ligament Injury. Am J Sports Med 2016;44(3):572–9.

72. Tripp DA, Stanish WD, Coady C, et al. The subjective pain experience of athletes following anterior cruciate ligament surgery. Psychol Sport Exerc 2004; 5(3):339–54.

73. Paterno MV, Flynn K, Thomas S, et al. Self-Reported Fear Predicts Functional Performance and Second ACL Injury After ACL Reconstruction and Return to Sport: A Pilot Study. Sports Health 2018;10(3):228–33.

74. Forsdyke D, Smith A, Jones M. Psychosocial factors associated with outcomes of sports injury rehabilitation in competitive athletes: a mixed studies systematic review. Br J Sport Med 2016;50:537–44.

75. Chmielewski TL, Jones D, Day T, et al. The association of pain and fear of movement/reinjury with function during anterior cruciate ligament reconstruction rehabilitation. J Orthop Sports Phys Ther 2008. https://doi.org/10.2519/jospt.2008. 2887.

76. Burland JP, Toonstra JL, Howard JS. Psychosocial Barriers After Anterior Cruciate Ligament Reconstruction: A Clinical Review of Factors Influencing Postoperative Success. Sports Health 2019. https://doi.org/10.1177/1941738119869333.

77. Padaki AS, Noticewala MS, Levine WN, et al. Prevalence of Posttraumatic Stress Disorder Symptoms Among Young Athletes After Anterior Cruciate Ligament Rupture. Orthop J Sport Med 2018;6(7):1–5.

78. Bolia IK, Haratian A, Bell JA, et al. Managing Perioperative Pain After Anterior Cruciate Ligament (ACL) Reconstruction: Perspectives from a Sports Medicine Surgeon. Open Access J Sport Med 2021;12:129–38.

79. Arthur-Cameselle J, Sossin K, Quatromoni P. A qualitative analysis of factors related to eating disorder onset in female collegiate athletes and non-athletes. Eat Disord 2017;25(3):199–215.

80. Matricciani L, Paquet C, Galland B, et al. Children's sleep and health: A meta-review. Sleep Med Rev 2019;46:136–50.

81. Vella SA, Swann C, Batterham M, et al. An Intervention for Mental Health Literacy and Resilience in Organized Sports. Med Sci Sports Exerc 2021;53(1):139–49.

82. Gouttebarge V, Bindra A, Blauwet C, et al. International Olympic Committee (IOC) Sport Mental Health Assessment Tool 1 (SMHAT-1) and Sport Mental Health Recognition Tool 1 (SMHRT-1): Towards better support of athletes' mental health. Br J Sports Med 2021;55(1):30–7.

83. Walter HJ, Abright AR, Bukstein OG, et al. Clinical Practice Guideline for the Assessment and Treatment of Children and Adolescents With Major and Persistent Depressive Disorders. J Am Acad Child Adolesc Psychiatry 2022;1–24. https://doi.org/10.1016/j.jaac.2022.10.001.

84. Walton CC, Rice S, Hutter RI, et al. Mental Health in Youth Athletes. Adv Psychiatry Behav Heal 2021;1(1):119–33.

85. Wilczyńska D, Qi W, Jaenes JC, et al. Burnout and Mental Interventions among Youth Athletes: A Systematic Review and Meta-Analysis of the Studies. Int J Environ Res Public Health 2022;19(17). https://doi.org/10.3390/ijerph191710662.

86. Ekelund R, Holmström S, Stenling A. Mental Health in Athletes: Where Are the Treatment Studies? Front Psychol 2022;13(July). https://doi.org/10.3389/fpsyg. 2022.781177.

87. Reardon CL, Factor RM. Sport psychiatry: A systematic review of diagnosis and medical treatment of mental illness in athletes. Sport Med 2010;40(11):961–80.

88. Jayanthi N, Pinkham C, Dugas L, et al. Sports Specialization in Young Athletes: Evidence-Based Recommendations. Sports Health 2013;5(3):251–7.

89. Brenner JS. Council on Sports Medicine and Fitness. Overuse injuries, overtraining, and burnout in child and adolescent athletes. Pediatrics 2007;119(6): 1242–5.

90. Post EG, Trigsted SM, Riekena JW, et al. The Association of Sport Specialization and Training Volume with Injury History in Youth Athletes. Am J Sports Med 2017;45(6):1405–12. https://doi.org/10.1177/0363546517690848.

91. Meeusen R, Duclos M, Foster C, et al. Prevention, diagnosis, and treatment of the overtraining syndrome: Joint consensus statement of the european college of sport science and the American College of Sports Medicine. Med Sci Sports Exerc 2013;45(1):186–205.

92. Bergmann P, Lucke C, Nguyen T, et al. Identification and Utility of a Short Form of the Pediatric Symptom Checklist-Youth Self-Report (PSC-17-Y). Eur J Psychol Assess 2020;36(1):56–64.
93. He JP, Burstein M, Schmitz A, et al. The strengths and difficulties questionnaire (SDQ): The factor structure and scale validation in U.S. Adolescents. J Abnorm Child Psychol 2013;41(4):583–95.
94. Rice S, Olive L, Gouttebarge V, et al. Mental health screening: Severity and cut-off point sensitivity of the Athlete Psychological Strain Questionnaire in male and female elite athletes. BMJ Open Sport Exerc Med 2020;6(1):1–6.
95. Kroenke K, Spitzer RL, Williams J. The PHQ-9: Validity of a brief depression severity measure. J Gen Intern Med 2001;16:606–13.
96. Freitag GF, Salem H, Conroy K, et al. The Patient-Reported Outcomes Measurement Information System (PROMIS) pediatric and parent-proxy short forms for anxiety: Psychometric properties in the Kids FACE FEARS sample. J Anxiety Disord 2023;94(July 2022):102677.
97. Nolte S, Coon C, Hudgens S, et al. Psychometric evaluation of the PROMIS® Depression Item Bank: an illustration of classical test theory methods. J Patient-Reported Outcomes 2019;3(1). https://doi.org/10.1186/s41687-019-0127-0.
98. Spitzer RL, Kroenke K, Williams JBW, et al. A brief measure for assessing generalized anxiety disorder: The GAD-7. Arch Intern Med 2006;166(10):1092–7.
99. Bender AM, Lawson D, Werthner P, et al. The Clinical Validation of the Athlete Sleep Screening Questionnaire: an Instrument to Identify Athletes that Need Further Sleep Assessment. Sport Med - Open 2018;4(1). https://doi.org/10.1186/s40798-018-0140-5.
100. Zulfiqar L, Chakrabarty B, Gulati S, et al. The Childhood and Adolescent Sleep Evaluation Questionnaire (CASEQ): Development and validation of an ICSD-3-based screening instrument, a community and hospital-based study. J Sleep Res 2022;31(2):1–13. https://doi.org/10.1111/jsr.13479.
101. Martinsen M, Holme I, Pensgaard AM, et al. The development of the brief eating disorder in athletes questionnaire. Med Sci Sports Exerc 2014;46(8):1666–75.
102. Couwenbergh C, Van Der Gaag RJ, Koeter M, et al. Screening for substance abuse among adolescents validity of the CAGE-AID in youth mental health care. Subst Use Misuse 2009;44(6):823–34.

Substance Misuse in Elite Athletes

Early Detection, Brief Intervention and Referral to Treatment

David R. McDuff, MD[a,b,c,*], Michelle Garvin, PhD[d,e],
Joy Chang, MD[a,f], Donald Thompson, MD[a,b]

KEYWORDS

- Substance misuse • Alcohol • Cannabis • Tobacco • Nicotine • Elite athletes
- Early detection

KEY POINTS

- Encounters with alcohol, cannabis, and nicotine/tobacco misuse is common.
- Early identification can reduce the negative consequences of misuse and prevent the progression to a substance use disorder.
- The use of screening instruments, negative consequences questionnaires, and urine testing can aid early identification.
- Brief motivational interventions with personalized feedback, social norming, goal setting, contingency management, and significant other involvement can change attitudes, beliefs, and use patterns.
- The simultaneous use of alcohol and marijuana (SAM) among athletes is increasing and is associated with increased adverse effects.

The authors declare no commercial or financial conflicts of interest and no funding sources were associated with this work.
[a] Department of Psychiatry, University of Maryland School of Medicine, 110 South Paca Street - 4th Floor, Baltimore, MD 21201, USA; [b] Baltimore Orioles, Major League Baseball, 333 West Camden Street, Oriole Park at Camden Yards, Baltimore, MD 21201, USA; [c] Maryland Centers for Psychiatry, 3290 North Ridge Road, Suite 320, Ellicott City, MD 21043, USA; [d] Detroit Lions, National Football League, 222 Republic Drive, Allen Park, MI 48101, USA; [e] Elite Performance Psychology, LLC, 205 Warrenton Drive, Silver Spring, MD 20904, USA; [f] University of Maryland, College Park, 8500 Paint Branch Drive, XFINITY Center, Room 2707, College Park, MD 20742, USA
* Corresponding author. Maryland Centers for Psychiatry, 3290 North Ridge Road, Suite 320, Ellicott City, MD 21043, USA
E-mail address: dmcduff52@gmail.com

INTRODUCTION

Sports medicine physicians and athletic trainers regularly encounter athletes who misuse substances that put them at risk for adverse social, interpersonal, academic, psychological, health and performance effects.[1-6] The most often encountered substances in collegiate and professional athletes are alcohol (binge drinking), cannabis (marijuana), and nicotine (oral tobacco/nicotine vaping).[7-15] Male athletes typically misuse substances at higher rates than female athletes and male and female athletes from certain sports (eg, lacrosse, ice hockey, swimming, rugby) have the highest rates of use and misuse.[16-19] Differences in use and misuse rates of some substances in athletes versus non-athletes can begin in high school where, for example, binge drinking rates for athletes is higher than in non-athletes by 9th grade.[8]

Alcohol and other substance use typically begins as recreational or social use in high school and increases from 8th to 12th grades in both athlete and general student populations.[19,20] In 2022 a national survey demonstrated that past year use rates were significantly higher for 12th graders than 8th graders for alcohol (51.9% vs 15.2%), cannabis (30.7% vs 8.3%), and nicotine vaping (27.3% vs 12%). For some athletes, substance use becomes more regular and heavier, progressing to misuse by the end of high school. Misuse is defined as using alcohol or other drugs in a manner, situation, amount, or frequency that could cause harm to a user or to those around them.[21] Common adverse effects vary somewhat by substance class, but include physical, social, legal, emotional, performance and academic consequences[2,11,16] (**Table 1**). If substance misuse is identified early, prompt intervention can prevent progression to a substance disorder with or without comorbid mental health symptoms and disorders.

Substances may be used individually or concurrently with an increasing trend for using two together such that their psychogenic and behavioral effects overlap. The simultaneous use of alcohol and marijuana (SAM) and alcohol and tobacco/nicotine is common among college students including student athletes.[22-25] When two substances are used simultaneously, additive adverse effects such as heavier and more frequent use, driving while impaired, academic and athletic underperformance, and an increased probability of developing comorbid substance use and mental health disorders are likely.[23]

The early identification of athletes who are misusing any of these substances, alone or in combination, is critical to prevent the range of negative consequences and/or progression to a substance use disorder. Behavioral observations, the longitudinal use of screening instruments and/or negative consequences questionnaires, and random urine testing are important mitigation strategies.[1,2,4] Given the amount of time that sports medicine physicians and athletic trainers spend with athletes, they are in the best position to pick up early behavioral signs and symptoms of increasing substance use or misuse (see **Table 1**). The regular use of screening instruments throughout the year, and especially pre-season, should be considered. Short screeners include the three question Alcohol Use Disorders Identification Test-Consumption Questions (AUDIT-C Appendix 1), the four question Cutting Down, Annoyance by Criticism, Guilty Feeling, and Eye Opener Adapted to Include Drugs (CAGE-AID Appendix 2), and the eight or three question Cannabis Use Disorder Screening Tool Revised or Short Form (CUDIT-R, CUDIT-SF Appendix 3).[26,27] For those who screen positive and/or have a positive urine test, a more detailed assessment documenting the current frequency of use, route of administration, and negative consequences using either the Brief Young Adult Alcohol Consequences Questionnaire (B-YAACQ) or the Brief Marijuana Consequences Questionnaire (B-MACQ) should be conducted.[28-30]

Table 1
Alcohol, cannabis, and tobacco/nicotine misuse: behavioral effects, intoxication, withdrawal, health and performance effects

Substance	Common Negative Behavioral Effects	Signs and Symptoms of Intoxication	Signs & Symptoms of Withdrawal	Negative Health Effects	Negative Performance Effects
Alcohol	Hangover, memory loss, passing out, embarrassing behaviors, lateness, low energy, interrupted/lost sleep, arguing or fighting, missing class, arrested (fight, DUI), unwanted sexual encounter, smell of alcohol on the breath, irritability	Sedation, slurred speech, poor balance, unpredictable behavior, blackouts, memory problems, lack of attention, dizziness, vomiting, flushing, fights, arrests, sexual inappropriateness, mood swings, self-harm	Sweating, increased heart rate, hand tremors, insomnia, nausea/vomiting, agitation, anxiety, fatigue, irritability, clammy skin, dilated pupils, mood swings, confused thinking, headache, loss of appetite, depression, seizures	Reduced bone density, impaired fracture healing, pancreatitis, myopathy, wasting, respiratory distress syndrome, pneumonia, stroke, hypertension, heart disease, oral cancers, hepatitis, cirrhosis, liver, and colorectal cancers	Dehydration, insomnia, impaired motor skills, reduced glycogen resynthesis, increased injury rates, impaired temperature regulation, weight gain, hangovers, accidents, lateness, missing important events
Cannabis	Reduced motivation, decline in school performance, tiredness/sluggishness, rudeness/irritability, trouble sleeping, regret of behaviors, driving while high, derealization, depersonalization, anxiety, paranoia, social isolation	Euphoria, bloodshot eyes, lack of motivation, dry mouth, increased appetite, paranoia, anxiety, cough, slowed reaction time, lethargy, drowsiness, impaired judgment, social withdrawal	Irritability, anger, aggression, anxiety, nervousness, insomnia, disturbing dreams, decreased appetite, weight loss, depressed mood, restlessness, headaches, fever, chills, sweating, abdominal pain	Impaired short-term memory and learning, inattention, impaired motor coordination and driving skills, increased risk of injury, altered judgment, anxiety, paranoia, psychosis, addiction, altered brain development, quitting school, cognitive impairment, decreased life satisfaction and achievement, chronic bronchitis.	Increased heart rate and blood pressure, slowed reaction time, impaired motor coordination, impaired concentration, decreased motor agility, reduced mental quickness

(continued on next page)

Table 1
(continued)

Substance	Common Negative Behavioral Effects	Signs and Symptoms of Intoxication	Signs & Symptoms of Withdrawal	Negative Health Effects	Negative Performance Effects
Tobacco/ Nicotine	External bulge in cheeks from moist snuff, spitting into a cup or on the ground, vaping pen in a locker or travel bag, using when ill or despite oral lesions, stained teeth and hands from nicotine, annoying other from smoking, vaping, spitting in public (eg, second-hand smoke or vapor)	Nausea, vomiting, headache, stomachache, loss of appetite, eye irritation, tremors, dizziness, anxiety, confusion, sweating, cough, increased heart rate, elevated blood pressure, excessive salivation	Irritability, anger, frustration, anxiety, cravings, restlessness, insomnia, depressed mood, difficulty concentrating, increased appetite, trouble sleeping	Heart disease, stroke, lung, gastrointestinal, and oral cancers, emphysema, chronic bronchitis, tooth loss, gum irritation, cataracts, rheumatoid arthritis, bone loss, chronic cough, erectile dysfunction, infertility, low birth weight babies, premature aging of the skin, delayed wound healing, decrease in taste and smell	Anxiety, insomnia, chronic respiratory infections, cough, shortness of breath, excess sputum production

Once alcohol, cannabis, and/or nicotine/tobacco misuse is identified and an in-depth assessment has been conducted, various interventions such as psychoeducation, direct or web-based individualized feedback, goal setting, support system involvement, contingency management and/or brief motivational interventions can be considered.[31–34] If these interventions are not effective in reducing substance use and/or its adverse effects, then referral to more targeted treatment (eg, outpatient, intensive outpatient, residential, inpatient detoxification) may be necessary.

This article will focus on alcohol, cannabis, and tobacco misuse and explore early detection, brief interventions, and referral to treatment. Additionally, a brief description of the available levels of care for the treatment of severe or intractable substance misuse or a substance use disorder will be presented.

ALCOHOL
Background

Binge drinking, with a range of adverse effects, is commonly encountered in US collegiate and professional athletes with certain sports (eg, lacrosse, rugby, ice hockey, swimming, baseball, field hockey) exhibiting higher rates than the general population. Binge drinking is defined as 4 or more standard drinks per drinking occasion for females and 5 or more drinks for males. Super binge drinking is defined as 10 or more drinks per drinking occasion and is seen more often in US male collegiate athletes (13%) than in female collegiate athletes (1.8%). Binge and super binge drinking are typically defined by the presence of one or more binge drinking episodes over the past two weeks.[16] For male collegiate athletes, certain sports have high rates for binge drinking ranging from 50% for wrestling to 64% and 69% for ice hockey and lacrosse respectively. For females, the sports with the highest rates range from 43% for volleyball to 56% and 57% for ice hockey and lacrosse respectively.[16] The most endorsed negative effects for binge drinking among collegiate athletes are hangover (52%), loss of memory of events (28.4%), regret of behaviors (25.4%), interrupted/lost sleep (20.7%), got into an argument or a fight (16.8%) and missed a class (14.2%).[16] Even though binge drinking rates for US collegiate athletes from all sports have declined from 2009 to 2017 (58% to 44% for men; 51% to 39% for women), the rates are still high in certain sports and the adverse consequences are serious (ie, physical injury (6.8%), poor academic performance (7.1%), and/or poor athletic performance (7.4%)).[16]

Very limited data exist on the rates of alcohol misuse (including heavy use and binge drinking) among current professional athletes, especially in the US. The data that exists from Europe and Australasia suggests that in general, rates of alcohol misuse are highly variable depending on the sport.[18,35–39] For example, a study of professional soccer players from five European countries found rates of current alcohol misuse that ranged from 6.0% in Sweden to 15.7% and 17% for Spain and Finland, respectively.[35] A study of professional rugby players from Australasian countries ranged from 22% misuse rates in one study[36] to much higher rates of 62.8% in another.[37] Rates among current and retired professional ice hockey players from four European countries were 7.6% for current players and 28.7% for retired ones.[38] Somewhat higher current rates were seen in active professional cricket players from South Africa (26%), while retired professional cricketers had rates of 22%.[39] Both of these studies included male athletes only. However, a study of male and female professional soccer players in Australia found the rate of alcohol misuse in the women athletes (43.8%) to be lower than that of males (50.7%).[18]

Early Detection

Athletic trainers and team physicians are in ideal positions to aid in the early detection of alcohol misuse. Proximity to, and time around athletes allows for frequent informal assessments and opportunities to learn about potential risky behaviors. Common behavioral signs of alcohol misuse that can be detected by athletic trainers, team physicians, and other support staff are detailed in **Table 1**.

Any athlete suspected of misusing alcohol or who has an adverse alcohol-related event (eg, blackout, fight, arrest, driving under the influence) should be assessed by the team physician or licensed mental health provider using motivational interviewing techniques and should receive the full 10-item Alcohol Use Disorders Inventory Test (AUDIT) adapted for use in the United States (USAAUDIT)[40,41] and the 24 item Brief Young Adult Alcohol Consequences Questionnaire.[42] USAAUDIT scores of 7 to 15 for women and 8 to 15 for men indicate hazardous drinking and should result in feedback and a brief intervention designed to reduce consumption and curb the adverse effects of alcohol misuse.

Another early detection strategy is to include alcohol urine testing as part of the panel for random screening of drugs of abuse and performance enhancers. Any level of alcohol in a morning urine test indicates heavy drinking the night before and should be assessed via motivational interviewing and administration of the USAAUDIT. Finally, because of the increasing likelihood of simultaneous use of alcohol and cannabis misuse, a cannabis use history (frequency, intensity, route of administration) and screening with the 8-item CUDIT-R or the 3-item CUDIT-SF (see Appendix 3) should occur. If SAM is present, there is an increased risk for comorbid mental health diagnoses and a screening for anxiety (Generalized Anxiety Disorder Screen-GAD-7), depression (Patient Health Questionnaire-PHQ-9), and sleep problems (Athlete Sleep Screening Questionnaire-ASSQ) should also be considered.[26]

Brief Interventions

Psychoeducation about the adverse effects of alcohol on sleep, energy, reaction time, emotional control, interpersonal relationships, and injury risk as well as its likelihood of reducing athletic and academic performance is a primary component of brief intervention strategies for alcohol misuse. Many athletes are unaware of the fixed metabolism of alcohol (only one drink an hour) which makes it unique among substances of misuse and increases the risk of heavy, rapid drinking. In addition, if alcohol is used simultaneously with cannabis or sedative/anxiety/depression medications (prescribed or over the counter) such as antihistamines, benzodiazepines, selective serotonin reuptake inhibitors (SSRIs), or sleeping pills, this potentiates the intoxicating effects of alcohol and makes adverse effects more likely.[1,2,4] Providing athletes with this information can help them make more educated decisions about their alcohol consumption.

For more serious alcohol misuse, as evidenced by a score of 16 to 24 on the USAAUDIT, a series of 1 to 4 brief motivational interviewing sessions should be implemented by a mental health provider working directly with the athlete/team or by an outpatient substance treatment program. These sessions should include personalized feedback, social norming, goal setting (academic, athletic, social), involvement of significant others (eg, peer, parent, coach), strategies for cutting down aimed at changing patterns of harmful use, and/or a trial of abstinence.

One example of such an intervention was created by Donohue and colleagues[32] for incoming first-year collegiate athletes. Following an assessment of the athletes' drinking behaviors, they created a one-session model (individual or group) with a follow-up assessment at 2 months that was led by a performance coach and included significant other involvement (typically a parent), goal setting and contingency contracting for goal achievement with an overall focus on alcohol as a potential barrier to sporting performance compared to a control group. Results showed that the brief intervention group, compared to controls, significantly reduced their alcohol consumption from baseline and experienced reductions in academic problems, injury concerns, dysfunctional thoughts, and stress.

Other interventions use on-line substance education modules (eg, *myPlaybook*) with personalized feedback and a focus on normative perceptions, behavioral expectancies, and harm prevention.[43] One such study using a revised version of *myPlaybook* and three iterative revision trials of 2000 to 3000 student athletes each was conducted by Rulison and colleagues.[34] While the first two trials did not result in reductions in alcohol and cannabis use at 30 days, the modified modules in the third trial had positive results. Results showed changes from baseline in normative views (ie, fewer athletes use substances regularly), positive alcohol expectancies (reduced), and negative marijuana expectancies (increased), but not on intentions to use behavioral strategies to reduce use.[34]

CANNABIS
Background

Self-reported rates of cannabis (marijuana) use and misuse among US collegiate and professional athletes are rising due to its expanded availability from medicalization/legalization and the decision by some professional sports (eg, Major League Baseball, National Football League) to reduce or discontinue random urine testing and eliminate sanctions in favor of evaluation and treatment.[10–12,16,44,45] Sports medicine providers should be aware of the prevalence rates, reasons for use, patterns of use, adverse effects, trends in potency, signs of misuse, and detection and intervention strategies for this substance.[2,4,6,16]

Studies of elite athletes in general show that approximately 1 in 4 use cannabis.[10,16,44] In US collegiate athletes, annual use rates are higher in: (1) men than women (26.3% vs 22.3%); (2) lacrosse, swimming, and wrestling for men (50%, 35%, 29% respectively), (3) lacrosse, ice hockey, field hockey, soccer and volleyball for women (34%, 29%, 29%, 27%, 27% respectively), (4) Division III than Division I (33% vs 18%) and in (5) states where it is legal than in those where it is not (39% vs 26%).[16] The most common reasons for use are socialization, pain control, well-being, stress reduction, and insomnia.[16,44]

Patterns of use range from episodic cannabidiol (CBD) alone and/or delta 9 tetrahydrocannabinol (THC with CBD simultaneously) to long-term regular use of higher potency THC with or without CBD and/or simultaneous use of alcohol and marijuana.[25,44] The most common routes of administration are inhaling (eg, smoking, vaping) or ingestion (edibles, tinctures)[16] and the most common short-term adverse behavioral effects are detailed in **Tables 1**.[46–48] When cannabis use becomes daily or near daily, the risk of additional adverse effects including the use of other illicit substances (eg, cocaine, methamphetamine), motor vehicle accidents, athletic injuries, permanent cognitive impairment, reduced life achievement, psychosis and/or progression to a cannabis use disorder becomes more likely.[46–50] In general, 1 out of 9 cannabis users progress to a use disorder; however, this increases to 1 in 6 if use starts in adolescence and to 1 in 4 for those that use daily.[46] Many of these adverse effects are due to the potency (THC level) of herbal US cannabis products which has risen over the past decade from approximately 10% in 2009 to 14% in 2019.[51] Similar increases have occurred in the United Kingdom, Central Europe, and New Zealand.[52] Cannabis levels are highest in cannabis concentrates (eg, ear wax, hash oil) with THC levels of 40% to 80%. Additional risks for concentrates include intoxication effects that are 3 to 4 times that of plant-based marijuana and the unknown risks of inhaling residual solvents.[53]

Early Detection

Annual preseason psychoeducational presentations on the patterns, prevalence, potency, and adverse effects of cannabis use and misuse to groups of athletes or teams with the distribution of a companion fact sheet or negative consequences questionnaire may prompt individuals to ask more questions about their use and review the pros and cons of continuing. Athletic trainers, team physicians, and sports mental health and performance providers should be educated regarding cannabis' early behavioral effects and typical signs and symptoms of intoxication and withdrawal (see **Table 1**).[54,55]

Random or surveillance urine testing is another way of identifying cannabis users or misusers. Random testing refers to testing small groups of athletes on a team each week with the intention of testing all team members over the season or the year. Surveillance testing refers to testing all members (or a representative sample – 50%) with or without the results being connected to a specific athlete's name to determine the point prevalence of use. This might be done for sports that are known to have the highest rates of use (eg, lacrosse, swimming, ice hockey, field hockey). High individual urine levels (ie, above 150 ng/mL) may indicate a daily or near daily user and warrant an evaluation.

Screening instruments such as the four question Cutting Down, Annoyance by Criticism, Guilty Feelings, Eye-opener modified to include cannabis/marijuana (CAGE-AID)[26] or the three question Cannabis Use Disorder Screening Tool-Short-Form (CUDIT-SF) which uses questions 3, 5, and 6 of the longer CUDIT-R[27] are recommended to identify misuse (see Appendices 2 and 3). A score of 2 or more indicates a positive screen for both the CAGE-AID and CUDIT-SF. A positive screen on one or both should result in a clinical assessment with a team physician or licensed mental health provider along with the administration of the 20-item Brief Marijuana Consequences Questionnaire.[30]

Brief Interventions

The literature on brief motivational interventions with personalized feedback for cannabis use and misuse in elite athletes is scarce. Like college students, young adult athletes at collegiate and professional levels are increasingly viewing cannabis use as safe and socially acceptable with a companion view that much higher percentages of their teammates are using than actually are.[24,25,56,57]

Given the documented adverse effects of both regular alcohol and cannabis use in athletes (see **Table 1**), brief interventions conducted by athletic trainers, team physicians, and/or sports mental health and substance providers are warranted.[24,50]

There is some evidence that brief motivational interventions with personalized feedback compared to assessment without intervention or psychoeducation alone can reduce positive expectancies and frequency of use, change attitudes about cannabis' safety and levels of normative use, and potentially prevent adverse consequences in non-athlete samples of adolescents and college students.[58–60] These motivational interventions are typically designed to encourage participants to change their behavior, teach behavioral coping and change skills, and connect to services using the FRAMES model (ie,: personalized *feedback*, *reinforcement* of personal responsibility, nonjudgmental *advice*, *menu* of strategies, *empathetic* listening, and activation of *self-efficacy*).[56]

Parisi and colleagues (2019) in a study of 12,150 students including 1233 student athletes found sufficient adverse effects of alcohol and cannabis use to recommend increased education and brief intervention skill development for athletic personnel (eg, coaches, athletic trainers, strength and conditioning staff).[24] They developed a 2-h training module with content on patterns and prevalence of use, risks for alcohol-related injury, risks for alcohol and cannabis-related academic difficulties, and skill building for motivational interviewing. The skill-building section of the module was designed to teach athletic personnel to have "meaningful conversations" about student athlete use and facilitate guiding help-seeking behaviors.

Another intervention mentioned earlier by Rulison and colleagues (2022)[34] used an iteratively modified version of *myPlaybook* during three trials of approximately 2000 to 3000 each Division I, II, and III athletes with content on norms of alcohol and cannabis use, expectancies of drug effects, harm reduction and life skills. For cannabis, they found reductions in views of teammates' levels of use and increased negative expectancies when using.

Finally, an alternative approach by Lee and colleagues (2021)[59] developed a novel Marijuana Consequences Checklist (26 items, MCC) in college undergraduates that attempted to more accurately document the common consequences of cannabis use of typical users. They discovered that for monthly or more frequent users, the top 6 "not so good" consequences over the past 30 days were: (1) had the munchies (83.9%); (2) experienced dry mouth (3) had trouble concentrating or paying attention (62.5%); (4) acted foolish or goofy (61.9%); (5) had trouble remembering things (57.4%); and (6) had low motivation (46.4%). They suggest using the MCC to generate a motivational discussion and deliver personalized feedback based on the response patterns from the 336 undergraduates that completed the checklist.

Based on the available evidence, coaches, athletic trainers, team physicians, and/or on-site mental health or substance use providers can use team-based presentations to present information on the adverse effects of cannabis use alone or in combination with alcohol and administer either the Brief Marijuana Consequences Questionnaire[30] or the Marijuana Consequences Checklist.[61] Those with regular or heavy patterns of cannabis use and a higher number of negative consequences can then receive individual personalized feedback with an open motivational discussion of the potential negative effects of cannabis on athletic and academic performance. Those who continue the use/misuse after this "open discussion" should have a formal assessment by a mental health provider and potential referral to an outpatient treatment program.

TOBACCO/NICOTINE
Background

The use and misuse of oral (spit) tobacco and other tobacco products (eg, cigars, cigarettes, hookah) and/or nicotine vaping is regularly encountered by sports medicine providers especially those that work in baseball, hockey, wrestling, golf, and lacrosse.[16,62] Overall annual use rates of the various tobacco products and nicotine vaping for US male collegiate athletes are: oral tobacco (21.8%); cigars (17%); cigarettes (14%); hookah (10%); and electronic cigarettes (8%) with 5% reporting daily use of oral tobacco.[16] There is substantial variation in annual male use rates by sports with far higher rates for annual oral tobacco use in ice hockey (46%), baseball (44%), lacrosse (35%) and wrestling (33%) and high rates for cigarettes in lacrosse (38%), golf (23%) and ice hockey (23%). Overall annual use rates for women collegiate athletes are far lower than for men for both cigarettes (5.3% vs 14%) and oral tobacco (0.6% vs 21.8%). However, just as for men, women's use rates vary significantly by sport with higher use rates of cigarettes in lacrosse (10%), ice hockey (9%) tennis (9%), and golf (8%) and higher use rates for oral tobacco in ice hockey (13%) and soft-ball (2%).[16]

One study of past 30-day use rates for 8617 collegiate athletes from the National College Health assessment II from 2011 to 2014 showed that oral tobacco use was 43% more likely in collegiate athletes for occasional use (1–19 days out of 30) and 152% more likely for frequent use (20 or more days out of 30) compared to non-athletes.[62] The same study showed that collegiate athletes were less likely to be occasional and frequent users of cigarettes and hookah (26% less for occasional hookah; 29% less for occasional cigarette use, and 52% less for frequent cigarette use) than their non-athlete counterparts. Overall male and female athlete use rates of nicotine vaping (electronic cigarettes) are daily (0.8%), weekly (0.8%), monthly (1.2%), and past year (5.4%).[16] These nicotine vaping rates however, are substantially lower than those seen in college students with 30-day use rates increasing from 6% in 2017 to 22% in 2019 and from 8% to 18% among 19-to-22-year-olds not in college.[63] The most common reason for tobacco and or nicotine vaping use in collegiate athletes are to fit in socially, for stress-relief, and to boost energy.[15] The most common adverse effects and signs and symptoms of intoxication and withdrawal are detailed in **Table 1**.[64]

There is far less information on tobacco or nicotine use among professional athletes. One study by Marclay and colleagues (2011) found overall rates in 2185 athletes from 43 different international professional sports of 15.3% using urine testing for nicotine and its metabolites.[65] When viewed by specific sports however, rates ranged from 26% to 56% depending on sport. Rates for the teams studied were as follows: American football (56%); ice hockey (32%); wrestling (32%); bobsleigh (31%); gymnastics (29%); rugby (28%); and skiing (26%).

Early Detection

Awareness of the high prevalence of tobacco use and nicotine vaping in certain sports (eg, ice hockey, baseball, American football, wrestling, golf) is one key to early detection. Questions about tobacco use and nicotine vaping should be included in the pre-season physical examination along with alcohol and cannabis. If use is endorsed, then additional screening with the 6-question Fagerstrom Dependence Scale (FDS - Appendix 4) should be considered.[66] A score of 5 or more indicates a significant dependence, while a score of 4 or less shows a low to moderate dependence. An additional approach is to have the team dentist do an oral exam at the time of the pre-season physical examination looking for signs of gum irritation or oral lesions (ie, leukoplakia). If the exam is positive, then more questions about the current and past pattern of use and desire to quit should be asked.

Brief Interventions

There are no recent studies of brief interventions for elite athletes who are using or misusing tobacco products or vaping nicotine. Older studies from 1999 to 2003 in high school, collegiate, and professional baseball players (where oral tobacco use rates in minor league and major league players ranged from 25% to 35%) have demonstrated the effectiveness of brief interventions in increasing the perception of risk and reducing levels of use.[67–70] Most of these studies included a dentist or dental assistant led, peer assisted brief intervention that occurred at the time of the preseason physical exam. The intervention provided personalized feedback regarding current, or future, oral health problems, level of nicotine dependence using the FDS, and provided strategies for quitting. In some of these dental-based interventions, the baseball team's athletic trainers continued the follow-up by encouraging continued abstinence and/or treatment seeking with a mental health professional skilled in tobacco or nicotine vaping cessation. In one randomized controlled trial of brief intervention of 307 high school baseball players, quit rates at 2 years were 23% compared to 13% in the control group.[70] In a similar brief intervention with professional baseball players from one organization conducted over ten successive years, oral leukoplakia declined, and the prevalence of oral tobacco use fell from 22.6% in 1991 to 9.4% in 2000.[71]

Based on the available evidence there seems to be merit in a dentist/dental technician-led oral preseason evaluation along with tobacco use screenings and assessment of dependence using the FDS followed by a brief motivational intervention with a provider experienced in tobacco/nicotine cessation. Another option is group-based brief motivational intervention with a tips-for-quitting guide along with one- and 3-month follow-ups. With advanced training in this domain, athletic trainers, team physicians, and team-based mental health providers could administer this intervention and conduct the follow-up.

REFERRAL TO TREATMENT

When an athlete is not responding to the brief intervention strategies described above, or is diagnosed as having a substance use disorder, they may benefit from referral to an addiction specialist for a more comprehensive evaluation to determine the next steps. Alternatively, if the athlete is already demonstrating medical signs and symptoms of withdrawal that indicate pending instability (ie, alcohol withdrawal-**Table 1**), they may require immediate medical detoxification in an outpatient or inpatient setting.

Treatment for a substance use disorder exists on a spectrum with the American Society of Addiction Medicine (ASAM) identifying 5 benchmark levels of care as a method of standardizing addiction treatment[80]. Level 0/0.5 includes prevention and early intervention and includes brief intervention strategies discussed above. Outpatient services are the focus of Level 1, while Level 2 is comprised of intensive outpatient and partial hospitalization services. Level 3 involves residential/inpatient services including clinically managed low-intensity and high-intensity residential services, and medically monitored intensive inpatient services. Level 4 is the highest level of care and is comprised of medically managed intensive inpatient services.[72]

The topical areas explored in the criteria for determining the appropriate level of care include (but are not limited to) medical complexity, behavioral health complexity, readiness to change, environmental instability, and previous experience in treatment settings. The process of determining the level of care and criterion match is best executed by a trained clinician and is typically completed upon initial intake and evaluation to a new treatment facility. Based upon this clinical assessment, the client enters treatment at a certain level best matched to address their level of instability and need, with the goal to progress to less clinically rigorous engagement as their needs evolve. Not every program is able to satisfy the definition of the full spectrum and may offer alternative referral if the individual demonstrates needs greater than what is available.

DISCUSSION

Sports medicine physicians and athletic trainers are in prime positions to help with the early identification, assessment, and brief intervention for substance misuse and abuse among athletes. Knowing utilization and misuse patterns of the sport you are working with can help enhance awareness of symptoms guide best questions to ask. Across all sports and competition levels, the most encountered substances of misuse are alcohol (binge drinking), cannabis (marijuana), and nicotine (oral tobacco/ nicotine vaping). While more detailed data exists for the collegiate population, there is limited data among professional athletes, especially current professional athletes in the US, making it more challenging to know prevalence rates for this population. Continued exploration of use and misuse patterns along with adverse consequences of use will help develop more effective prevention, assessment, and intervention processes for this population.

Development of an organizational plan for training, identification, intervention, and treatment prior to the start of the season will help sports medicine staff know when and how to assess for misuse of alcohol, cannabis, and nicotine. Pre-participation physicals is an ideal time for sports medicine staff to begin asking questions and assessing behaviors via self-report screeners, open-ended questioning, medical exams, and urine screens. Following transitions and acute events (ie, injury, trade, transfer, and so forth) is another time to screen for changes in behaviors and substance use patterns. While discrete transitions provide ideal times for screening, sports medicine staff have frequent interactions and access to players that allows for ongoing informal screening and behavior monitoring throughout the year.

While geared toward sports medicine physicians and athletic trainers, many other athlete-facing staff may be in roles to help facilitate prevention, identification, and early intervention depending on the organization and individual athlete relationships. Coaches, player engagement/development staff, dieticians, strength and conditioning, and equipment staff are a few of the groups that may be in positions to identify signs and symptoms of misuse/abuse. Training with all athlete-facing staff can help with identification and referral to the sports medicine staff for further assessment and evaluation when warranted.

Training for sports medicine staff on early identification, motivational interviewing, and brief interventions for alcohol, cannabis, and nicotine use is recommended. Partnering with licensed mental health providers can aid in this training and provide an easy transition from brief intervention to higher levels of ongoing care. The ASAM levels of care outline the continuum of treatment based on patterns of use and symptoms. It is important for sports medicine staff to develop relationships with addiction specialists in the community along with local area treatment facilities providing the full spectrum of care. These relationships will help facilitate access to, and transition of care when higher levels of treatment is warranted.

CLINICS CARE POINTS

- Screening for alcohol, cannabis, and tobacco/nicotine misuse prior to each season can lead to early detection and brief intervention.
- The simultaneous use of alcohol with either cannabis or tobacco/nicotine is associated with increased adverse effects.
- Brief Motivational Intervention training for substance misuse should become a part of the ongoing education of athletic trainers and team physicians.

REFERENCES

1. McDuff D, Stull T, Castaldelli-Maia JM, et al. Recreational and ergogenic substance use and substance use disorders in elite athletes: a narrative review. Br J Sports Med 2019;53(12):754–60.

2. Stull T, Morse E, McDuff DR. Substance Use and Its Impact on Athlete Health and Performance. Psychiatr Clin North Am 2021;44(3):405–17.
3. Exner J, Bitar R, Berg X, et al. Use of psychotropic substances among elite athletes - a narrative review. Swiss Med Wkly 2021;151:w20412.
4. McDuff D, Garvin M, Thompson D. In: Reardon CL, editor. Substance use and use disorders in *mental health Care for elite athletes*. Springer Nature Switzerland AG; 2022. p. 131. https://doi.org/10.1007/978-3-031-08364-8_14.
5. Dougherty JW 3rd, Baron D. Substance Use and Addiction in Athletes: The Case for Neuromodulation and Beyond. Int J Environ Res Public Health 2022;19(23):16082.
6. Walters P, Hillier B, Passetti F, et al. Diagnosis and Management of Substance Use Disorders in Athletes. Advances in Psychiatry and Behavioral Health 2021;1(1):135–43.
7. Pitts M, Chow GM, Donohue B. Relationship between General and Sport-Related Drinking Motives and Athlete Alcohol Use and Problems. Subst Use Misuse 2019;54(1):146–55.
8. Doumas DM, Mastroleo N. Heavy Drinking among High School Student Athletes and Non-Athletes: Do Differences Emerge as Early as the Ninth Grade? Subst Use Misuse 2022;57(5):799–805.
9. Marzell M, Morrison C, Mair C, et al. Examining Drinking Patterns and High-Risk Drinking Environments Among College Athletes at Different Competition Levels. J Drug Educ 2015;45(1):5–16.
10. Docter S, Khan M, Gohal C, et al. Cannabis Use and Sport: A Systematic Review. Sports Health 2020;12(2):189–99.
11. Kennedy M. Cannabis, cannabidiol and tetrahydrocannabinol in sport: an overview. Internal Medicine Journal of Australasia 2022. https://doi.org/10.1111/imj.15724.
12. Ware MA, Jensen D, Barrette A, et al. Cannabis and the Health and Performance of the Elite Athlete. Clin J Sport Med 2018;28(5):480–4.
13. Ford JA, Pomykacz C, Veliz P, et al. Sports involvement, injury history, and nonmedical use of prescription opioids among college students: an analysis with a national sample. Am J Addict 2018;27:15–22.
14. Mündel T. Nicotine: sporting friend or foe? A review of athlete use, performance consequences and other considerations. Sports Med 2017;47:2497–506.
15. Deck S, Nagpal TS, Morava A, et al. Tobacco use among varsity athletes - why do they do it and how do we make it stop: a brief report. J Am Coll Health 2021;1–5. https://doi.org/10.1080/07448481.2021.1897014 [published online ahead of print, 2021 Mar 24].
16. NCAA. National study on substance abuse habits of college student-athletes, 2018. Available: https://ncaaorg.s3.amazonaws.com/research/substance/2018RES_SubstanceUseFinalReport.pdf Accessed 2 January 2023.
17. Du Preez EJ, Graham KS, Gan TY, et al. Depression, anxiety, and alcohol use in elite rugby league players over a competitive season. Clin J Sport Med 2017;27:530–5.
18. Kilic Ö, Carmody S, Upmeijer J, et al. Prevalence of mental health symptoms among male and female Australian professional footballers. BMJ Open Sport Exerc Med 2021;7(3):e001043.
19. Mountjoy M, Edwards C, Cheung C, et al. Implementation of the International Olympic Committee Sport Mental Health Assessment Tool 1: Screening for Mental Health Symptoms in a Canadian Multisport University Program 2022. Clin J Sport Med 2022. https://doi.org/10.1097/JSM.0000000000001077.

20. NIDA. Most reported substance use among adolescents held steady in 2022. National Institute on Drug Abuse website. https://nida.nih.gov/news-events/news-releases/2022/12/most-reported-substance-use-among-adolescents-held-steady-in-2022. December 15, 2022 Accessed January 2, 2023.

21. Substance Abuse and Mental Health Services Administration (US). Office of the surgeon general (US). *Facing Addiction in America: the surgeon general's Report on alcohol, drugs, and health.* Washington (DC): US Department of Health and Human Services; 2016.

22. Yurasek AM, Aston ER, Metrik J. Co-use of Alcohol and Cannabis: A Review. Curr Addict Rep 2017;4(2):184–93.

23. White HR, Kilmer JR, Fossos-Wong N, et al. Simultaneous Alcohol and Marijuana Use Among College Students: Patterns, Correlates, Norms, and Consequences. Alcohol Clin Exp Res 2019;43(7):1545–55.

24. Parisi CE, Bugbee BA, Vincent KB, et al. Risks associated with alcohol and marijuana use among college student athletes: The case for involving athletic personnel in prevention and intervention. J Issues Intercoll Athl 2019;12:343–64.

25. Michael Orsini Muhsin, Milroy Jeffrey J, Wyrick David L, et al. Polysubstance Use Among First-Year NCAA College Student-Athletes. J Child Adolesc Subst Abuse 2018;27(3):189–95.

26. Gouttebarge V, Bindra A, Blauwet C, et al. International Olympic Committee (IOC) Sport Mental Health Assessment Tool 1 (SMHAT-1) and Sport Mental Health Recognition Tool 1 (SMHRT-1): towards better support of athletes' mental health. Br J Sports Med 2021;55(1):30–7.

27. Bonn-Miller MO, Heinz AJ, Smith EV, et al. Preliminary Development of a Brief Cannabis Use Disorder Screening Tool: The Cannabis Use Disorder Identification Test Short-Form. Cannabis Cannabinoid Res 2016;1(1):252–61.

28. Riordan BC, Flett JAM, Hunter J, et al. Fear of missing out (FoMO): the relationship between FoMO, alcohol use, and alcohol-related consequences in college students. Annals of Neuroscience and Psychology, 2015, 2:7. Available at: http://www.vipoa.org/neuropsychol. Accessed January 30, 2023

29. Simons JS, Dvorak RD, Merrill JE, et al. Dimensions and severity of marijuana consequences: development and validation of the Marijuana Consequences Questionnaire (MACQ). Addict Behav 2012;37(5):613–21.

30. Bravo AJ, Pearson MR, Pilatti A, et al, Cross-Cultural Addictions Study Team. Negative marijuana-related consequences among college students in five countries: measurement invariance of the Brief Marijuana Consequences Questionnaire. Addiction 2019;114(10):1854–65.

31. Hennessy EA, Tanner-Smith EE, Mavridis D, et al. Comparative Effectiveness of Brief Alcohol Interventions for College Students: Results from a Network Meta-Analysis. Prev Sci 2019;20(5):715–40.

32. Donohue B, Loughran T, Pitts M, et al. Preliminary Development of a Brief Intervention to Prevent Alcohol Misuse and Enhance Sport Performance in Collegiate Athletes. J Drug Abuse 2016;2:3.

33. Agley J, Walker BB, Gassman RA. Adaptation of alcohol and drug screening, brief intervention and referral to treatment (SBIRT) to a department of intercollegiate athletics: The COMPASS project. Health Educ J 2013;72(6):647–59.

34. Rulison KL, Milroy JJ, Wyrick DL. A randomized iterative approach to optimizing an online substance use intervention for collegiate athletes. Transl Behav Med 2022;12(1):ibab119.

35. Gouttebarge V, Backx FJ, Aoki H, et al. Symptoms of Common Mental Disorders in Professional Football (Soccer) Across Five European Countries. J Sports Sci Med 2015;14(4):811–8.
36. Gouttebarge V, Hopley P, Kerkhoffs G, et al. A 12-month prospective cohort study of symptoms of common mental disorders among professional rugby players. Eur J Sport Sci 2018;18(7):1004–12.
37. Du Preez EJ, Graham KS, Gan TY, et al. Depression, Anxiety, and Alcohol Use in Elite Rugby League Players Over a Competitive Season. Clin J Sport Med 2017; 27(6):530–5.
38. Gouttebarge V, Kerkhoffs GMMJ. A prospective cohort study on symptoms of common mental disorders among current and retired professional ice hockey players. Phys Sportsmed 2017;45(3):252–8.
39. Schuring N, Kerkhoffs G, Gray J, et al. The mental wellbeing of current and retired professional cricketers: an observational prospective cohort study. Phys Sportsmed 2017;45(4):463–9.
40. Babor TF, Higgins-Biddle JC, Robaina K. The Alcohol Use Disorders Identification Test, Adapted for Use in the United States: A Guide for Primary Care Practitioners SAMHSA 2016 https://sbirt.webs.com/USAUDIT-Guide_2016_final-1.pdf#page21 retrieved on 7 March 2023.
41. Higgins-Biddle JC, Babor TF. A review of the Alcohol Use Disorders Identification Test (AUDIT), AUDIT-C, and USAUDIT for screening in the United States: Past issues and future directions. Am J Drug Alcohol Abuse 2018;44(6):578–86.
42. Zamboanga BL, Wickham RE, George AM, et al. The Brief Young Adult Alcohol Consequences Questionnaire: A cross-country examination among university students in Australia, New Zealand, Canada, Argentina, and the United States. Drug Alcohol Depend 2021;227:108975.
43. myPlaybook Alcohol and Other Drugs Education (AOD) for Collegiate Athletes, National Institute on Drug Abuse. https://preventionstrategies.com/myplaybook-collegiate-program/.
44. Zeiger JS, Silvers WS, Fleegler EM, et al. Cannabis use in active athletes: Behaviors related to subjective effects. PLoS One 2019;14(6):e0218998.
45. Where it stands: Weed policies by U.S. sports league. Jeff Tracy, Axios Sports, 20 Oct 2021https://www.axios.com/2021/10/20/weed-policies-sports-leagues-nba-mlb-nfl-nhl retrieved 13 February 2023.
46. Volkow ND, Baler RD, Compton WM, et al. Adverse health effects of marijuana use. N Engl J Med 2014;370(23):2219–27.
47. Hasin D, Walsh C. Cannabis Use, Cannabis Use Disorder, and Comorbid Psychiatric Illness: A Narrative Review. J Clin Med 2020;10(1):15.
48. Crocker CE, Carter AJE, Emsley JG, et al. When Cannabis Use Goes Wrong: Mental Health Side Effects of Cannabis Use That Present to Emergency Services. Front Psychiatry 2021;12:640222.
49. Di Forti M, Quattrone D, Freeman TP, et al. The contribution of cannabis use to variation in the incidence of psychotic disorder across Europe (EU-GEI): a multicentre case-control study. Lancet Psychiatr 2019;6(5):427–36.
50. NCAA Emerging Science on Cannabis/Marijuana: Implications for Student Athletes by Jason Kilmer, 10 October 2019https://www.ncaa.org/news/2019/10/10/emerging-science-on-cannabis-marijuana-implications-for-student-athletes.aspx accessed 13 February 2023.
51. ElSohly MA, Chandra S, Radwan M, et al. A Comprehensive Review of Cannabis Potency in the United States in the Last Decade. Biol Psychiatry Cogn Neurosci Neuroimaging 2021;6(6):603–6.

52. Freeman TP, Craft S, Wilson J, et al. Changes in delta-9-tetrahydrocannabinol (THC) and cannabidiol (CBD) concentrations in cannabis over time: systematic review and meta-analysis. Addiction 2021;116(5):1000–10.
53. NIDA. Cannabis (Marijuana) Concentrates DrugFacts. National Institute on Drug Abuse website. https://nida.nih.gov/publications/drugfacts/cannabis-marijuana-concentrates. June 25, 2020 Accessed February 13, 2023.
54. Takakuwa KM, Schears RM. The emergency department care of the cannabis and synthetic cannabinoid patient: a narrative review. Int J Emerg Med 2021; 14(1):10.
55. Diagnostic and Statistical Manual of Mental Disorders: DSM-5. 5th edition, American Psychiatric Association, 2013. DSM-V, doiorg.db29. linccweb.org/10.1176/appi.books.9780890425596.dsm02.
56. Halladay J, Petker T, Fein A, et al. Brief interventions for cannabis use in emerging adults: protocol for a systematic review, meta-analysis, and evidence map. Syst Rev 2018;7(1):106.
57. 10 professional athletes who use marijuana. Insider Jackson Thompson, 2022, https://www.insider.com/10-professional-athletes-who-use-marijuana-2022-1.
58. D'Amico EJ, Parast L, Shadel WG, et al. Brief motivational interviewing intervention to reduce alcohol and marijuana use for at-risk adolescents in primary care. J Consult Clin Psychol 2018;86(9):775–86.
59. Lee CM, Kilmer JR, Neighbors C, et al. Indicated prevention for college student marijuana use: a randomized controlled trial. J Consult Clin Psychol 2013;81(4): 702–9.
60. Calomarde-Gómez C, Jiménez-Fernández B, Balcells-Oliveró M, et al. Motivational Interviewing for Cannabis Use Disorders: A Systematic Review and Meta-Analysis. Eur Addiction Res 2021;27(6):413–27.
61. Lee CM, Kilmer JR, Neighbors C, et al. A Marijuana Consequences Checklist for Young Adults with Implications for Brief Motivational Intervention Research. Prev Sci 2021;22(6):758–68.
62. Clarest J, Grandner M, Turner R, et al. Substance Use Among Collegiate Athletes Versus Non-Athletes. Athl Train Sports Health Care 2021;13(6):443–52.
63. Sherburne M. Dramatic increases in vaping marijuana, nicotine among US college students, young adults. Results from the University of Michigan Monitoring the Future Annual Survey.Published September 15, 2020. https://news.umich.edu/dramatic-increases-in-vaping-marijuana-nicotine-among-us-college-students-young-adults/retrieved 20 February 2023.
64. Mündel T. Nicotine: Sporting Friend or Foe? A Review of Athlete Use, Performance Consequences and Other Considerations. Sports Med 2017;47(12): 2497–506.
65. Marclay F, Grata E, Perrenoud L, et al. A one-year monitoring of nicotine use in sport: frontier between potential performance enhancement and addiction issues. Forensic Sci Int 2011;213(1–3):73–84.
66. Heatherton TF, Kozlowski LT, Frecker RC, et al. The Fagerstrom Test for Nicotine Dependence: A revision off the Fagerstrom Tolerance Test. Br J Addict 1991;86: 1119–27.
67. Severson HH, Klein K, Lichtensein E, et al. Smokeless tobacco use among professional baseball players: survey results, 1998 to 2003. Tobac Control 2005; 14(1):31–6.
68. Walsh MM, Greene JC, Ellison JA, et al. A dental-based, athletic trainer-mediated spit tobacco cessation program for professional baseball players. J Calif Dent Assoc 1998;26(5):365–76.

69. Gansky SA, Ellison JA, Rudy D, et al. Cluster-Randomized Controlled Trial of An Athletic Trainer-Directed Spit (Smokeless) Tobacco Intervention for Collegiate Baseball Athletes: Results After 1 Year. J Athl Train 2005;40(2):76–87.

70. Gansky SA, Ellison JA, Kavanagh C, et al. Oral screening and brief spit tobacco cessation counseling: a review and findings. J Dent Educ 2002;66(9):1088–98.

71. Sinusas K, Coroso JG. A 10-yr study of smokeless tobacco use in a professional baseball organization. Med Sci Sports Exerc 2006;38(7):1204–7.

72. Mee-Lee D, Shulman GD, Fishman MJ, et al, editors. The ASAM criteria: treatment criteria for addictive, substance-related, and Co-occurring conditions. 3rd edition. Carson City, NV: The Change Companies; Copyright 2013 by the American Society of Addiction Medicine; 2013.

APPENDIX
AUDIT- C

The following questions are about alcohol use. Please respond to each question by circling the number from "0" to "4" that represents your alcohol use.

1. How often do you have a drink containing alcohol?
   Never (0) monthly or less (1) 2 to 4 times a month (2) 2 to 3 times a week (3) 4 or more times a week (4)
2. How many standard drinks containing alcohol do you have on a typical day when you drink?
   1 to 2 (0) 3 to 4 (1) 5 to 6 (2) 7 to 9 (3) 10 or more (4)
3. How often do you have six or more drinks on one occasion?
   Never (0) less than monthly (1) monthly (2) weekly (3) daily or almost daily (4)

   Calculate the score by summing up the answers on the 3 items. A score of ≥ 4 for men & ≥ 3 for women is a positive screen.

CAGE-AID (alcohol, cannabis/marijuana, tobacco/nicotine, other drug(s))

The following questions are about alcohol, cannabis/marijuana tobacco/nicotine use in the last 3 months. Please respond to each question by circling "yes" or "no."

1. In the last 3 months, have you felt you should cut down or stop using alcohol, cannabis, tobacco/nicotine or other drugs?
   Alcohol Yes (1) No (0); *Cannabis* Yes (1) No (0) *Tobacco/nicotine* Yes (1) No (0) *Other drugs* Yes (1) No(0)
2. In the last 3 months, has anyone annoyed you or gotten on your nerves by telling you to cut down or stop using alcohol, cannabis, tobacco/nicotine, other drugs ?
   Alcohol Yes (1) No (0); *Cannabis* Yes (1) No (0) *Tobacco/nicotine* Yes (1) No (0) *Other drugs* Yes (1) No(0)
3. In the last 3 months, have you felt guilty or bad about how much you use alcohol, cannabis, tobacco/nicotine, other drugs?
   Alcohol Yes (1) No (0); *Cannabis* Yes (1) No (0) *Tobacco/nicotine* Yes (1) No (0) *Other drugs* Yes (1) No(0)
4. In the last 3 months, have you been waking up wanting to use alcohol, cannabis, tobacco/nicotine, other drugs?
   Alcohol Yes (1) No (0); *Cannabis* Yes (1) No (0) *Tobacco/nicotine* Yes (1) No (0) *Other drugs* Yes (1) No(0)

   Calculate the total score for each substance by summing up the answers on the four items. A score of >2 is a positive screen for men and women.

CUDIT-SF

Do you currently use cannabis? YES or NO; If YES

1. How often during the past 6 months did you find that you were not able to stop using cannabis once you had started?
   Never (0) Less than monthly (1) monthly (2) Weekly (3) Daily or almost daily (4)
2. How often in the past 6 months have you devoted a great deal of time getting, using, or recovering from cannabis?
   Never (0) Less than monthly (1) monthly (2) Weekly (3) Daily or almost daily (4)
3. How often in the past 6 months have you had a problem with you memory or concentration after using cannabis?
   Never (0) Less than monthly (1) monthly (2) Weekly (3) Daily or almost daily (4)

Calculate the total score by summing up the answers on the 3 items. A score of >2 is a positive screen for women and men.

Fagerstrom Test for Nicotine Dependence

Do you currently use tobacco products? No Yes
If "yes," read each question listed. For each question, circle the answer choice which best describes your response.

1. How soon after you wake up do you smoke your first cigarette?
   Within 5 minutes (3) 6 to 30 minutes (2) 31 to 60 minutes (1) After 60 minutes (0)
2. Do you find it difficult to refrain from smoking in places where it is forbidden (for example, in church, at the library, in the cinema)? No (0) Yes (1)
3. Which cigarette would you hate most to give up?
   The first one in the morning (1) Any other (0)
4. How many cigarettes per day do you smoke?
   10 or less (0) 11 to 20 (1) 21 to 30 (2) 31 or more (3)
5. Do you smoke more frequently during the first hours after waking than during the rest of the day? No (0) Yes (1)
6. Do you smoke when you are so ill that you are in bed most of the day? No (0) Yes (1)

Scoring Instructions: Add up the responses to all items. A score of 5 or more indicates a significant dependence, while a score of 4 or less shows a low to moderate dependence.

Attention-Deficit / Hyperactivity Disorder in Athletes

Collin Leibold, MD, MS[a],*, Racheal M. Smetana, PsyD[b],
Siobhán M. Statuta, MD[c]

KEYWORDS

- ADHD • Sports medicine • Athletes • Mental health

KEY POINTS

- Attention-deficit/hyperactivity disorder (ADHD) is a relatively common neurodevelopmental disorder that, if not managed appropriately, can have profound negative influence on functioning in school, work, and relationships.
- ADHD may be more common among athletes compared with the general population.
- Diagnosing ADHD requires a thorough history from the patient and often from parents and coaches.
- First-line treatment for all patients 6 years and older with ADHD is stimulant medication.
- Regulation of stimulant medications varies among sports federations and frequently requires rigorous documentation of how the diagnosis was attained.

HISTORY

ADHD, or attention-deficit/hyperactivity disorder, is a neurodevelopmental disorder that is defined as a persistent pattern of inattention and/or hyperactivity/impulsivity that interferes with functional development per the most recent edition of the Diagnostic and Statistical Manual of Mental Disorders (DSM-5-TR).[1] ADHD is characterized as predominantly inattentive, predominantly hyperactive, or mixed. Matthews, Nigg, and Fair (2014) trace this condition's history as far back as the 1700s when a syndrome of "attention deficit" was described.[2] ADHD was further studied in the early 20th century among children who demonstrated defiance and hyperactivity behavior patterns after encephalitis and subsequently were reported to respond

[a] Department of Family Medicine, University of Virginia, 1215 Lee Street, Charlottesville, VA 22903, USA; [b] Psychiatry & Neurobehavioral Sciences, University of Virginia Health, PO Box 800203, Charlottesville, VA 22903, USA; [c] Primary Care Sports Medicine Fellowship, Family Medicine and Physical Medicine & Rehabilitation, UVA Sports Medicine, University of Virginia Health System, PO Box 800729, Charlottesville, VA 22908-0729, USA
* Corresponding author.
E-mail address: CML3SC@uvahealth.org

Clin Sports Med 43 (2024) 145–157
https://doi.org/10.1016/j.csm.2023.06.013
0278-5919/24/© 2023 Elsevier Inc. All rights reserved.

well to stimulant medications. These observations were consolidated into the diagnosis of "hyperkinetic reaction of childhood" in the DSM-II.[3] The diagnosis was renamed Attention Deficit Disorder (ADD) in the DSM-III and subsequently Attention Deficit Hyperactivity Disorder in the DSM-III revision in 1987, with emphasis on attention deficit as the definitive feature of the diagnosis.[4,5] It was not until DSM-IV that ADHD was acknowledged to occur in adults; the previous theory being that it was a disorder of childhood that patients outgrew by mid-adulthood.[6] Although adult-onset ADHD has been proposed as its own unique sub-category of ADHD, DSM-5-TR criteria currently still require symptoms to have been present prior to age 12 years.[7]

EPIDEMIOLOGY

As a relatively recently described diagnosis, it is difficult to determine the prevalence of ADHD. A 2007 cross-national comparison study using the DSM-IV criteria estimated that 5.2% of adults in the United States (US) had ADHD.[8] Given that the newer DSM-5-TR criteria is less restrictive, it is likely that the current rate of ADHD among adults is higher. Among pediatric populations, the prevalence of ADHD has been increasing over the past 20 years. National Health Interview Survey data estimated ADHD prevalence in US children as 6% in 1997 and 10% in 2017.[9] This was corroborated in a systematic review describing childhood ADHD prevalence of 5% −10%, and increasing.[10] Internationally, rates appear to be similar with a global prevalence of pediatric ADHD of 7.2%.[11]

Theories to the increasing prevalence vary but mainly align with better education regarding the condition and broader diagnostic definition with DSM iterations. As ADHD has become more recognized, it has yielded earlier symptom recognition by parents, teachers, and physicians. Improved access to health care and general destigmatization of the disorder has allowed for more expeditious diagnosis and treatment.[9] However, with improved recognition of the disorder, it has been posited that changes to diagnostic thresholds, patient or physician misinformation, and/or insufficient diagnostic practices may contribute to over-diagnosis of ADHD in children and adults, which could inflate prevalence rates.

Historically, ADHD was more commonly diagnosed in boys than in girls; however, this ratio of boys to girls has been narrowing.[12] In the US, there is considerable variance in the geographic distribution of ADHD diagnoses. Data from the National Survey of Children's Health from 2016 to 2019 revealed ADHD prevalence ranged from a low of 6.6% in Hawaii to a high of over 15% in Mississippi and Louisiana.[13] In general, rates were lower in the western states and higher in the southeast and Appalachian regions of the country, with a notable disparity between metropolitan (lower rates) and non-metropolitan (higher rates) areas. Socioeconomic factors and higher potential for exposure to adverse childhood experiences in rural areas are associated with higher prevalence rates and seem to account for some regional differences.[14]

Prevalence rates also differ by race. Clinical identification of ADHD is lower in Black and Latinx populations as compared to White populations.[15] A number of reasons seem to underlie these differences in prevalence rates and include: 1) Underdetection may come from clinician bias in labeling symptoms as oppositional rather than a result of ADHD; 2) Socially oppressed and marginalized groups may not have access to health care resources to obtain accurate diagnosis; 3) Symptom rating scales may be culturally biased and fail to pick up on ADHD symptoms in racially and ethnically diverse groups.[16]

Estimates of the prevalence of ADHD in athletes are at least equal to, if not higher than, general population estimates, ranging from 4.2% to 8.1% across studies.[17] College athletes are likely overrepresented among ADHD diagnoses; at Texas A&M during the 2009 to 2010 academic year, between 7% and 9% of athletes reported taking stimulant or non-stimulant medications for diagnosed ADHD.[18] Prevalence among elite athletes has not been well documented, but also seems higher than general population studies. Major League Baseball (MLB) provides support for this assertion through data on therapeutic use exemptions (TUEs), a process by which an athlete is permitted to use a medication on the World Anti-Doping Agency's Prohibited List (WADA). In the 2019 to 2020 season, the MLB reported that 90 athletes were granted TUEs for an ADHD diagnosis.[19] Beyond these known cases, it can be ascertained that not all MLB players with ADHD have been diagnosed, and not all who have been diagnosed have been prescribed a stimulant; therefore, the actual prevalence of ADHD among MLB players is likely higher.[20]

Why could the prevalence of ADHD be higher among athletes compared with the general population? One explanation is that sports are therapeutic for people with ADHD. For example, in teenagers with diagnoses of ADHD and no history of medical treatment, a randomized clinical trial showed that 6 weeks of methylphenidate plus exercise was superior to 6 weeks of methylphenidate plus education in decreasing reported clinical symptoms.[21] In this explanation, adolescents are naturally drawn to sports as therapy for their ADHD symptoms. Olympic marathoner Molly Seidel has narratively described the similarity she feels between exercise and stimulants this way: "[Adderall gave me the] quiet, functioning brain in my day-to-day life that I was previously only able to get with intense physical activity."[22]

Another complementary theory is that those with ADHD have an intrinsic advantage in sports. The symptom of impulsivity may lend itself toward quicker decision making in the sporting arena proving to be an advantage for the athlete. Additionally, Parr proposes an interesting distinction between 2 neural circuits: the sustained attention circuit, which is deficient in ADHD, and the "fascination" circuit, which is intact.[18] Athletes, such as Seidel, are able to capitalize on their "fascination" with sport, thus allowing them an ability to hyperfocus in a way that gives them a competitive advantage.

PATHOPHYSIOLOGY

ADHD is a neurobiological disorder that results in neuropsychological deficits and behavioral symptoms.[23] ADHD is associated with structural differences in the frontal brain regions, in that gray matter in the frontal cortex appears to develop later and persistently remain smaller in patients with ADHD compared with the general population.[24] Neurobiological underpinnings are mediated by the relationship between the frontal lobe and the basal ganglia–a relationship governed by dopamine–in which the basal ganglia can exert inhibitory or excitatory control over the frontal lobe.[24] When people with ADHD are given tasks that require them to inhibit motor activity, they have hypoactive functioning of the network between the frontal lobe and the basal ganglia.[25] This evidence mirrors the clinical finding of a deficit in inhibitory control among people with ADHD. Functional neuroimaging studies reveal a reversal in neural network activation during restful waking states and states with high cognitive load in people with ADHD.[23] Examples of restful waking states include walking in the woods or cooking dinner. During these states, the attentional load is low, and the mind can wander; neural networks most active at these times are the default mode networks. During times of high cognitive load–such as taking a math test or studying football plays–the prominent neural networks are cognitive control networks. In people without ADHD, when cognitive load increases, there is an inverse relationship between the default mode network and the cognitive control network. The part of the brain associated with mind wandering becomes less active and the part of the brain associated with focus becomes more active. This inverse association is less prominent in people with ADHD, in whom the default mode network remains active even as the cognitive control network increases, which could lead to inattention when rigid attention is expected.

Differences in dopaminergic control of behavior in people with ADHD versus those without could underlie the reversal in neural network states. It has been hypothesized that people with ADHD have tonically low levels of dopamine, which predisposes them to prefer immediate reward.[25] An alternative theory states that people with ADHD have deficient increases in dopamine associated with imagining a future reward.[26] Both theories explain why stimulant medications improve symptoms of people with ADHD, as stimulants produce acute increases in dopamine in the brain.

DIAGNOSIS: DSM-5-TR CRITERIA, COMORBIDITIES

Based on the epidemiology of ADHD, sports health providers will be confronted with athletes with diagnosed or undiagnosed ADHD. It is important, therefore, to have a process to screen for and make the diagnosis of ADHD, especially among athletes who present with comorbid conditions.

To make the diagnosis, look to the DSM-5-TR, which differentiates 3 categories of ADHD: predominantly hyperactive/impulsive, predominantly inattentive, and combined. These categories are based on the type and number of specific symptoms. Patients must have 6 or more symptoms of hyperactivity/impulsiveness or inattentiveness (**Table 1**)[27] that are present for a minimum of 6 months and interfere with social, academic, or occupational function. At least some symptoms must be present in more than one area of functioning (eg, school, home, social life), and at least some symptoms must have been present prior to age 12. Symptoms cannot be better explained by another mental health condition.

Since diagnosis relies on symptoms being present in more than one domain of functioning, obtaining collateral information is recommended in children and adolescents.[15] Tools are available to obtain collateral information, including the Vanderbilt and Conners assessments. In adults, obtaining collateral information can be more challenging, and it is possible to make the diagnosis with a thorough history complemented by a self-rating scale such as the Adult ADHD Self-Report Scale.

Practically speaking, if a student-athlete complains of symptoms of inattention or hyperactivity that interfere with school, work, or sports, a reasonable next step would be to ask them to fill out the Adult ADHD Self-Report Scale. If the athlete reports more than 5 symptoms of either hyperactivity or inattention, a thorough history can determine whether these symptoms are present in more than one area of functioning and were present at least before the age of 12. In some cases, symptoms prior to age 12 may have been subtle or managed through behavioral strategies (eg, organizational structure from a parent, therapeutic effect of participation in sport), and it is only when those supports no longer mitigate ADHD symptoms that functional challenges become more apparent, thus necessitating an evaluation as an adult. A detailed history should also address comorbid conditions to determine whether these symptoms are better explained by another mental health condition. If questions remain after the screening tool and a history, collateral interview with a parent or the athlete's coach could be obtained–with the athlete's permission.

Table 1 ADHD symptoms	
Inattentive	**Hyperactive/impulsive**
Often:	Frequently:
1. Struggles with details.	1. Fidgets or taps hands/feet when seated.
2. Makes careless mistakes in work, schoolwork, or other activities.	2. Impulsive.
	3. Leaves seat when inappropriate.
3. Struggles with sustained attention in tasks or play.	4. Unable to play or take part in leisure activities quietly.
4. Does not complete tasks or follow through on instructions.	5. Struggles with planning.
5. Has difficulty organizing activities or assignments or activities.	6. Is "on the go" as if there is endless energy.
6. Avoids tasks requiring sustained concentration or mental effort.	7. Talks excessively.
	8. Blurts out answers to questions prematurely.
7. Loses necessary items.	9. Has difficulty waiting his/her turn.
8. Easily distractible.	10. Interrupts or intrudes on others' conversations or activities.
9. Unable to multitask.	
10. Forgetful in daily activities.	
11. Inattention when spoken to directly.	

At least 6 symptoms in the following table must have been present since age 12, must be present in two or more settings, and must interfere with functioning for the diagnosis of ADHD to be considered. Symptoms cannot occur exclusively during the course of schizophrenia or other psychotic disorder and they cannot be better explained by another DSM-V diagnosis. An ADHD diagnosis can be described as predominantly inattentive, predominantly hyperactive, or combined; diagnoses should also be specified as to whether symptoms are in partial remission and whether symptoms are mild, moderate, or severe.

From: CDC website: Symptoms and Diagnosis of ADHD. https://www.cdc.gov/ncbddd/adhd/diagnosis.html. Accessed June 26, 2023.

Perhaps the most challenging part of making the diagnosis of adult ADHD is the final sentence in the DSM-5-TR criteria: "the symptoms are not better explained by another mental disorder (such as mood disorder, anxiety disorder, dissociative disorder, or a personality disorder)."[1] ADHD is often comorbid with other mental disorders. In a study that assessed adult ADHD and comorbidities by in-depth clinical assessments, Kessler, and colleagues (2006) found strong associations between ADHD and any mood disorder (OR 5.0, 95% CI 3.0–8.2), any anxiety disorder (OR 3.7, 95% CI 2.4–5.5), and any substance use disorder (OR 3.0, 95% CI 1.4–6.5).[28] These findings were replicated in a study assessing ADHD comorbidities among first-year college students in the US.[29] Using clinical information gathered from a semi-structured clinical interview, it was found that 55% of students who met criteria for ADHD had at least one non-ADHD mental health diagnosis and 31% had at least 2 non-ADHD mental health diagnoses. These rates were higher than the population of students without ADHD, for whom the corresponding rates were 11% and 4%, respectively. One practical question that arises from the high prevalence of comorbid conditions in ADHD is whether an athlete's ADHD symptoms are better explained by another mental health condition. For example, how can a clinician distinguish between a person with comorbid anxiety and ADHD versus a person with anxiety whose symptoms of inattention mimic ADHD? Again, an in-depth history is key. If a student-athlete without any known history of ADHD symptoms is now currently experiencing inattention, but also endorses an onset of general worry, ruminative thoughts, or difficulty controlling their worry, then inattention may be more related to anxiety. In this case, it would be reasonable to refer for the treatment of anxiety and reassess inattention when anxiety is managed. If the same-student athlete has at least some ADHD symptoms prior to age 12, it would be reasonable to treat both conditions at the same time, though emphasis should always be placed on treating the more functionally impairing condition. The American Association of Pediatrics (AAP) acknowledges there exist system-level barriers to successfully implementing a process for screening for comorbid conditions.[15] As noted previously, Black and Latinx children are less likely to have ADHD diagnosed and treated compared with other populations, thus culturally competent practices in diagnosing and treating ADHD are necessary. In situations in which a diagnosis of ADHD cannot be confidently disentangled from another comorbid condition based on symptom screening and a thorough history, referral for psychological evaluation may be considered.

TREATMENT: MEDICATION; THERAPEUTIC USE EXEMPTION REQUIREMENTS IN DIFFERENT SPORTS

Once a diagnosis is attained, management must be considered. First-line treatment for ADHD among children and adults is stimulant medication, supported by a long history of use among patients with ADHD and recent clinical trials. A randomized controlled trial of 430 adults with ADHD found that methylphenidate was superior to placebo at all time points, and a follow-up study found persistent benefits from prior treatment with methylphenidate even after study conditions were relaxed.[30,31] For children, the AAP has a grade A recommendation for FDA (Food and Drug Administration) approved medications for patients ages 6 to 18 who are diagnosed with ADHD.[15]

In practice, a stimulant can be initiated and titrated over the course of 1 week. A low dose should be started, followed by subsequent regular assessments for clinical improvement. The dose should be titrated up to find the dose at which maximal clinical benefit is achieved without adverse effects.[15] At least 90% of patients with ADHD will respond to one or both common stimulant medications (amphetamine and methylphenidate); however, the response can be idiosyncratic, meaning it is impossible to predict to which stimulant or at what dose a given patient will respond.[32] Also, up to 25% of patients may only respond to one of the 2 common stimulants, thus prescribers may need to switch classes if a medication remains ineffective.[32]

All stimulant medications have an FDA warning for high potential for abuse and dependence, therefore the FDA recommends assessing the risk of abuse prior to prescribing as well as regularly monitoring for abuse and diversion. The AAP similarly recommends screening patients for substance use disorder prior to starting a stimulant medication with referral to a sub-specialist if a patient screens positive for active substance use.[15] See **Table 2** for contraindications and cautions to treatment with methylphenidate.[33]

Table 2 Contraindications and cautions to treatment with Ritalin Hydrochloride (methylphenidate hydrochloride)	
Absolute Contraindications	**Cautions**
Hypersensitivity to methylphenidate or any component of formulation	Cardiovascular: hypertension, serious arrhythmias, peripheral vasculopathy, coronary artery disease, structural heart disease, cardiomyopathy
Use during or within 14 d after MAO-I therapy	Neurologic: seizure disorder (may lower seizure threshold)
	Psychiatric: bipolar disorder (may lead to manic episode), stimulant use disorder

Management of ADHD among elite athletes is further complicated by reporting requirements among different levels of competition. The World Anti-Doping Agency's (WADA) prohibited list states all stimulants are banned in-competition.[34] For an athlete to take a stimulant during competition adhering to WADA's code, a health care professional must apply for a Therapeutic Use Exemption (TUE) to the local anti-doping agency. The process for obtaining a TUE is extensive, requiring proper detailed medical documentation and rigorous review to ensure the medication allows the athlete to compete in a suitable state of health without conveying any competitive advantage.

In the US, a doctor prescribing a stimulant for an Olympic-level athlete must submit a thorough application to the US Anti-Doping Agency (USADA) based on required checklist items. Specifically, USADA states that enough information must be included such that a USADA psychiatrist or psychologist could make the diagnosis of ADHD without ever seeing the patient. This is a high bar, and it requires the following:

- copies of self-report scales (eg, Adult ADHD Clinical Diagnostic Scale),
- a discussion of differential diagnoses,
- a list of comorbidities (including how they have been diagnosed and managed),
- a note about how the physician is sure that symptoms are due to ADHD and not to exhaustion or over-training,
- testimonials from the athlete, a parent/caregiver, and a coach/teacher that symptoms have been present from prior to age 12, have been present in more than one domain of functioning, and have interfered with daily function. The testimonials must also describe symptoms on and off stimulant medications.

USADA also notes the psychological evaluation must be completed by a psychiatrist if the athlete is planning to use the TUE in a competition sanctioned by an International Federation. The National Collegiate Athletic Association (NCAA) also bans stimulant medications in and out of competition if a medical exemption form is not in place. Documentation does not need to be submitted prior to a collegiate athlete using a stimulant medication, but prescribing providers are required to complete an ADHD Medical Exemption form, which must be maintained on file in the athletic department.[35] The form must include clinic notes from a comprehensive clinical evaluation that specifically includes individual and family history of mental health conditions, DSM-5-TR criteria for ADHD, and supportive clinical evaluation scales (eg, Connors', Adult ADHD Self-report Scale). Data from a neuropsychological or psychoeducational evaluation often supplement the aforementioned criteria to support medical necessity of stimulant use. In the event that an athlete tests positive for a stimulant, the athletic department then sends the completed ADHD Medical Exemption form to Drug-Free Sport International. The exemption request is evaluated by the NCAA Committee on Competitive Safeguards and Medical Aspects of Sports.

Stimulant medications are the first-line treatment for ADHD, but non-stimulant medications can be considered. and include atomoxetine, a selective norepinephrine reuptake inhibitor, and the alpha-2 agonists guanfacine and clonidine.[12] The AAP Clinical Practice Guideline states that non-stimulant medications have a lower effect size compared with stimulant medications–0.7 versus 1[15] and therefore are considered second-line treatment for ADHD. Clonidine and guanfacine can be used as adjunct treatment; atomoxetine is more commonly used as stand-alone treatment although some evidence suggests it can be safe and effective when used as an adjunct.[15] Although non-FDA approved, medications that are used off-label for the treatment of ADHD include tricyclic antidepressants, bupropion, and some high blood pressure medications. Non-stimulant medications for ADHD have not been approved in the preschool age group.

Psychosocial interventions for ADHD generally play a secondary role to medications, largely due to the findings of the Multimodal Treatment Study of ADHD.[36] The exception to this rule is pre-school children, for whom Parent and Teacher Behavioral Modification is first-line.[15] The Multimodal Treatment Study of ADHD evaluated children, most of whom had a comorbid condition, comparing 4 interventions: community care, behavioral treatment, medication management, and combined medication and behavioral treatment. The main finding of the study was that medication management had a similar effect to combined treatment on ADHD symptoms (as assessed by parent and teacher ratings). Both medication and combined treatment were superior to behavioral treatment and community care alone. The combined treatment was occasionally superior (though with small effect sizes) than medication or behavioral treatment alone.

Student-athletes in particular would likely benefit from learning compensatory and organizational strategies to help manage symptoms (eg, disorganization, forgetfulness). Further, student-athletes are often eligible for academic accommodations, including additional time on exams or preferential seating in the classroom, to provide additional classroom support to address symptoms of inattention and/or hyperactivity. A neuropsychological or psychoeducational evaluation can help inform appropriate academic accommodations or behavioral intervention needs.

MONITORING: ADVERSE EFFECTS, REASONS FOR DISCONTINUATION, CAUSES FOR CONCERN RE: NEUROTOXICITY, CONCUSSION IN ATHLETES WITH ATTENTION-DEFICIT/HYPERACTIVITY DISORDER

Although stimulants have been deemed safe and effective treatment for ADHD, they are not without risk. Stimulants carry an FDA black box warning due to the high risk of abuse and dependence. As above, patients should be carefully screened for substance use disorder prior to starting a stimulant. Once initiated, patients must be regularly monitored for signs of misuse, abuse, or dependence, which can include behaviors like taking more medication than prescribed, asking for refills too early, and multiple requests to escalate doses. The full DSM-5-TR criteria for stimulant use disorder is included in **Box 1** as a reference.

The anticipated effects of stimulants include decreased appetite and possible weight loss. This effect can be a concern in athletes with risk factors for relative energy deficiency in sports (RED-s), especially in distance runners and gymnasts. In patients with a documented history of an eating disorder, the decision to start a stimulant should be carefully weighed against the possibility that the medicine could worsen the athlete's caloric state or eating pattern.

The decision of when to take a stimulant medication is unique to each individual athlete. The primary purpose for prescribing stimulants for student-athletes with ADHD is to reduce the detrimental effect of ADHD on academic or professional performance and/or social relationships, a fact that must be made clear to patients. Taking the medication prior to competition with the goal of improving performance, although not specifically disallowed by the NCAA or WADA if appropriate documentation is completed, appears to violate the spirit of anti-doping regulations and should be discouraged.

Stimulant medications pre-competition likely violates the spirit of anti-doping rules, but are they also medically contraindicated pre-competition? A large retrospective cohort study compared the rate of serious cardiovascular events (eg, sudden cardiac death, heart attack, stroke) between individuals (2 - 24 year old) prescribed a stimulant for ADHD to controls who were not prescribed a stimulant medication.[37] Although

---

Box 1
DSM-5-TR criteria for stimulant use disorder

A pattern of amphetamine-type substance, cocaine, or other stimulant use leading to clinically significant impairment or distress, as manifested by at least two of the following, occurring in a 12-month period.

1. Stimulant is often taken in larger amounts and/or over a longer period than the patient intended.

2. Persistent attempts or one or more unsuccessful efforts made to cut down or control stimulant use.

3. A great deal of time is spent in activities necessary to obtain the stimulant, use the stimulant, or recover from efforts.

4. Craving or strong desire or urge to use the stimulant.

5. Recurrent stimulant use resulting in a failure to fulfill major role obligations at work, school, or home.

6. Continued stimulant use despite having persistent or recurrent social or interpersonal problems caused or exacerbated by the effects of the substance.

7. Important social, occupational, or recreational activities given up or reduced because of stimulant use.

8. Recurrent stimulant use in situations in which it is physically hazardous.

9. Stimulant use is continued despite knowledge of having a persistent or recurrent physical or psychological problem that is likely to have been caused or exacerbated by the substance.

10. Tolerance[a], as defined by either of the following:
    a. Markedly increased amounts of the substance in order to achieve intoxication or desired effect.
    b. Markedly diminished effect with continued use of the same amount.

11. Withdrawal[a], as manifested by either of the following

[a]Tolerance and withdrawal criteria should not be used in patients taking stimulants medications only under appropriate medical supervision.

---

event rates were low, this study did not find an association between prescriptions for stimulants and serious cardiovascular events.

Considerable attention has been paid to concussion incidence, recovery, and management in athletes with ADHD. When an athlete sustains a concussion, research does not support pausing or stopping a stimulant medication; therefore, athletes with ADHD should continue to be treated for ADHD while recovering from a concussion (unless another medical comorbidity raises concern for ongoing treatment with stimulant medication).

Baseline testing, a common practice in high school, collegiate, and elite athletics, may be affected by ADHD. Alsalaheen, and colleagues (2016) found that individuals with ADHD were more likely to have invalid baseline ImPACT scores compared with individuals without ADHD.[38] This finding was supported in a recent meta-analysis, which found that baseline ImPACT scores are lower among athletes with ADHD compared with athletes without ADH.[39] This study further found evidence that low baseline scores are mitigated among athletes with treated ADHD.

Whether athletes with ADHD demonstrate a longer recovery or worse outcomes from a concussion has been highly debated. Data from a systematic review did not find a clear association between longer recovery from concussion and ADHD.[40]

Similarly, a large cohort study demonstrated that adolescents with ADHD do not take longer to recover from a concussion, and recovery times did not differ based on treatment type or prior history of concussion.[41]

Some evidence suggests an association between ADHD and concussion risk. A retrospective data analysis of over 32,000 adolescent athletes found that a developmental history of ADHD was associated with a greater prevalence of concussion.[42] Similarly, Maietta, and colleagues (2022) found that athletes with ADHD were more likely to self-report a history of concussion compared with athletes without ADHD.[39] The underlying factors to these findings are not well known, though it has been suggested that ADHD symptoms (eg, impulsiveness)[43] or neurocognitive deficits (eg, deficits in attention or executive functioning) could be risk factors for concussion. This is an area of additional future study.

Summary

ADHD is common among the general population and may be slightly more common among athletes. Diagnosis requires six or more DSM-5-TR symptoms to have been present prior to age 12 and to have an effect on functioning in multiple settings. Different sporting organizations have varying requirements on documentation when making a diagnosis. Stimulant medications are the mainstay of treatment; psychosocial interventions, exercise, and non-stimulant medications can serve as adjuncts. All patients started on stimulants should be screened for substance use disorder. Taking stimulants prior to competition with the intention of improving athletic performance likely violates the spirit of anti-doping rules. Future directions in research on ADHD in sports include determining whether ADHD is overrepresented among the population of elite athletes and parsing out the relationship between ADHD and concussion risk and recovery.

CLINICS CARE POINTS

- Recognize potential ADHD in student-athletes with relevant symptoms and functional impairment.
- Diagnose ADHD based on a thorough personal and family history after ruling out alternative conditions.
- Screen all patients who are being considered for stimulant therapy for substance use disorder. Regularly monitor patients on stimulants for signs of stimulant use disorder.
- Do not withhold stimulant therapy from patients with the clear diagnosis of ADHD and no history of substance use disorder.

DISCLOSURE

The authors have no financial or commercial disclosures.

REFERENCES

1. American Psychiatric Association. (2022). Diagnostic and statistical manual of mental disorders (5th ed., text rev). Available at: https://doi.org/10.1176/appi.books.9780890425787
2. Matthews M, Nigg JT, Fair DA. Attention deficit hyperactivity disorder. Curr Top Behav Neurosci 2014;16:235–66.

3. American Psychiatric Association. (1968). Diagnostic and statistical manual of mental disorders (2nd ed.).

4. American Psychiatric Association. (1980). Diagnostic and statistical manual of mental disorders (3rd ed.).

5. American Psychiatric Association. (1994). Diagnostic and Statistical Manual of Mental Disorders (4th ed.).

6. McGough JJ, McCracken JT. Adult attention deficit hyperactivity disorder: moving beyond DSM-IV. Am J Psychiatry 2006;163(10):1673–5.

7. Taylor LE, Kaplan-Kahn EA, Lighthall RA, et al. Adult-Onset ADHD: A Critical Analysis and Alternative Explanations. Child Psychiatry Hum Dev 2022;53(4): 635–53.

8. Fayyad J, De Graaf R, Kessler R, et al. Cross-national prevalence and correlates of adult attention-deficit hyperactivity disorder. Br J Psychiatry 2007;190:402–9.

9. Xu G, Strathearn L, Liu B, et al. Twenty-year trends in diagnosed attention-deficit/ hyperactivity disorder among US children and adolescents, 1997–2016. JAMA Netw Open. NLM (Medline) 2018;1:e181471.

10. Sayal K, Prasad V, Daley D, et al. ADHD in children and young people: prevalence, care pathways, and service provision. Lancet Psychiatr 2018;5(2):175–86.

11. Thomas R, Sanders S, Doust J, et al. Prevalence of attention-deficit/hyperactivity disorder: a systematic review and meta-analysis. Pediatrics 2015;135(4). Available at: www.pediatrics.org/cgi/content/full/135/4/e994.

12. Posner J, Polanczyk GV, Sonuga-Barke E. Attention-deficit hyperactivity disorder. Lancet 2020;395(10222):450–62.

13. "State-Based Prevalence of ADHD Diagnosis and Treatment 2016-2019." Centers for Disease Control and Prevention, Centers for Disease Control and Prevention, 14 Oct. 2022, Available at: https://www.cdc.gov/ncbddd/adhd/data/diagnosis-treatment-data.html. Accessed June 1, 2023.

14. Zgodic A, McLain AC, Eberth JM, et al. County-level prevalence estimates of ADHD in the United States. Ann Epidemiol 2023;79:56–65.

15. Wolraich ML, Hagan JF, Allan C, et al. SUBCOMMITTEE ON CHILDREN AND ADOLESCENTS WITH ATTENTION-DEFICIT/HYPERACTIVE DISORDER; Clinical Practice Guideline for the Diagnosis, Evaluation, and Treatment of Attention-Deficit/Hyperactivity Disorder in Children and Adolescents. Pediatrics 2019; 144(4):e20192528.

16. Fadus MC, Ginsburg KR, Sobowale K, et al. Unconscious Bias and the Diagnosis of Disruptive Behavior Disorders and ADHD in African American and Hispanic Youth. Acad Psychiatry 2020;44(1):95–102.

17. Poysophon P, Rao AL. Neurocognitive Deficits Associated With ADHD in Athletes: A Systematic Review. Sports Health 2018;10(4):317–26.

18. Parr JW. Attention-deficit hyperactivity disorder and the athlete: new advances and understanding. Clin Sports Med 2011;30(3):591–610.

19. Martin, Thomas M. Major League Baseball, 2020 Public Report of Major League Baseball's Joint Drug Prevention and Treatment Program. Available at: https://img.mlbstatic.com/mlb-images/image/upload/mlb/ylj7vghznkikcpolyiu3.pdf. Accessed 7 Mar. 2023.

20. Han DH, McDuff D, Thompson D, et al. a/Attention-deficit/hyperactivity disorder in elite athletes: a narrative review. Br J Sports Med 2019;53:741–5.

21. Choi JW, Han DH, Kang KD, et al. Aerobic exercise and attention deficit hyperactivity disorder: brain research. Med Sci Sports Exerc 2015;47(1):33–9.

22. Molly Seidel Instagram post. June 8, 2022.

23. Drechsler R, Brem S, Brandeis D, et al. ADHD: Current Concepts and Treatments in Children and Adolescents. Neuropediatrics 2020;51(5):315–35.
24. Ambrosino S, de Zeeuw P, Wierenga LM, et al. What can cortical development in attention-deficit/hyperactivity disorder teach us about the early developmental mechanisms involved? Cereb Cortex 2017;27(09):4624–34.
25. Sagvolden T, Aase H, Johansen E, et al. A dynamic developmental theory of attention-deficit/hyperactivity disorder (ADHD) predominantly hyperactive/impulsive and combined subtypes. Behavioral and Brain Sciences 2005;28:397–468.
26. Tripp G, Wickens JR. Dopamine transfer deficit: a neurobiological theory of altered reinforcement mechanisms in ADHD. JCPP (J Child Psychol Psychiatry) 2008;49:691–704.
27. CDC website: Symptoms and Diagnosis of ADHD. Available at: https://www.cdc.gov/ncbddd/adhd/diagnosis.html. Accessed June 26, 2023.
28. Kessler R. The prevalence and correlates of adult adhd in the United States: results from the National Comorbidity Survey Replication. Am J Psychiatry 2006;163–716.
29. Anastopoulos AD, DuPaul GJ, Weyandt LL, et al. Rates and Patterns of Comorbidity Among First-Year College Students With ADHD. J Clin Child Adolesc Psychol 2018;47(2):236–47.
30. Philipsen A, Jans T, Graf E, et al. Effects of Group Psychotherapy, Individual Counseling, Methylphenidate, and Placebo in the Treatment of Adult Attention-Deficit/Hyperactivity Disorder: A Randomized Clinical Trial. JAMA Psychiatr 2015;72(12):1199–210.
31. Lam AP, Matthies S, Graf E, et al. Comparison of Methylphenidate and Psychotherapy in Adult ADHD Study (COMPAS) Consortium. Long-term Effects of Multimodal Treatment on Adult Attention-Deficit/Hyperactivity Disorder Symptoms: Follow-up Analysis of the COMPAS Trial. JAMA Netw Open 2019;2(5):e194980.
32. Solanto MV. Neuropsychopharmacological mechanisms of stimulant drug action in attention-deficit hyperactivity disorder: a review and integration. Behav Brain Res 1998;94(1):127–52.
33. Ritalin hydrochloride package insert. US Food and Drug Administration.
34. "The Prohibited List." World Anti Doping Agency, 3 Jan. 2023, Available at: https://www.wada-ama.org/en/prohibited-list. Accessed June 1, 2023.
35. "Medical Exceptions Procedures." NCAA Sport Science Institute. Available at: https://www.ncaa.org/sports/2015/1/23/medical-exceptions-procedures.aspx. Accessed June 1, 2023.
36. Jensen PS, Hinshaw SP, Swanson JM, et al. Findings from the NIMH Multimodal Treatment Study of ADHD (MTA): implications and applications for primary care providers. J Dev Behav Pediatr 2001;22(1):60–73.
37. Cooper WO, Habel LA, Sox CM, et al. ADHD drugs and serious cardiovascular events in children and young adults. N Engl J Med 2011;365(20):1896–904.
38. Alsalaheen B, Stockdale K, Pechumer D, et al. Validity of the Immediate Post Concussion Assessment and Cognitive Testing (ImPACT). Sports Med 2016;46(10):1487–501.
39. Maietta JE, Renn BN, Goodwin GJ, et al. A systematic review and meta-analysis of factors influencing ImPACT concussion testing in high school and collegiate athletes with self-reported ADHD and/or LD. Neuropsychology 2023;37(2):113–32.
40. Cook NE, Iaccarino MA, Karr JE, et al. Attention-Deficit/Hyperactivity Disorder and Outcome After Concussion: A Systematic Review. J Dev Behav Pediatr 2020;41(7):571–82.

41. Cook NE, Iverson GL, Maxwell B, et al. Adolescents With ADHD Do Not Take Longer to Recover From Concussion. Front Pediatr 2021;8:606879.
42. Iverson GL, Wojtowicz M, Brooks BL, et al. High School Athletes With ADHD and Learning Difficulties Have a Greater Lifetime Concussion History. J Atten Disord 2020;24(8):1095–101.
43. Pujalte GGA, Maynard JR, Thurston MJ, et al. Considerations in the Care of Athletes With Attention Deficit Hyperactivity Disorder. Clin J Sport Med 2019;29(3): 245–56.

Review of Media Representation of Sport Concussion and Implications for Youth Sports

Aaron S. Jeckell, MD[a,*], R. Shea Fontana, DO[a,b,1],
Rolando Gonzalez, MD[a,c,d,2]

KEYWORDS

- Sport-related concussion • Media • Removal from sport
- Chronic traumatic encephalopathy • Youth sport

KEY POINTS

- Many individuals learn about sport-related concussion (SRC) through various forms of media (newspaper, online news, social media, film, and so forth)
- Popular media does not always portray SRC accurately and there are many examples of misinformation in reporting.
- Knowledge about SRC varies considerably based on several factors, but accurate understanding of the injury does not always correlate to appropriate action.
- Given the high utility of various forms of media usage, this presents an opportunity to convey accurate SRC information.

INTRODUCTION

Participation in youth sport confers numerous mental health and physical benefits.[1] Nonetheless, participating in physical activity comes with inherent risks. Sport-related concussion (SRC), a type of mild traumatic brain injury (mTBI), is a risk associated with any physical activity. The impact of SRC and the potential long-term neurocognitive effects have been a mainstay in media over the past 2 decades. This has been driven by cases in which the postretirement declines of high-profile athletes have been attributed to SRC and repetitive brain impacts sustained during playing

[a] International Society for Sport Psychiatry; [b] University of South Carolina School of Medicine – Greenville; [c] Golisano Children's Hospital of Southwest Florida; [d] Florida State University College of Medicine
[1] Present address: 10 Patewood Drive, Street 130, Greenville, SC 29615.
[2] Present address: 12310 Coconut Creek Court, Fort Myers, FL 33908.
* 1601 23rd Avenue, South Nashville, TN 37212.
E-mail address: aaron.jeckell.md@gmail.com

Clin Sports Med 43 (2024) 159–172
https://doi.org/10.1016/j.csm.2023.06.012
0278-5919/24/© 2023 Elsevier Inc. All rights reserved.
sportsmed.theclinics.com

careers. Press coverage of these events has likely had a significant impact on public opinion regarding SRC and participation in youth sport. Rates of participation in some high school (HS) sports such as football and basketball have decreased in recent years for the first time in decades, notwithstanding the COVID-19 pandemic. Athlete and parent concern about SRC is frequently cited as a driving factor, and for those who do remain engaged in sport, fear of SRC remains high. Other beliefs about the short- and long-term impact of SRC are not always consistent with up-to-date science.[2] As varying forms of media remain major sources of SRC-related information, an exploration of its impact is worthwhile. Here, the authors examine some of the ways that media has represented SRC and how this representation may continue to influence youth sport participation today.

HISTORICAL PERSPECTIVE OF MEDIA AND SPORT-RELATED CONCUSSION

The first "Concussion Crisis" took place in the late nineteenth and early twentieth centuries. American Football was popular at that time, especially in the Ivy League colleges. The sport had few rules or regulations, and participants wore little protective equipment. Injuries abounded and team physicians were becoming increasingly aware of the hazards associated with play. The injury that we know today as concussion gained special notice. Popular media did not shy away from using colorful language to convey the risks of injury to their readers. In 1893, The New York Times noted that the sport incurred, "nearly the same risk that a soldier [assumes] on the battle field,"[3] and that, "an ordinary rebellion in the South American or Central American states is as child's play compared with the destructiveness of a day's game."[4]

Public alarm grew along with the understanding that SRC was a more nuanced and dangerous injury than previously thought. Physicians were beginning to appreciate that SRC might actually be difficult to detect and was occurring at a higher rate than previously believed.[5] Nichols and Smith noted that "A player might automatically run through a considerable series of plays before his fellows noticed that he was mentally irresponsible."[6]

Amid this fear and uncertainty, popular opinion called for change. In the 1900s, new rules made the game safer and it became more common for athletes to wear padding or other equipment.[7] Concerns persisted though, in particular regarding the long-term consequences of head injury. Harrison Martland published "Punch Drunk" in 1928 examining the long-term effect of head injury on boxers.[8] The public urgency to address the issue waned over the years, with much of the focus shifting to head injuries that were affecting the soldiers of World War I and II. It was not until the early twenty-first century that SRC was once again thrust into the spotlight.

Dr Bennett Omalu and colleagues reignited concern about SRC with his case reports on former National Football League (NFL) players with chronic traumatic encephalopathy (CTE).[9] In 2007, Boston University partnered with the Sports Legacy Institute to create the Boston University Center for the Study of Traumatic Encephalopathy, a group that has been on the frontline of concussion research since then. With this new wave of research, the popular media once again seized on SRC. The film *Concussion* was released in 2015, a semi-fictionalized take on Dr Omalu's research and the controversy surrounding the NFLs response. The film was criticized by much of the scientific community for oversimplifying the science and suggesting that football alone was the cause of death for athletes found to have CTE. Other contemporary headlines declared, "111 N F L. Brains, All But One Had CTE."[10,11] Recent publications have created an impression that nearly all professional football players will experience CTE, regardless of experiencing an identified concussion. Despite the tremendous amount of research that has taken place in recent years, many knowledge gaps persist, and media portrayal of scientific understanding of SRC is not always accurate.

CURRENT UNDERSTANDING OF SPORT-RELATED CONCUSSION: A BRIEF SUMMARY

An SRC is a type of mTBI induced by a biomechanical force that is transmitted to the brain. This impact leads to a constellation of neuropsychiatric symptoms (physical signs, behavioral, cognitive, or somatic changes) that typically resolve over the course of days or weeks. Recovery is characterized by an initial period of rest followed by a graded series of physical and cognitive steps that increase in difficulty and culminate in return to physical and academic activity.[12]

The impact that causes SRC leads to a cascade of events resulting in disruption of neurochemical homeostasis as well as increases in free radicals and other regulators of neuroinflammation. The energy required to reestablish homeostasis is believed to cause the hallmark symptoms seen during SRC recovery.[13] These changes take place on the microscopic level, and macroscopic changes (hemorrhage, fracture, gross lesions) are not consistent with SRC. Readily available neuroimaging (commuted tomography, MRI, x-ray) is unable to detect concussion and is used to rule out more severe injury.[14]

Concussion has historically accounted for 3% to 8% of all sport-related injuries that present to the emergency department.[15] Sports that involve athletes moving at a high velocity, interaction with an object (ball, puck, bat, and so forth), and/or intentional contact/tackling put participants at higher risk for injury.[16] Younger individuals may be more susceptible to SRC due to factors including mechanical features and being in a period of ongoing and rapid neurologic, cognitive, and emotional development.[17] However, Pierpoint and colleagues found that collegiate athletes had higher rates of SRC than HS athletes.[16] Overall, rates of concussion seem to be on the rise. This may be due to improved recognition and detection of SRC, improved awareness and appreciation of the importance of proper treatment and management, and changes in sport rules, equipment, and playing styles.[18]

The disease known as CTE is considered to be a result of repetitive concussions or sub-concussive impacts, the latter being a term with no consensus definition. It is diagnosed by pathologic findings of hyperphosphorylated tau proteins in perivascular locations at the depths of the cortical sulci.[19] These findings, only diagnosable on postmortem histopathological examination, are felt to be distinct from other neurodegenerative diseases. The number and severity of head impacts necessary to impart CTE has not been established. The degree to which CTE may cause neuropsychiatric symptoms, which are not required for diagnosis, is unknown. Although CTE has largely been studied in professional contact sport athletes and military personnel, it is likely present in many other individuals and the links to other factors such as age, medical issues, substance exposure, and genetics are unknown.[20]

Representation of Sport-Related Concussion in Popular Media

We sought to recreate the experience of a lay person looking to learn more about SRC. We used Google to search for "concussion in sport" and limited our results to material produced between January 2012 and December 2022 (**Fig. 1**). Browsing history was cleared to avoid any potential bias from past searches and we only used the News section of Google. The search resulted in approximately 116,000 articles. A random sampling from the first 10 pages (first 100 articles) resulted in 25 articles from reputable media outlets being selected. Five were excluded due to the requirement of a subscription or membership. Twenty articles were used for this examination (**Table 1**).

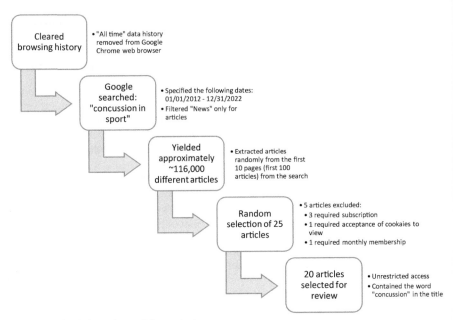

Fig. 1. Methodology for article analysis.

The term "concussion" was mentioned in all 20 articles. The terms "brain injury" appeared in 13/20 articles and "head injury" and/or "head impact" appeared in 13/20 articles. CTE appeared in 13/20 articles, and dementia was represented in 10/20 articles. CTE and dementia were typically mentioned as potential long-term risks associated with sustaining concussions or "repeated head injuries." The words "retirement," "retired," or "retire" were found in 9/20 articles. Both retirement and CTE/dementia reports were mostly seen after 2016 which correlates with several events covered in the media (NFL lawsuit and the movie *Concussion* in 2015). "Minor" or "mild" was used in 7/20 articles to discuss the severe brain injury. Other terms that were noted to recur: "subconcussive," "repetitive hits to the head," "repeat head trauma," and "cognitive decline." No idioms for SRC, such as "bell rung," were found in this sample, but "head clash" was used once in the sampled articles.

Our findings corroborate data found in several recent studies looking at the impact of social media has on SRC representation. The investigators from an analysis looking at mTBI-related press releases between January 2012 and December 2019 found a considerable amount of misrepresentation; 83% of 66 press releases reviewed exhibited at least one manifestation of "spin," of misleading titles (58%), reporting (74%), claims (67%), and inappropriate extrapolation (38%).[21] Another study revealed the frequent use of misleading terms reporting on SRC such as "mild concussion," "minor concussion," "slight concussion," and terms such as "concussion," "head injury," "brain injury," "head clash," and "brain trauma" being used interchangeably as descriptors.[22]

Eighty three percent of sports fans check a social media platform while watching an event on television.[23] A 2011 study (data collected for 1 week in 2010) revealed that Twitter is an active source for concussion-related information ranging from "news-related tweets" to "sharing personal information/situation" and "inferred management" of concussions.[24] Similarly, TikTok has gained significant traction since its inception in 2005. Carter and colleagues identified 157 TikTok videos that met inclusion criteria for concussion-related content—only two of the videos included

Table 1
Data collection looking at the frequency of the below buzzwords related to concussion within each article (*n* = 20)

Media Source	Year	Concussion: Total[a]	Concussion: Filtered[b]	Head Injury and/or Head Impact	Brain Injury	Mild/Minor[c]	Chronic Traumatic Encephalopathy/CTE[d]	Retire, Retired, or Retirement[e]	Dementia
The Guardian	2022	22	13	1	0	0	7	0	0
CNN	2022	18	16	4	2	0	6	0	1
Futurity	2021	16	9	0	0	0	0	0	0
RTE	2020	24	18	5	4	3	14	1	5
ABC News	2019	19	10[f]	0 ("head clash" = 1)	0	0	3	1	0
ABC News	2019	40	28	4	0	1	1	0	0
Los Angeles Times	2019	18	15[f]	1	1	1	0	1	1
CNN Health	2019	46	34	0	2	0	0	0	1
ESPN	2019	45	38	4	1	0	1	1	0
News Medical Life Sciences	2019	24	20	14	0	0	7	3	2
NPR	2018	28	20	6	2	1	16	0	1
Healthline	2018	12	11	2	1	0	1	2	1
The Sport Journal	2016	81	60	1	1	0	8	3	1

(continued on next page)

Table 1
(continued)

Media Source	Year	Concussion: Total[a]	Concussion: Filtered[b]	Head Injury and/or Head Impact	Brain Injury	Mild/Minor[c]	Chronic Traumatic Encephalopathy/CTE[d]	Retire, Retired, or Retirement[e]	Dementia
The Sport Journal	2016	106	73[f]	25	2	1	3	0	1
The Conversation	2016	17	12	0	3	0	7	1	7
NPR	2016	31	20	0	3	1	0	0	0
Healthline	2015	24	17	2[f]	0	0	0	0	0
Bleacher Report	2015	12	9	0	3	0	0	0	0
National Academies	2013	43	39[f]	2	2	2	1	2	0
CNN Health	2013	22	17	0	0	2	0	0	0

[a] The number of times concussion appears on the Web site; inclusive of advertisements, picture headings, and title of article/subheadings.

[b] The number of times concussion appears within the body of the text; excluded the above from (1) and concussion pertaining to the title of the movie *Concussion* or any concussion work group or foundation.

[c] "Mild" or "minor" used to describe the severity of concussion or traumatic brain injury.

[d] Did not duplicate the count when this term was followed by chronic traumatic encephalopathy (CTE) as a descriptor. For example, CTE counted as 1.

[e] Articles described retirement as an outcome or referenced retired players in the context of concussion.

[f] Sport(s)-related concussion used at least once in the article.

"educational content" with one being viewed greater than 1 million times.[25] Videos that came from a verified account tended to be the most viewed, and the vast majority of the videos reviewed took on a "light-hearted approach" to the topic of concussion.[25] Social media and personalized search engines use algorithms to increase the likelihood that users will continue to engage with their platform. Developers advertise stories or posts based off the relevancy of previous interactions. This can amplify risk of confirmation bias, especially when the content is scientific in nature. Post after post from similar sources or authors can potentiate the spread of misinformation and essentially change the algorithm for the user to remain in this perpetual cycle with limited interaction from opposing views or newer publications that may debunk past findings.

Media and Removal from Sport

Chris Borland was 24 year old when he retired from the NFL, citing "fear of concussions" as the primary factor for his decision. He had sustained an SRC in training camp yet kept playing immediately after and throughout the rest of the season. News outlets and articles referred to Borland as having experienced a "ding," "minor concussion," or his "bell rung." It was emphasized that he was in his first season as a linebacker when he made this decision to retire. He reported reading extensively about concussions and talking to teammates and family members about these fears. Articles quote him saying that reactions from his teammates were "mixed," some of whom cited money as a reason not to retire.

Borland is one example out of numerous who have retired from the NFL and expressed concerns about SRC and the long-term impacts.[26] Social media has been an integral source in spreading this information. Online responses have been mixed with some fans supporting Borland's decision, whereas others have suggested that he would be easy to replace.

This concern has been mirrored in youth sport populations. Rates of participation in youth sport have varied over the past decades, particularly in the past several years due to the COVID-19 pandemic. In 2021, 78% of children ages 6 to 12 years participated in a team or individual sport. However, only 37% regularly participated in a team sport on a regular basis, a decrease from previous years (45% in 2008). In the 13 to 17-year-old demographic, 74% participated in a team or individual sport, though only 42% participated on a regular basis.[27] American Football, lacrosse, ice hockey, and wrestling have shown persistent declines relative to a decade ago.[28] Early specialization, lack of access, time/financial costs, diminishing interest among participants, and concern about injury are all factors contributing to these shifts. Of note, participation in tackle football for children aged 6 to 12 year old declined 29% from 2016 to 2021, whereas participation in flag football increased 15%.[27]

Retirement from sport after SRC is complicated, with no consensus as to when this should be considered.[29] This decision should be highly individualized and take into account various factors including age, level of play, medical and psychiatric history, and family history. The biological, psychological, and social factors that influence a professional athlete to retire are considerably different than those impacting a youth athlete. The degree to which media representation of professional athletes retiring from sport may influence youth athletes or their parents to do the same is not yet known.

COLLEGE ATHLETE OPINIONS OF SPORT-RELATED CONCUSSION

Collegiate athletes have been found to have a relatively high level of understanding regarding SRC.[30] Attitudes are described as positive with athletes indicating that notifying medical staff and reporting injuries is important. Although contact/combat-sport athletes are more likely to receive education regarding SRC, they are less likely to report symptoms per one study, and data suggest that knowledge does not necessarily translate to positive reporting behaviors.[31] Underreporting behaviors are a significant concern with 15% to 45% of collegiate athletes electing not to report suspected or hypothetical concussive symptoms.[32,33] Across multiple studies, collegiate athletes often cited concussion nondisclosure to fear of missed playing time, fear of missing a game, fear of letting down teammates, or at the time, did not believe they suffered a concussion.[30–34] Athletes have cited medical professionals (73.2%) and school-based professionals (68.4%) as sources of SRC education, and nearly one-third cited books, movies, social media, or sporting news outlets as an SRC resource.[32]

HIGH SCHOOL AND YOUTH ATHLETE OPINIONS OF SPORT-RELATED CONCUSSION

Although youth HS athletes may possess some accurate knowledge regarding SRC, there remain significant gaps in understanding and application of this knowledge. General SRC knowledge and attitudes are variable with SRC knowledge ranging widely (39%–80%).[35–40] One study found that 12% of youth English rugby players adhered to the recommended return to play (RTP) guidelines.[37] Miyashita and colleagues surveyed a variety of HS athletes and found that 95.6% agreed to the statement that "there are long term effects" from SRC, yet 50.9% also described believing that "the importance of the game should affect RTP decisions."[35] A study of New Zealand rugby players found considerable differences in SRC knowledge and attitudes with similar declines in reporting behaviors toward the end of season when competition needs were higher.[36]

Doucette and colleagues found that female athletes had higher SRC knowledge scores, and soccer players scored higher than collision athletes.[40] Athletes from in lower socioeconomic areas scored lower in knowledge and attitudes toward SRC.[36] Bloodgood and colleagues surveyed 252 HS athletes with most viewing SRC as a "critical issue." The younger athletes were more likely to believe concussions were a "critical issue" compared with the older athletes of this study (ages 16–18 years; 34%). More than half of the youth athletes disagreed with the statement "I am fearful that my circle of friends would think I was dumb for caring about concussion."[41] Approximately half of HS athletes would not report SRC symptoms.[40,42] A 2020 systematic review of SRC reporting behaviors found evidence for underreporting behaviors in all 26 studies.[43] Reasons for underreporting included: "not wanting to leave the game, not thinking their injury was serious enough, and wanting to avoid letting the team down." High levels of concussion knowledge (>80% correct on concussion fact knowledge) did not correlate with increased reporting of SRC, similar to that of collegiate athletes in other studies.[34,43]

Seventy one percent of New Zealand soccer players identified their coaches as a primary source on SRC information.[36] Youth athlete concussion knowledge was positively influenced by higher parental SRC knowledge, history of prior SRC, and older athlete age.[44] Most of the Canadian HS athletes identified their parents or guardians as a primary source of SRC information,[45] whereas 22% of South Korean athletes had heard of SRC from media.[46]

Parental Opinion of Sport-Related Concussion

Adults displayed high knowledge regarding concussions, often scoring $\geq$75% on SRC-related questionnaires.[38,47] Despite this, parents frequently answered incorrectly believing that neuroimaging studies are capable of detecting SRC.[38] Parents also tend to be concerned about permanent brain damage due to SRC.[47] Ninety-six percent of parents reported belief that there are long-term effects of SRC.[48] Parents of children who play contact sports (37%) are more likely to be concerned their child will develop CTE as compared with those who do not (21%).[49] In comparison surveys, parents were more likely to express concern for long-term consequences of SRC, whereas the youth athletes were more concerned about RTP.[50] Kroshus and colleagues found that more than half of parents were somewhat or very worried about concussion.[51] Nearly 87% reported worry about injury risk with concussion as the injury cited most according to a recent survey.[27] Parents acquire their information from a variety of sources, the primary of which are doctors (35%) and popular media (12.8%). Other studies have found that nearly half of adults obtain SRC information from news media, 36% from sports media, and 34% from physicians.[38]

Fear of SRC and potential long-term sequelae is a common driver for voluntary removal from sport. Hibshman and colleagues found that 49% of parents would prohibit their children from participation in a collision sport, primarily listing safety concerns.[52] Twenty-six percent of parents that previously allowed their child to play football indicated that they would no longer allow them to continue.[38] Nearly half of American parents reported that they would encourage their child to play a sport other than tackle football due to fear of concussion, up 8% from 4 years prior.[53] There are adult factors that support youth contact sports participation including being a female parent, older parent, having an older eldest child, or personal prior participation in contact sports.[39] Adults (with and without children) were less likely to allow daughters to participate in contact sports.[39]

DISCUSSION

Over the past several decades, both youth athletes and parents have become keenly aware of SRC and the potential impact the injury can have. Researchers continue to expand our understanding of SRC, exploring the factors that can predict injury, detection and diagnosis, recovery, treatment, long-term impact, and the links between head impacts and CTE. Despite ongoing questions in the medical community, many lay individuals are under the impression that science has established a consensus answer for these issues. A likely factor for this is how these issues are being reported. In addition to medical professionals, popular media, including entertainment and social media, is the most common source of information for many individuals, with certain demographic factors influencing this. Communities with less access to medical professionals may fill that void with media as their primary source for SRC guidance. This can be problematic, as popular media has been demonstrated to frequently misrepresent SRC data.

Misinformation, spin, omissions, or inaccurate conclusions are unfortunately common issues.[21] Measured and evidence-based reporting of credible research may run secondary to attention grabbing headlines. Our media search found that CTE was mentioned in 65% of articles reviewed and retirement/retired athlete in 50%. Only 25% did not contain a mention of CTE, dementia, or retirement, and those articles tended to be older. If a parent or athlete was to have a similar search experience, it is likely that the idea of CTE and retirement would be suggested to them. Many individuals do not have the scientific background to ascertain whether their risk for these issues is significant or indicates a change in their activity or sport of interest.

Other headlines might have a similar anxiety-inducing effect. The media portrayal of the work done by Mez and colleagues is a notable example.[11] In a paper supplied by a convenience sample of brains from former football players donated for CTE research, they found that a high percentage had the neuropathological findings of CTE. A New York Times article later reported that all but one of the brains from 111 former NFL players had CTE. A casual reader might easily interpret this to mean that participation in a high level of football is all but a guarantee to develop CTE, something that cannot be established based on the data presented in that study. The biological, psychological, and social factors that so often impact retired athletes are often minimized. Retired athletes can be subject to financial, personal, social, and injury/pain medication-related stressors, all of which can mimic the behavioral and cognitive features associated with CTE. Factors like those rarely impact amateur or youth athletes. Reporting, including all these issues, may shift parental concerns about participation in youth sport.

Journalists can also ensure the accurate use of concussion-related terminology. Descriptors such as mild, moderate, or severe are inaccurate, and colloquialisms such as a "ding" or having ones "bell rung" should be avoided.[22] When reporting on the personal experiences of concussed athletes, factors such as level of play, biological and medical attributes, and social circumstances can be mentioned to avoid extrapolating their decisions or the risks that they face onto other individuals.

Mass media and news communications play a pivotal role in the dissemination of public health information. Popular media is intentionally forming not only what is shared, but the context in which information is shared and distributed to consumers. Regardless of scientific accuracy, this material has the potential to reach millions of people and influence public perception of a topic almost instantaneously. There is a tremendous amount of potential that various social media platforms have when it comes to using entities (ie, National Collegiate Athletic Association [NCAA] and NFL) or "influencers" such as pro-athletes, to help promote concussion awareness and management and to stop the spread of misinformation. Media also has the power to educate a wide audience, which can positively influence concussion awareness and knowledge through factual reporting and advocacy.

Another concerning factor is that an accurate understanding of SRC does not always lead to appropriate response. Despite appropriate SRC knowledge, many youth athletes admit that they would not report concussion symptoms, or feel that preemptive return to activity would be appropriate given an important enough game. Youth athletes will often cite fear of missing playing time or letting down their coaches as major contributors as to why they would not report their injury. Another theory is that appropriate SRC education may in effect "coach" athletes as to how to hide symptoms or feign recovery, a response that could be disastrous.[54] Athletes do get a great deal of SRC information from news and social media, presenting an opportunity to shine a focus on the need for immediate and accurate reporting of symptoms after injury.

Parental anxiety regarding risk of SRC should be measured against the countless benefits of participation in sport. In particular, team sports are proved to increase confidence, decrease depression and anxiety, and enhance feelings of interconnectedness with peers, in addition to the physical benefits of activity.[1] Although no one should be encouraged to engage in any sport that they do not feel safe in, a consideration of the risks and benefits, as well as safe alternatives, should be given. Rarely would complete removal from all sport be necessary.

SUMMARY

The risk of SRC is real and should not be taken lightly. However, it should be emphasized that with appropriate treatment, this is an injury from which recovery is very likely. Further research regarding the long-term risks of participation in sport and repetitive head injury is needed. The benefits of sport participation should be measured against the risks, and every effort should be made to make sport accessible, equitable, and safe for all involved to maximize the psychosocial benefits of sport. To that end, media representation should emphasize an accurate representation of the current consensus of SRC. In doing so, we can hope to equip athletes, parents, and coaches with the appropriate information with which to make important decisions about participating in sport.

CLINICS CARE POINTS

- Clinicians should be aware of where their patients acquire sport-related concussion (SRC) information from, misunderstandings they may have, and provide appropriate education regarding this injury.

- Ensure that your patients and athletes have an accurate understanding of SRC and appropriate responsiveness to injury.

- Stress the importance of a full recovery and return to baseline before full return to sport.

- Participation in youth sport confers many benefits such as improved confidence and feelings of interconnectedness, and the inherent risks associated with play should be weighed against the benefits.

DISCLOSURE

The authors have nothing to disclose.

REFERENCES

1. Eime RM, Young JA, Harvey JT, et al. A systematic review of the psychological and social benefits of participation in sport for children and adolescents: informing development of a conceptual model of health through sport. Int J Behav Nutr Phys Act 2013;10:98 [published Online First: Epub Date]|.
2. Roberts SD, Schatz P, Register-Mihalik J, et al. Parent knowledge of and attitudes towards youth sport-related concussion and associations with child and parent factors. Concussion 2021;6(4):Cnc93 [published Online First: Epub Date]|.
3. Change the football rules: the rugby game as played now is a dangerous pastime. New York Times; 1893.
4. Yale again triumphant. New York Times; 1894.
5. Harrison EA. The first concussion crisis: head injury and evidence in early American football. Am J Public Health 2014;104(5):822–33 [published Online First: Epub Date]|.
6. Nichols EH, Smith HB. The physical aspect of American football. Boston Med Surg J 1906;1.
7. Nichols EH, Richardson FL. Football Injuries of the Harvard Squad for Three Years under the Revised Rules. Boston Med Surg J 1909;160(2):33–7 [published Online First: Epub Date]|.
8. Martland HS. Punch Drunk. Journal of the American Medical Association 1928; 91(15):1103–7.
9. Omalu BI, DeKosky ST, Minster RL, et al. Chronic traumatic encephalopathy in a National Football League player. Neurosurgery 2005;57(1):128–34.

10. Ward J, Williams J, Manchester S. 111 N.F.L. Brains, all but one had CTE. The New York Times; 2017.
11. Mez J, Daneshvar DH, Kiernan PT, et al. Clinicopathological Evaluation of Chronic Traumatic Encephalopathy in Players of American Football. JAMA 2017;318(4): 360–70 [published Online First: Epub Date]|.
12. McCrory P, Meeuwisse W, Dvořák J, et al. Consensus statement on concussion in sport-the 5(th) international conference on concussion in sport held in Berlin, October 2016. Br J Sports Med 2017;51(11):838–47 [published Online First: Epub Date]|.
13. Giza CC, Hovda DA. The new neurometabolic cascade of concussion. Neurosurgery 2014;75(0 4):S24–33 [published Online First: Epub Date]|.
14. McCullough BJ, Jarvik JG. Diagnosis of concussion: the role of imaging now and in the future. Phys Med Rehabil Clin N Am 2011;22(4):635–52.
15. Kelly KD, Lissel HL, Rowe BH, et al. Sport and recreation-related head injuries treated in the emergency department. Clin J Sport Med 2001;11(2):77–81 [published Online First: Epub Date]|.
16. Pierpoint L, Collins C. Epidemiology of Sport-Related Concussion. Clin Sports Med 2021;40:1–18 [published Online First: Epub Date]|.
17. Sim A, Terryberry-Spohr L, Wilson KR. Prolonged recovery of memory functioning after mild traumatic brain injury in adolescent athletes. Journal of Neurosurgery JNS 2008;108(3):511–6 [published Online First: Epub Date]|.
18. Lincoln AE, Caswell SV, Almquist JL, et al. Trends in Concussion Incidence in High School Sports:A Prospective 11-Year Study. Am J Sports Med 2011;39(5): 958–63 [published Online First: Epub Date]|.
19. McKee AC, Cairns NJ, Dickson DW, et al. The first NINDS/NIBIB consensus meeting to define neuropathological criteria for the diagnosis of chronic traumatic encephalopathy. Acta Neuropathol 2016;131(1):75–86 [published Online First: Epub Date]|.
20. Noy S, Krawitz S, Del Bigio MR. Chronic Traumatic Encephalopathy-Like Abnormalities in a Routine Neuropathology Service. J Neuropathol Exp Neurol 2016; 75(12):1145–54 [published Online First: Epub Date]|.
21. Choi AR, Feller ER. Misrepresentation of mild traumatic brain injury research in press releases. Pm r 2022;14(7):769–78 [published Online First: Epub Date]|.
22. Ahmed OH, Hall EE. "It was only a mild concussion": Exploring the description of sports concussion in online news articles. Physical Therapy in Sport 2017;23: 7–13 [published Online First: Epub Date]|.
23. Hull K, Schmittel A. A Fumbled Opportunity? A Case Study of Twitter's Role in Concussion Awareness Opportunities During the Super Bowl. J Sport Soc Issues 2014;39(1):78–94 [published Online First: Epub Date]|.
24. Sullivan SJ, Schneiders AG, Cheang C-W, et al. 'What's happening?' A content analysis of concussion-related traffic on Twitter</em&gt. Br J Sports Med 2012;46(4):258–63 [published Online First: Epub Date]|.
25. Carter PN, Hall EE, Ketcham CJ, et al. Not Just for Dancing? A Content Analysis of Concussion and Head Injury Videos on TikTok. Frontiers in Sports and Active Living 2021;3. https://doi.org/10.3389/fspor.2021.692613 [published Online First: Epub Date]|.
26. Winterburn C. 5 NFL players who were forced to retire after suffering concussions Sportskeeda, 11/8/2022.
27. Jewett R, Kerr G, MacPherson E, et al. Experiences of bullying victimisation in female interuniversity athletes. Int J Sport Exerc Psychol 2020;18(6):818–32 [published Online First: Epub Date]|.

28. Associations TNFoSHS. High School Athletics Participation Survey, 2022.
29. Laker SR, Meron A, Greher MR, et al. Retirement and Activity Restrictions Following Concussion. Phys Med Rehabil Clin N Am 2016;27(2):487–501 [published Online First: Epub Date]|.
30. Conway FN, Domingues M, Monaco R, et al. Concussion Symptom Underreporting Among Incoming National Collegiate Athletic Association Division I College Athletes. Clin J Sport Med 2020;30(3):203–9 [published Online First: Epub Date]|.
31. Chizuk H, Haider M, Solomito M, et al. Concussion reporting behaviors in student athletes across sexes and levels of contact. Journal of Concussion 2021;5. 205970022110150.
32. Beidler E, Wallace J, Alghwiri AA, et al. Collegiate Athletes' Concussion Awareness, Understanding, and -Reporting Behaviors in Different Countries With Varying Concussion Publicity. J Athl Train 2021;56(1):77–84 [published Online First: Epub Date]|.
33. Davies SC, Bird BMM. Motivations for Underreporting Suspected Concussion in College Athletics. J Clin Sport Psychol 2015;9:101–15.
34. Bretzin AC, Anderson M, Bhandari N, et al. Concussion Nondisclosure in Youth Sports. J Athl Train 2022;57(7):688–95 [published Online First: Epub Date]|.
35. Miyashita TL, Diakogeorgiou E, Hellstrom B, et al. High School Athletes' Perceptions of Concussion. Orthop J Sports Med 2014;2(11). 2325967114554549.
36. Salmon DM, Romanchuk J, Sullivan SJ, et al. Concussion knowledge, attitude and reporting intention in rugby coaches and high school rugby players. Int J Sports Sci Coach 2020;16(1):54–69 [published Online First: Epub Date]|.
37. Kearney PE. See J. Misunderstandings of concussion within a youth rugby population. J Sci Med Sport 2017;20(11):981–5 [published Online First: Epub Date]|.
38. Taranto E, Fishman M, Garvey K, et al. Public Attitudes and Knowledge About Youth Sports Participation and Concussion Risk in an Urban Area. J Natl Med Assoc 2018;110(6):635–43 [published Online First: Epub Date]|.
39. Memmini AK, Van Pelt KL, Wicklund A, et al. Evaluating Adult Decision-Making Modifiers in Support of Youth Contact-Sport Participation. J Athl Train 2022; 57(1):44–50 [published Online First: Epub Date]|.
40. Doucette MM, Du Plessis S, Webber AM, et al. In it to win it: Competitiveness, concussion knowledge and nondisclosure in athletes. Phys Sportsmed 2021; 49(2):194–202 [published Online First: Epub Date]|.
41. Bloodgood B, Inokuchi D, Shawver W, et al. Exploration of awareness, knowledge, and perceptions of traumatic brain injury among American youth athletes and their parents. J Adolesc Health 2013;53(1):34–9 [published Online First: Epub Date]|.
42. Wallace J, Covassin T, Nogle S, et al. Knowledge of Concussion and Reporting Behaviors in High School Athletes With or Without Access to an Athletic Trainer. J Athl Train 2017;52(3):228–35 [published Online First: Epub Date]|.
43. Ferdinand Pennock K, McKenzie B, McClemont Steacy L, et al. Under-reporting of sport-related concussions by adolescent athletes: a systematic review. Int Rev Sport Exerc Psychol 2020;1–27. https://doi.org/10.1080/1750984X.2020.1824243 [published Online First: Epub Date]|.
44. Beidler E, Bretzin AC, Schmitt AJ, et al. Factors associated with parent and youth athlete concussion knowledge. J Safety Res 2022;80:190–7 [published Online First: Epub Date]|.
45. Hunt C, Michalak A, Johnston E, et al. Knowledge, Attitudes and Concussion Information Sources Among First Nations in Ontario. Can J Neurol Sci 2018;45(3): 283–9 [published Online First: Epub Date]|.

46. Lee H, Resch J, Han T, et al. Sport-Related Concussion Knowledge and Occurrence: A Survey of High School and College Athletes in South Korea. Int J Athl Ther Train 2016;21:53–60 [published Online First: Epub Date]|.
47. Kim S, Connaughton DP. Youth Soccer Parents' Attitudes and Perceptions About Concussions. J Adolesc Health 2021;68(1):184–90.
48. Schatz P, Corcoran M, Kontos AP, et al. Youth Soccer Parents' Perceptions of Long-Term Effects of Concussion Developmental. Neuropsychology 2020;45(3): 110–7 [published Online First: Epub Date]|.
49. Daugherty J, Sarmiento K. Chronic traumatic encephalopathy: what do parents of youth athletes know about it? Brain Inj 2018;32(13–14):1773–9 [published Online First: Epub Date]|.
50. Nanos KN, Franco JM, Larson D, et al. Youth Sport-Related Concussions: Perceived and Measured Baseline Knowledge of Concussions Among Community Coaches, Athletes, and Parents. Mayo Clin Proc 2017;92(12):1782–90 [published Online First: Epub Date]|.
51. Kroshus E, Qu P, Chrisman SPD, et al. Parental concern about concussion risk for their children. Soc Sci Med 2019;222:359–66.
52. Hibshman N, Yengo-Kahn A, Wiseman A, et al. Child participation in collision sports and football: what influences parental decisions? Phys Sportsmed 2022; 50(2):171–80.
53. Poll Murray M. Nearly half of parents would discourage football due to concussions. NBC News/Wall Street Journal 2018;4:38.
54. Mrazik M, Dennison CR, Brooks BL, et al. A qualitative review of sports concussion education: prime time for evidence-based knowledge translation. Br J Sports Med 2015;49(24):1548–53.

Athlete Maltreatment in Sport

Carla D. Edwards, MSc, MD, FRCPC

KEYWORDS

• Maltreatment • Athletes • Harassment • Abuse • Mistreatment • Sports

KEY POINTS

- Early studies of maltreatment in sports were plagued by inconsistent definitions and concepts.
- Forms of maltreatment in sports include harassment, abuse, neglect, bullying, hazing, and discrimination.
- Victims of maltreatment can experience significant consequences to mental health, physical health, and athletic career.
- Blind loyalty, indifference, ignorance, protectionism, and denial can lead to intentional or unintentional complicity and perpetuation of maltreatment.
- Survivors of abuse, sport organizations, law enforcement bodies, and governments often reach an impasse regarding investigation, consequence, and change.

INTRODUCTION

The celebrated side of sports is the high-intensity display of athleticism and competition that draws spectators to the stands, televisions, and streaming services. That version of sports is presented as the hotly contested, highly sought-after glory that the competitors sacrifice their time and bodies to pursue. The competitive passion for sport can be observed at every level of sport: from youth sports leagues to elite and professional sports competitions.

This chapter will peel back the layers of sports to expose the elements that are not glamorous or celebrated. It will explore the staggering costs under the surface: to athletes, members of the athlete's entourage, and teammates when maltreatment occurs. It will also outline the role of the team physician in providing a safe clinical environment and tools to navigate disclosure and beyond.

Department of Psychiatry and Behavioural Neurosciences, McMaster University, St. Joseph's Healthcare, Hamilton West 5th Campus, Administration B3, 100 West 5th Street, Hamilton, Ontario L8N 3K7, Canada
E-mail address: edwardcd@mcmaster.ca
Twitter: @Edwards10Carla (C.D.E.)

Clin Sports Med 43 (2024) 173–186
https://doi.org/10.1016/j.csm.2023.06.004
0278-5919/24/© 2023 Elsevier Inc. All rights reserved.

PART 1: MALTREATMENT DEFINED

The incidence of athlete mistreatment in sports has been identified for several decades. Early research in the area was plagued with inconsistency in definition and conceptual framework.[1,2] By 2008, several significant publications established key benchmarks which provided a foundation for understanding the major components of mistreatment experienced by athletes. A review of these definitions is provided in the following section.

Maltreatment defined broadly as "volitional acts that result in or have the potential to result in physical injuries and/or psychological harm"[3] can be experienced in many different ways and involve various individuals in the athletic environment. This author holds that all forms of mistreatment, including harassment, abuse, neglect, bullying, discrimination, and hazing can be characterized as forms of maltreatment. Most forms of maltreatment occur when there is a power differential or imbalance in the relationship of perpetrator and victim. Essentially anyone involved in sport, from the athlete to their entourage, support team, personal supports, coaches, parents, administrators, officials, organization, fans (physically present as well as remote), social media contributors, peers, teammates, and sponsors, all represent both potential victims and perpetrators of maltreatment. This transactional relationship, viewed as a "maltreatment web," is illustrated in **Fig. 1**.

1. Abuse: In the sport setting, abuse has been defined in terms of psychological, physical, and sexual abuse.
    a. Psychological abuse: A pattern of deliberate, prolonged, repeated noncontact behaviors within a power-differentiated relationship. The behaviors that constitute psychological abuse target a person's inner life in all its profound scope.[4-6] Specific example of psychological abuse described by athletes include belittling, humiliating, shouting, scapegoating, rejecting, isolating, and threatening

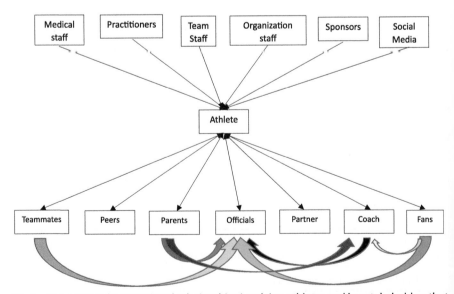

Fig. 1. The potential transactional relationships involving athletes and key stakeholders that create a "maltreatment web." Relationships more likely to feature unidirectional maltreatment are represented along the top of the diagram, while relationships that can feature bidirectional and complex multidimensional maltreatment are represented along the bottom.

behaviors, as well as being ignored or denied attention and support.[5,7–10] This term is often used interchangeably with emotional abuse.

b. Physical abuse: intentional trauma or physical injury caused by punching, beating, kicking, biting, burning, or otherwise harming an athlete. This could include forced or mandated inappropriate physical activity (eg, age-inappropriate or physique-inappropriate training loads, when injured or in pain), forced alcohol consumption, or systematic doping practices.[4] Other forms of physical abuse have also been identified, including excessive intensive training and physical violence by adults—including corporal punishment.[11]

c. Sexual abuse: Any conduct of a sexual nature with person(s) of any age that is perpetrated against the victim's will, without consent or in an aggressive, exploitative, manipulative, or threatening manner, including noncontact, contact, or penetrative, where consent is coerced/manipulated or is not or cannot be given.[7,12–15] Nontouching sexual abuse includes indecent exposure, unwanted or coerced observation of masturbation, masturbation in front of an athlete, sexually oriented comments, jokes or sexual innuendoes made to/about an athlete or other staff, taking or possessing revealing photos of an athlete, and coach discussing their sex life with an athlete.[1]

2. Harassment: Forms of harassment in sport include, but are not limited to, physical harassment, sexual harassment, psychological/emotional harassment, and harassment targeting gender, gender identity, race, and sexual orientation.[1] It involves unwanted or coerced behaviors that are in violation of an individual's human rights. Harassing behaviors can be directed toward an individual or a group and are considered to be based upon an abuse of power and trust by a person in a position of authority[1,16]; however, harassing behaviors can also be seen between other groups.

a. Psychological/emotional harassment: Harassing behaviors include any comment, conduct, or gesture directed toward an individual or a group of individuals, which is insulting, intimidating, humiliating, malicious, degrading, or offensive.[17] Individuals can experience harassment because of their race or ethnic origin, socio-economic status, culture, age, disability, gender, sexuality, or religious beliefs.[1] This can include put-downs or jokes about an individual; embarrassing/upsetting stories told about an individual; unwelcome, offensive, or hostile facial expressions or body gestures; and written or graphically derogatory material about the athlete.[1]

b. Physical harassment: Physically intimidating behaviors such as pushing, shoving or purposely bumping into a person, or other threatening or intimidating actions.[1]

c. Sexual harassment: Any unwanted and unwelcome conduct of a sexual nature, whether verbal, nonverbal, or physical.[4] This may include vulgar or lewd sexual comments, forcing an individual to wear sexually revealing attire, inappropriate/unwanted physical touching or fondling, repeated suggestions or propositions to engage in sexual conduct, and quid pro quo (ie, making an athlete's opportunities contingent on engagement in a particular sexual activity).[1]

d. Gender-based harassment: Reference to someone's gender in negative, vulgar, or derogatory terms, or exclusion of an individual based on gender.[1]

e. Race-based harassment: Reference to someone's race in negative, vulgar, or derogatory terms or exclusion of an individual based on race.[1] A component of racism.

f. Homophobia: Reference to someone's sexuality in negative, vulgar, or derogatory terms or exclusion of an individual based on sexual orientation.[1] Antipathy, contempt, prejudice, aversion, or hatred toward lesbian, gay, or bisexual individuals.[4]

3. Neglect: It is represented by a lack of reasonable care[18] and an all-round deprivation of attention,[19] which can be undertaken by coaches, athlete entourages, or senior leaders of the team. It has been characterized as passive or passive-aggressive inattention to an individual's needs, nurturing, or well-being.[20] Omissions in care can result in significant harm (physical or psychological) or risk of significant harm. Neglect is conceptualized into categories of physical, educational, emotional, and social neglect.[1] This definition equally applies to coaches and athlete entourages.

   a. Physical neglect: Including refusal or delay of health care, denying an athlete appropriate recovery time, and delaying medical assessment or treatment of a sport injury until the completion of a competition. Additional examples include abandonment of an athlete as punishment for poor performance; inadequate supervision during travel, training, or competition; inadequate spotting of an athlete on skills of foreseeable risk; inadequate nutrition, clothing, or hygiene; and prescribed dieting or other weight-control methods (eg, weigh-ins, caliper tests) without regard for the nutritional well-being and health of the athlete.[1]

   b. Educational neglect: Encouraging an athlete to miss classes for training or competition, encouraging an athlete to cease education for training and competition, and inattention to special education needs.[1]

   c. Psychological/emotional neglect: The concept of inadequate nurturing or affection or an unintentional chronic lack of attention or performance feedback that would be reasonably expected by an athlete (eg, ignoring lesser-performing athletes during training or competition, refusal of, or interference with, psychological care).[1]

   d. Social neglect: Inattention to social needs, chronic exclusion of an athlete from team social events, discouraging an athlete from having friendships with teammates/persons outside sport, chronic rejection, chronic unrealistic performance expectations, permitted maladaptive behavior (where the care giver has reason to be aware of the existence and seriousness of the problem and does not intervene).[1]

4. Bullying: Unwanted, repeated and intentional, aggressive behavior usually among peers and can involve a real or perceived power imbalance. Bullying can include actions such as making threats, spreading rumors or falsehoods, attacking someone physically or verbally, and deliberately excluding someone (4). It can include physical, verbal, or psychological attacks or intimidations that are intended to cause fear, distress, or harm to the victim. Bullying is based on an imbalance of power, with a more powerful individual oppressing the less-powerful one. It includes an absence of provocation by the victim and repeated incidents between the same individuals over a prolonged period of time.[1,21]

   a. Cyberbullying: Willful and repeated harm inflicted through the use of computers, cell phones, and other electronic devices.[22]

   b. Physical bullying: These behaviors include theft, hitting, kicking, punching, shoving, slapping, biting, and preventing a person from going somewhere.[1]

   c. Psychological/emotional bullying: It includes teasing, spreading rumors, threatening comments, name-calling, humiliation, and ridicule.[1]

   d. Social bullying (including hazing): Includes isolation from social activities or nonacceptance in a peer group, intentional exclusion of an athlete from postcompetition celebrations, and hazing or initiation rituals. Hazing is defined as "any humiliating or dangerous activity expected of someone to join a group regardless of willingness to participate."[23] Hazing activities in sport include being yelled at, cursed at, forced to associate with specific people, acting as a personal servant, being forced to drink excessively, destruction or theft of property, and simulation of sexual acts.[24]

5. Discrimination: Consists of making a distinction between groups or individuals, and treating those individuals or groups differently based on unjustified or illegal criteria.[25] Discrimination in sport frequently involves stigmatization on the basis of external characteristics such as skin color, body shape, and gender. The most common types of discrimination in sports are racism and homophobia, while religious and disability-related discrimination are also encountered.[25] Common expressions of discrimination are verbal, behavioral, direct, and indirect. Racism-based discrimination in sports is well described by Begel and includes physical violence, racial profiling, systemic/institutional racism, discriminatory decision-making, and microaggressions.[26]

PART 2: MALTREATMENT IN SPECIFIC SPORT POPULATIONS

Athlete maltreatment may be experienced by any athlete at any age in any sport at any level from any nation at any time; in other words, at any stage of the sport journey.[27–30] Despite the ubiquitous risk, some populations may have greater vulnerability due to specific characteristics of the athlete population in which they belong. Having an awareness of the risk of maltreatment among specific athlete groups can assist with screening, detection, and support.

Four groups of athletes have been identified to be at higher risk of maltreatment in sport: the child athlete,[31–33] the elite athlete,[33,34] athletes with a disability,[35] and athletes who identify as LGBTQ (lesbian, gay, bisexual, trans-sexual, queer).[36,37]

Youth Sports

Young athletes may be at exceptional risk of all types of maltreatment due, in part, to the youth sport environment in which the drive for extraordinary success is often prioritized.[33,38] Competitive sports have unique structures, cultures, and environments that create conditions that are conducive for maltreatment to occur. These include participation from a young age, significant power differentials between coaches and athletes, male-dominated gender ratios, authoritarian leadership, rewards for participation and performance, and special attention for the athletes whose skill clearly separates them from the rest.[39–42]

In addition to the risk of abuse, neglect, and boundary violations, youth athletes are vulnerable to commodification because of their exceptional skill and sport potential. Through "by proxy" ambitions, athletes become objects upon which perpetrators project their own ambitions and are tools used by the perpetrator (either consciously or unconsciously) to achieve what they perceive to be their own success.[33] Potential perpetrators of "achievement by proxy" can include anyone in positions of authority or influence in the athlete's life and career, including parents, coaches, mentors, agents, and others in the sports system.[33]

Numerous studies have explored the prevalence of various types of mistreatment in youth sports. One study involving elite Canadian athletes reported a prevalence rate of sexual abuse prior to the age of 16 years at 1.9%,[43] while a retrospective study of elite Australian athletes identified a prevalence rate of sexual abuse prior to the age of 18 years as 9.7%.[44] Among more than 60,000 youth athletes in a large UK study, prevalence rates of 3% for sexual abuse and 29% for sexual harassment were reported.[45] Another study surveying Canadian youth athletes in 2015 reported that 14% of the cohort experienced bullying in sport.[46] A retrospective survey of 4000 adults in Belgium and the Netherlands revealed that almost half (44%) experienced at least one form of harassment and abuse as youth athletes, including 14% of respondents who experienced sexual abuse, 11% of whom experienced physical abuse, and 33% of whom experienced psychological abuse.[47]

The origins of safe sport were rooted in the recognition of the vital need to protect children in sports. Many of the foundational documents emphasizing the rights of individuals to an environment free from harassment and abuse are grounded in the United Nations Convention on the Rights of the Child (1989), specifically in articles 19 and 31.[48] While this document does not specifically address youth sport, it identifies the rights of children that should be protected from maltreatment in all aspects of life, including recreational activities. Publications describing the importance of upholding human rights to prevent discrimination and violence in sport were first published in 1998[49] and 2004[50] by the former Secretary of the Committee on the Rights of the Child in the UN Office of the High Commission. A fundamental document published by the United Nations Children's Fund (UNICEF) in 2010[51] reported the lack of child protection policies against harassment and abuse in sport from 119 countries surveyed despite the previous call to action in the UN World Report on Violence against Children.[52]

High-Performance Sports

Evidence demonstrates that the elite athletes are at elevated risk of maltreatment relative to athletes who compete at the recreational level.[29,33,34,53] In fact, the risk of experiencing various types of maltreatment rises as the level of talent and competition increases.[29,30,34,39,53,54] The competitive sport environment can increase vulnerability to maltreatment when the focus on winning overshadows health or other reasons for sport participation.[55] For many athletes and parents, maltreatment is accepted as the price of success, and a form of cultural acquiescence occurs.[1,56] In an online survey of nearly 1000 current and former national team athletes, 75% endorsed experiencing at least one form of maltreatment, and at least one physically harmful behavior was reportedly experienced by 14.3%. The most commonly endorsed form of harmful behavior was psychological, with 24% of athletes reportedly experiencing an average of 2.6 psychologically harmful behaviors, and 23.7% of athletes reported experiencing neglectful behaviors. Lower numbers of sexually harmful behaviors (4.7%) and physically harmful behaviors (3.4%) were reported.[57]

Professional Sports

Maltreatment can also be experienced by adult professional athletes irrespective of size, race, or gender. The National Football League franchise Miami Dolphins made headlines in 2013 when reports of bullying, hazing, and homophobic slurs emerged from their locker room.[58] Professional hockey team Chicago Blackhawks of the National Hockey League (NHL) settled a lawsuit with a former player in 2021 following an investigation regarding sexual abuse by a coach.[59] Widespread systemic abuse within the United States Women's Soccer Team and the National Women's Soccer League was exposed in a detailed report from an independent investigation that was commissioned by US Soccer.[60–62] Women's soccer also made headlines after three big-name players left the French National Team due to conditions that were described as harmful for their mental health. Various types of maltreatment were alleged.[63] In Sierra Leone, the women's soccer team sustained poor conditions, neglect, sexual harassment and abuse, psychological abuse, bullying, and exclusion.[64]

Disabled Athletes

Studies have demonstrated elevated rates of maltreatment among disabled athletes.[35,36] Estimations suggest that individuals with disabilities are at a four-times higher risk of being victimized than individuals without a disability,[65] with those with an intellectual disability in the highest risk group.[66] A comparison of victimization rates between children with and without disabilities indicated that children with disabilities are victimized at higher rates than those without disabilities (31% vs 9%).[67] In sport, youth athletes with disabilities are reported to experience double to triple the risk of psychological, physical, and sexual abuse and harassment when compared with youth athletes in general.[34]

Several individual and sport factors contribute to specific vulnerabilities to maltreatment faced by this group. These include uninformed assumptions being made about their care needs, exploiting the athlete's dependence for personal care (including communication, travel, competition management, assistance with getting into the competition attire [including bathing suits]), and blurring of roles, responsibilities, and boundaries in the coach-[68] and caregiver-relationships with the athlete.[36,69,70]

LGBTQIA2S+

Another group identified as having higher rates of discrimination, marginalization, persecution, maltreatment, oppression, and overt violence include those who identify as LGBTQIA2S+ (lesbian, gay, bisexual, transgender, queer and/or questioning, intersex, asexual, two-spirit, and other affirmative ways in which people choose to self-identify).[71] In many countries, this group is vulnerable to arrest, extortion, and even the death penalty where discriminatory laws criminalize consensual same-sex relationships.[71,72] Globally, trans individuals do not have a pathway for legal recognition of their gender identity, and in some countries, they are unable to access gender-affirming health care of any type. Intersex children and adults may be forced to undergo medically unnecessary interventions.[71] Athletes who identify with this group are also at a higher risk of maltreatment.[36,37] In an international survey of nearly 10,000 people in sport, it was reported that 80% of respondents either witnessed or experienced homophobia in sport.[37] Sport-based homophobia can manifest in several different ways, including systemically through employment conditions,[37,73] team selection, career duration,[74,75] and marginalization in the sport environment.[76] Several professional sports leagues have introduced "Pride" events in an attempt to promote inclusivity, reduce stigma, and create safe environments for players, staff, and fans. This promotion resulted in controversy in the NHL when several players refused to participate in Pride activities, stating that it did not align with their beliefs.[77] Inclusion of trans athletes in the current global sports structure has been a lightning rod for debate and will likely continue in this fashion for several years as elements of human rights, inclusivity, medical science, and sports science collide.

PART 3: OUTCOMES OF MALTREATMENT IN SPORTS

Maltreatment in sports has been associated with many negative outcomes in mental health, physical health, and sport involvement. Specific mental health effects include self-harm,[78] eating disorders,[13,14] depression, anxiety, avoidance, dependence, low self-esteem, substance abuse,[79] somatic manifestations of psychological disturbance, and suicide.[33,42,80] Elements of maltreatment such as grooming and gaslighting can have chronic impacts on relationships, self-esteem, confidence, and the ability for the victim to identify when they are at risk or experiencing maltreatment. Grooming is characterized by perpetrators slowly gaining trust before systematically breaking down interpersonal barriers.[13] Athletes may feel trapped into compliance because of trust, loyalty, and affinity or affection for their abuser. Grooming is often motivated by the abuser's quest for power and control, using threats, rewards, privileges, or special attention to ensure cooperation and manipulate the victims to maintain secrecy.[13] Gaslighting is characterized by the abuser causing the victim to question their own thoughts, beliefs, feelings, instincts, and sanity, which shifts the power balance to the abuser.[81] Perpetrators of gaslighting use techniques such as withholding, countering, blocking/diverting, trivializing, and denial to "break down" their victims. In sport, athletes who question perpetrator behavior in the grooming process may then experience gaslighting, as the abuser attempts to make the athlete question the veracity of their experiences and manipulate them into not sharing their suspicions with others.

Physical outcomes of maltreatment can include physical injury, urogenital trauma and infections, traumatic brain injury, unwanted pregnancy, and death.[44,82–84]

Maltreatment can lead to loss of opportunity and curtail an athlete's career in sport. Studies have demonstrated long-lasting effects of maltreatment on athletes including performance detriment, loss of sponsorship, and sport drop out.[4,8–10,73,76]

PART 4: SAFEGUARDING ATHLETES

The responsibility of safeguarding athletes falls on everyone involved in the athletes' lives and sport experience, including their parents, teammates, coaches, physicians, interdisciplinary support team (including sport scientists and allied health professionals), organizations, and governments. Safety is intricately associated with culture, expectations, codes of conduct, accountability, and consequences. Maltreatment occurs when there is a power imbalance and an abuse of power. These dynamics facilitate maltreatment and perpetuate silence and protectionism. Across all levels of sport athletes, parents, teammates, and staff fear repercussions for reporting maltreatment that is experienced, witnessed, or suspected. Comprehensive recommendations for action at the levels of the athlete, team, organization, sports medicine and allied health practitioners, and sports science researchers are described in detail elsewhere and are beyond the scope of this chapter.[4] However, it is recommended that the readers approach each athlete, particularly those in higher risk groups, with consideration of the potential for maltreatment; and approach each individual with a safe, open, empathetic exploration that can facilitate disclosure. It is important to be aware of personal bias, loyalties, and conflicts of interest when supporting athletes. Blind loyalty, indifference, ignorance, protectionism, and denial can lead to intentional or unintentional complicity and perpetuation of maltreatment.

PART 5: THE GREAT IMPASSE

Since the USA gymnasts became an unwitting force against maltreatment and organizational complicity,[85] dozens of groups of high-performance athletes have reported experiences of maltreatment to sports organizations, governments, and media.[86] Canadian athletes from several national sport organizations testified before a governmental committee about their experiences of maltreatment and organizational inaction and repeatedly requested a judicial inquiry into abuse in the Canadian sport system. Their requests were repeatedly denied by the government-appointed panel, and alternative suggestions from panel members included restorative justice.[87] Transformational justice was suggested by a group of Canadian scholars as an approach that would pursue systemic change by "situating survivors and abusers within social structures, past and present."[88] The process of transformational justice would address the root causes of violence to facilitate reimagining systems to "allow for more supportive, safe, and accountable communities."[88]

Athlete survivors of maltreatment are frequently silenced by the harassment and abuse process.[29,89] Conflicts of interest and organizational risk mitigation may prevent acknowledgment of maltreatment and acceptance of responsibility. This can lead to an impasse between survivors, sport organizations, and governments.

SUMMARY

Maltreatment in sport can take many forms and can be experienced by any athlete at any time. Maltreatment can have serious and long-lasting effects on the mental health, physical health, and athletic careers of victims. Certain athlete groups are at higher risk of maltreatment. Perpetrators and facilitators of maltreatment can include other athletes, coaches, staff, practitioners, sport administrators, parents, fans, and other members of the athlete entourage. Prevention and systemic change are only effective if structures and policies are established and enforced at every level of the sport. Safe, independent reporting and investigative pathways are necessary elements for safeguarding athletes. Conflicts of interest, denial, indifference, and protectionism facilitate maltreatment and prevent justice, accountability, and systemic change.

CLINICS CARE POINTS

- Maltreatment in sport can take many forms and can be experienced by any athlete at any time.
- Maltreatment can have serious and long-lasting effects on the mental health, physical health, and athletic careers of victims.
- Certain athlete groups are at higher risk of maltreatment. Perpetrators and facilitators of maltreatment can include other athletes, coaches, staff, practitioners, sport administrators, parents, fans, and other members of the athlete entourage.
- Each athlete, particularly those in higher risk groups, should be approached with consideration of the potential for maltreatment, and approach each individual with a safe, open, empathetic exploration that can facilitate disclosure.
- It is important to be aware of personal bias, loyalties, and conflicts of interest when supporting athletes.

DISCLOSURE

The author has nothing to disclose.

REFERENCES

1. Stirling AE. Definition and constituents of maltreatment in sport: establishing a conceptual framework for research practitioners. Br J Sports Med 2009;43: 1091–9.
2. Porter MR, Antonishak J, Reppucci ND. Policy and applied definitions of child maltreatment. In: Feerick MM, Knutson JF, Trickett PK, et al, editors. Child abuse and neglect: definitions, classifications, and a framework for research. Baltimore: Brooks Publishing; 2006. p. 331–41.
3. Crooks CV, Wolfe DA. Child abuse and neglect. In: Mash EJ, Barkley RA, editors. Assessment of childhood disorders. 4th edition. New York: Guilford Press; 2007. p. 1–17.
4. Mountjoy M, Brackenridge C, Arrington M, et al. International Olympic Committee consensus statement: harassment and abuse (non-accidental violence) in sport. Br J Sports Med 2016;50:1019–29.

5. Stirling AE, Kerr GA. Defining and categorizing emotional abuse in sport. Eur J Sport Sci 2008;8:173–81.

6. Stirling AE, Kerr GA. The perceived effects of elite athletes' experiences of emotional abuse in the coach-athlete relationship. Int J Sp Exerc Psychol 2013; 11:87–100.

7. Leahy T, Pretty G, Tenenbaum GA. Perpetrator methodology as a predictor of traumatic symptomatology in adult survivors of childhood sexual abuse. J Interpers Viol 2004;19:521–40.

8. Stafford A, Alexander K, Fry D. 'There was something that wasn't right because that was the only place I ever got treated like that': children and young people's experiences of emotional harm. Childhood 2015;22:121–37.

9. Gervis M, Dunn N. The emotional abuse of elite child athletes by their coaches. Child Abuse Rev 2004;13:215–23.

10. Pinheiro MC, Pimenta N, Resende R, et al. Gymnastics and child abuse: an analysis of former international Portuguese female artistic gymnasts. Sport Educ Soc 2014;19:435–50.

11. David P. Human rights in youth sport: a critical review of children's rights in competitive sports. New York: Routledge; 2005. p. 31–51.

12. Johansson S. Coach–athlete sexual relationships: if no means no does yes mean yes? Sport Educ Soc 2013;18:678–93.

13. Brackenridge C, Fasting K. The Grooming Process in Sport: Narratives of Sexual Harassment and Abuse. Auto/Biography 2005;13(1):33–51. https://doi.org/10.1191/0967550705ab016oa.

14. Owton H, Sparkes AC. Sexual abuse and the grooming process in sport: Learning from Bella's story. Sport Educ Soc 2017;22(6):732–43. https://doi.org/10.1080/13573322.2015.1063484.

15. Ryan GD, Lane SL. Juvenile sexual offending: causes, consequences, and correction. San Francisco (CA): Jossey-Bass; 1997. p. 3–9.

16. Ljungqvist A, Mountjoy M, Brackenridge C, et al. Consensus statement: sexual harassment and abuse in sport, 2007. http://multimedia.olympic.org/pdf/en_report_1125.pdf. Accessed March 20, 2023.

17. Skate Canada. Professional coaches' code of ethics. 2005. http://www. mbskates.ca/PDF/Coaches/Coaching%20Code%20of%20Ethics%20- %20as%20of%20Setember%202005.pdf. Accessed March 25, 2023.

18. Glaser D. Emotional abuse and neglect (psychological maltreatment): a conceptual framework. Child Abuse Neglect 2002;26:697–714.

19. Iwaniec D. Identifying and dealing with emotional abuse and neglect. Child Care Pract 2003;9:49–61.

20. American Humane Association. Definitions of the national study data items and response categories: technical report #3. Denver: American Humane Association; 1980.

21. Ferrington DP. Understanding and preventing bullying. Crime Justice 1993;17: 381–458.

22. Hinduja S, Patchin J. Cyberbullying: identification, prevention and response. Cyberbullying Research Center; 2022. https://cyberbullying.org/Cyberbullying-Identification-Prevention-Response-2022.pdf. Accessed March 26, 2023.

23. Hoover NC, Pollard N. Initiation rites in American high schools: a national survey. New York: Alfred University; 2000.

24. Hinkle SL. Cognitive dissonance in athletic hazing: the roles of commitment and athletic identity. Unpublished doctoral dissertation. University of Northern Colorado, Greeley, Colorado: United States of America, 2005.

25. European parliament in history briefing: fighting discrimination in sport. European Union; 2020. www.europarl.europa.eu/RegData/etudes/BRIE/2021/696163/EPRS_BRI(2021)696163_EN.pdf. Accessed March 26, 2023.
26. Begel Dan. Tackling racism in sports psychiatry. Sports Psychiatry 2023;1–10. https://doi.org/10.1024/2674-0052/a000041.
27. Edwards C, Claussen MC, Schmidt RE. Mental health impacts of interpersonal violence in sports [Editorial]. Sports Psychiatry: Journal of Sports and Exercise Psychiatry 2023;2(1):1–2.
28. Parent S, Fortier K. Prevalence of interpersonal violence against athletes in the sport context. Curr Opin Psychol 2017;16:165–9.
29. Leahy T, Pretty G, Tenenbaum G. Prevalence of sexual abuse in organised competitive sport in Australia. J Sex Aggress 2002;8(16–36):548.
30. Fasting K, Brackenridge C, Knorre N. Performance level and sexual harassment prevalence among female athletes in the Czech Republic. WSPAJ 2010;19: 26–32.
31. LSEPS. European Union kids online report. London: Science LSoEaP; 2014.
32. Council of Europe. Start to talk, 2019. Available: https://www.coe.int/en/web/sport/start-to-talk Accessed 1 Nov 2021.
33. Tofler IR, Knapp PK, Lardon MT. Achievement by Proxy Distortion in Sports: A Distorted Mentoring of High-achieving Youth. Historical Perspectives and Clinical Intervention with Children, Adolescents and their Families. Clin Sports Med 2005; 24:805–28.
34. Vertommen T, Schipper-van Veldhoven NHMJ, Hartill MJ, et al. Sexual harassment and abuse in sport: the NOC*NSF helpline. Int Rev Sociol Sport 2015;50: 822–39.
35. Tuakli-Wosornu YA, Sun Q, Gentry M, et al. Non-accidental harms ('abuse') in athletes with impairment ('para athletes'): a state-of-the-art review. Br J Sports Med 2020;54(3):129.
36. Kirby SL, Demers G, Parent S. Vulnerability/prevention: Considering the needs of disabled and gay athletes in the context of sexual harassment and abuse. Int J Sport & Exerc Psych 2008;6(4):407–26.
37. Denison E, Kitchen A. Out on the fields, the first international study on homophobia in sport. Nielsen, Bingham Cup Sydney 2014, Australian Sports Commission, Federation of Gay Games. 2015. Available: http://www.outonthefields.com/wp-content/uploads/2016/04/Out-on-the-Fields-Final-Report.pdf Accessed March 28, 2023.
38. Mountjoy M and Edwards C. (2022). Athlete mental health impacts of harassment and abuse in sport. 10.1007/978-3-031-08364-8_16.
39. Alexander K, Stafford A, Lewis R. The experiences of children participating in organised sport in the UK. Edinburgh: Dunedin Academic Press; 2001.
40. Brackenridge CH. Violence and abuse prevention in sport. In: Kaufman K, editor. The prevention of sexual violence: a practitioners' sourcebook. Holyoke, MA: NEARI Press; 2010. p. 401–13.
41. Cense M, Brackenridge CH. Temporal and developmental risk factors for sexual harassment and abuse in sport. Eur Phys Educ Rev 2001;7(1):61–79.
42. Kirby S, Greaves L, Hankivsky O. The dome of silence: sexual harassment and abuse in sport. Halifax: Fernwood Publishing; 2000.
43. Raakman E, Dorsch K, Rhind D. The development of a typology of abusive coaching behaviours within youth sport. Int J Sports Sci Coach 2010;5:503–15.
44. Timpka T, Spreco A, Dahlstrom, et al. Suicidal thoughts (ideation) among elite athletics (track and field) athletes: cross-sectional study of associations with

sexual and physical abuse victimization, aspects of sports participation, and psychological and behavioural resourcefulness. Br J Sports Med 2021 Feb;55(4): 198–205.

45. Alexander K, Stafford A, Lewis R. The experiences of children participating in organised sport in the UK. London: NSPCC; 2011.

46. Evans B, Adler A, Macdonald D, et al. Bullying victimization, and perpetration among adolescent sport teammates. Pediatr Exerc Sci 2016;28(2):296–303.

47. Vertommen T, Schipper-van Veldhoven N, Wouters K, et al. Interpersonal violence against children in sport in the Netherlands and Belgium. Child Abuse Negl 2016; 51:223–36.

48. UN Article. UNCRC. United nations Convention on the rights of the child: Resolution adopted by the general assembly. Geneva (Switzerland): United Nations; 1989. Available: https://www.unicef.org/child-rights-convention/convention-text#. Accessed April 1, 2023.

49. David P. Children's Rights and Sport. Olympic review: Revue Olympique. 24. Lausanne: International Olympic Committee; 1998. p. 36–45.

50. David P. Human rights in youth sport: a critical review of Children's rights in competitive sport. Taylor & Francis; 2004.

51. Brackenridge C, Fasting K, Kirby S, et al. Protecting children from violence in sport: a review with a focus on industrialized countries. UNICEF Innocenti Research Centre; 2010. ISBN: 978-88-89129-96-8 Available at: https://www.unicef-irc.org/publications/pdf/violence_in_sport.pdf. Accessed 28 March 2023.

52. Pinheiro PS. United Nations Secretary-General's World report on violence against children. (2006) United Nations. Available: http://www.violencestudy.org/IMG/pdf/English.pdf Accessed 28 Mar 2023.

53. Fasting K, Brackenridge C, Sundgot-Borgen J. Experiences of sexual harassment and abuse among Norwegian elite female athletes and nonathletes. Res Q Exerc Sport 2003;74(1):84–97.

54. Douglas K, Carless D. Life story research in sport: understanding the experiences of elite and professional athletes through narrative. London: Routledge; 2014.

55. Tofler I, DiGeronimo TF. Keeping your kids out front without kicking them from behind: how to nurture high-achieving athletes, scholars, and performing artists. San Francisco (CA): Jossey-Bass; 2000.

56. Stirling AE, Kerr GA. Elite female swimmers' experiences of emotional abuse across time. J Emot Abuse 2007;7:89–113.

57. Willson E, Kerr G, Stirling A, et al. Prevalence of Maltreatment Among Canadian National Team Athletes. J Interpers Violence 2022;37(Issue 21–22). https://doi.org/10.1177/08862605211045096.

58. ESPN.com ESPN News Service. Incognito, others tormented Martin. 2014. https://www.espn.com/nfl/story/_/id/10455447/miami-dolphins-bullying-report-released-richie-incognito-others-responsible-harassment. Accessed March 29, 2023.

59. ESPN.com ESPN News Service. Chicago Blackhawks, Kyle Beach reach settlement on lawsuit. December 15, 2021. https://www.espn.com/nhl/story/_/id/32878093/chicago-blackhawks-kyle-beach-reach-settlement-lawsuit. Accessed March 29, 2023.

60. Gregory S. Time. 'Horrified and Heartbroken.' Allegations of Abuse Shake U.S. Women's Soccer https://time.com/6219654/us-womens-soccer-abuse/October 5, 2022. Accessed March 29, 2023.

61. Yates S. Report of the Independent Investigation to the U.S. Soccer Federation Concerning Allegations of Abusive Behavior and Sexual Misconduct in Women's Professional Soccer OCTOBER 3, 2022. https://www.documentcloud.org/documents/23117289-king___spalding_-_full_report_to_ussf?responsive=1&title=0. Accessed March 29, 2023.

62. Tennery A. Inquiry shows abuse, misconduct 'systemic' in U.S. National Women's Soccer League. October 3, 2022. https://www.reuters.com/lifestyle/sports/inquiry-shows-abuse-misconduct-systemic-us-top-flight-nwsl-2022-10-03/.

63. AFP. France football mutiny as three stars quit national women's team. February 24, 2023. https://www.france24.com/en/live-news/20230224-france-football-mutiny-as-three-stars-quit-national-women-s-team. Accessed March 30, 2023.

64. Aarons E, Molina R and Cizmic A. The Guardian. Sun 26 Mar 2023. 'I've seen hell': the allegations rocking women's football in Sierra Leone. https://www.theguardian.com/football/2023/mar/26/ive-seen-hell-the-allegations-rocking-womens-football-in-sierra-leone. Accessed March 30, 2023.

65. Sobsey D. Violence and abuse in the lives of people with disabilities: the end of silent acceptance? Baltimore (MD): Paul H. Brooks; 1994.

66. Sobsey D, Doe T. Patterns of sexual abuse and assault. Sex Disabil 1991;9: 243–59.

67. Sullivan PM, Knutson JF. Maltreatment and disabilities: a population based epidemiological study. Child Abuse Negl 2000;24:1257–73.

68. Valenti-Hein D, Schwartz L. The sexual abuse interview for those with developmental difficulties. Santa Barbara (CA): James Stanfield Company; 1995.

69. CPSU. International safeguards for children in sport. NSPCC; 2014.

70. Kerr A. Protecting disabled children and adults in sport and recreation—the guide. Leeds (United Kingdom): The National Coaching Foundation; 1999.

71. UN Human Rights Office of the High Commissioner. Human Rights Topics: LGBTI People https://www.ohchr.org/en/topic/lgbti-people?gclid=CjwKCAjwrJ-hBhB7EiwAuyBVXVhNPvV72-vqWrDPKftF_BYZk2Md3xjwaD-_ulsSw7vqmFh1WlR0JRoCoQIQAvD_BwE. Accessed April 1, 2023.

72. Everett C. South Africa progressive on LGBT rights but gays still battle for social reform. Int Bus 2014;2011.

73. CAAWS. Seeing the invisible, speaking about the unspoken: a position paper on homophobia. Ottawa (Ontario): Canadian Association for the Advancement of Women in Sport and Physical Activity; 2012.

74. Griffin P. Strong women, deep closets—lesbians and homophobia in sport. Champaign (IL): Human Kinetics; 1998.

75. Gall D. Play fair. Sportsnet, 2015.

76. Demers G. Homophobia in sport: fact of life, taboo subject. Can J Women Coaching 2006;6:1–13.

77. Logan N. As NHL teams, players opt out of Pride Night events, concerns grow about league's commitment to change. CBC News; 2023. https://www.cbc.ca/news/canada/nhl-hockey-pride-lgbtq-1.6790930. Accessed April 1, 2023.

78. Chaplo SD, Kerig PK, Bennett DC, et al. The roles of emotion dysregulation and dissociation in the association between sexual abuse and self-injury among juvenile justice–involved youth. J Trauma & Dissociation 2015;16:272–85.

79. Brennan C. USA Today. October 7, 2022. Former figure skater Bridget Namiotka dead at 32 after coming forward as victim of sexual abuse. https://www.usatoday.com/story/sports/olympics/2022/10/07/former-us-pairs-figure-skater-bridget-namiotka-dies/8207385001/Accessed April 1, 2023.

80. Human Rights Watch. "I was hit so many times, I can't count." July 20, 2020. https://www.hrw.org/report/2020/07/20/i-was-hit-so-many-times-i-cant-count/ abuse-child-athletes-japan Accessed April 1, 2023.
81. National Domestic Violence Hotline. What Is Gaslighting? https://www.thehotline.org/resources/what-is-gaslighting/. Accessed April 1, 2023.
82. Burke M. Obeying until it hurts: coach-athlete relationships. J Philos Sp 2001;28: 227–40.
83. Marks S, Mountjoy M, Marcus M. Sexual harassment and abuse in sport: the role of the team doctor. Br J Sports Med 2012;46:905–8.
84. Matza, Max. BBC. Settlement after US student athlete Grant Brace died begging for water. March 17, 2023. https://www.bbc.com/news/world-us-canada-64985192. Accessed April 1, 2023.
85. Rahal S, Kozlowski K. 204 impact statements, 9 days, 2 counties, a life sentence for Larry Nassar. Detroit News; 2018. Available: https://www.detroitnews.com/story/news/local/michigan/2018/02/08/204-impact-statements-9-days-2-counties-life-sentence-larry-nassar/1066335001/. Accessed April 1, 2023.
86. Hall M. The Guardian. 'Tip of the iceberg': why abuse in Canadian sport is worse than it seems. January 27, 2023. https://www.theguardian.com/sport/2023/jan/27/abuse-canada-sport-inquiry-hockey-gymnastics-soccer. Accessed April 1, 2023.
87. Kerr G. The Globe and Mail. February 2, 2023. https://www.theglobeandmail.com/opinion/article-instead-of-another-judicial-inquiry-we-should-use-restorative-justice/. Accessed April 1, 2023.
88. Giannitsopolous S, Ross M, Dennie M, et al. The Conversation. How transformative justice can address abuse in Canadian sport. February 20, 2023. https://theconversation.com/how-transformative-justice-can-address-abuse-in-canadian-sport-198122. Accessed April 1, 2023.
89. Moushey B, Dvorchak B. Game over: jerry sandusky, penn state, and the culture of silence. New York: William Morrow; 2012.

Media's Effect on Athletes' Mental Health

Tammy Ng, MD[a], Howard Sanders, MD[a], Sarah Merrill, MD[b],
Marcia Faustin, MD[c,d],*

KEYWORDS

- Mental health • Traditional media • Social media • Diversity • Females • Athletes

KEY POINTS

- Athletes potentially face punitive measures for not complying with their sports media obligations.
- Compared to the general population, athletes have additional incentives to benefit from social media use.
- Athletes of diverse and minoritized backgrounds may be subject to marginalizing media coverage.
- Although media attention for athletes has various positive impacts, it can also serve as a profound source of stress and lead to negative mental health consequences.
- Understanding the potential negative impact of media on athletes' mental health may lead sports medicine medical staff to create ways to support the athlete's interactions with media through policies and procedures.

INTRODUCTION

In addition to being held as models of physical prowess, elite athletes are also expected to demonstrate mental and emotional "strength." Vulnerability about mental health has historically been stigmatized among competitive athletic culture, due in part to emotions being perceived as a weakness.[1–3] In recent years, sports medicine organizations across the world, including the American Medical Society for Sports Medicine (AMSSM), National Collegiate Athletics Association (NCAA), and the

[a] Department of Pediatrics, University of California, Davis, School of Medicine, 2516 Stockton Boulevard, Sacramento, CA 95817, USA; [b] Department of Family Medicine, University of California, San Diego, School of Medicine, 402 Dickinson Street, San Diego, CA 92103, USA; [c] Department of Family & Community Medicine, University of California, Davis, School of Medicine, 3301 C Street, Suite 1600, Sacramento, CA 95816, USA; [d] Department of Physical Medicine & Rehabilitation, University of California, Davis, School of Medicine, 3301 C Street, Suite 1600, Sacramento, CA 95816, USA
* Corresponding author. Department of Family & Community Medicine, University of California, Davis, School of Medicine, 3301 C Street, Suite 1600, Sacramento, CA 95816.
E-mail address: mfaustin@ucdavis.edu

Clin Sports Med 43 (2024) 187–198
https://doi.org/10.1016/j.csm.2023.06.022
0278-5919/24/© 2023 Elsevier Inc. All rights reserved.

International Olympic Committee (IOC) have acknowledged the importance of an athlete's mental health and made efforts to better identify mental health challenges in sport.[2,4-10] Although extensive research demonstrates that participating in sports positively impacts an athletes' mental health,[11-14] both the AMSSM and IOC have published statements acknowledging that the athletic environment has the potential to precipitate or exacerbate mental health issues.[4,5] Media exposure is a significant environmental element that can have a both a positive and negative impact on an athlete's performance.[2]

Media comes in many forms and fundamentally serves as a means of mass communication. Traditional media includes broadcast television, radio, and printed mediums such as newpapers and magazines.[15,16] Compared to newer forms of media, traditional media relies more heavily on objective third party reporters to share information, such as newscasters, radio hosts, or journalists.[17] The emergence of digital media, including social media, enables users to both consume and create content through a variety of formats, including text, photographs, video, and audio.[16,18] Popular social media platforms include Twitter, Facebook, Instagram, TikTok, Reddit, and Snapchat. Each social media platform has its unique features. For instance, Twitter messages are currently limited to 280 characters, and photos and videos shared on Snapchat auto-delete after a set time period. Several social media platforms, such as Instagram and Snapchat, boast appearance-enhancing filters that users can apply to their photos and videos. TikTok is popular for its short-form videos, many of which last less than a minute. Although Facebook and Reddit are structured differently, both platforms provide users the opportunity to join forums based off of their interests.

ATHLETES' TRADITIONAL MEDIA OBLIGATIONS

Athletes may begin to interact with traditional media starting at the high school level and above, although elite-level athletes may begin to interact with media at a younger age, at both local, national, and international levels. Professional athletes interact with traditional media on a regular basis, and most professional sports have agreements with media press organizations.[19] The following is a brief overview of media obligations at each level of play and within the governing bodies of major professional sports.

At the high school level, there are typically no obligations for athletes to interact with the media. However, it is often sought after by players and coaches to generate collegiate and professional interest.[20,21] Some high school teams have policies and procedures in place that require formal media requests to gain sideline media access. To our knowledge, there are no easily identifiable cases in which high school administrators have placed restrictions on high school athlete-media interactions, although this may vary by individual schools or school districts.

At the collegiate level, athletes are viewed by their schools as representatives of their institution and often require administrative approval prior to speaking to journalists or participating in media appearances. A 2020 study performed by the University of Florida College of Journalism and Communications found that 50 of 58 student-athlete handbooks from public universities "explicitly forbade athletes from speaking to journalists without permission from the athletic department."[22] This practice is controversial and viewed by some as the restriction of free speech.[22] Many college and universities provide introductory media training for their athletes.[23]

Professional athletes' media obligations are typically set forth in written player agreements developed jointly by players associations, their respective league, and the league's primary sports journalism organization(s).[24–26] In general, professional athletes are required to interact with the traditional media on a regular basis, typically anywhere from 10 to 20 minutes following the conclusion of the game.[19] Some professional sports organizations, such as the National Football League (NFL) prepare athletes by providing media training, including on-set workshops with broadcast networks, and brand management.[24,27]

In the past decade, there have been several high profile cases of athletes who have refused media participation, resulting in fines and, ironically, attention-grabbing news stories. For example, in 2015, Seattle Seahawks star running back Marshawn Lynch was threatened with a $500,000 fine for not participating in the Super Bowl XLIX media day.[28] In response, Lynch gave an interview at the media day, famously repeating, "I'm just here so I won't get fined."[28] In 2021, the NBA fined the Brooklyn Nets and star player Kyrie Irving $35,000 over Irving's "repeated refusal to participate in postgame media availability."[29] At the 2021 French Open, 2nd seed ranked Naomi Osaka announced that she would not participate in required post-match news conferences, citing mental health concerns. She incurred a $15,000 fine and withdrew from the tournament.[30] Similarly, in 2016, Venus Williams was fined $5,000 for skipping a post-match press conference at the Australian Open.[31]

Olympic level athletes are also subject to required interaction with media. To prepare, training courses that provide education regarding media interaction, sponsorship attraction, as well as image and crisis management are required by the International Olympic Committee.[32] Victorious Olympic athletes often participate in press tours following high-profile medal victories to capitalize on fan excitement, maximize visibility immediately following events, and optimize monetary gains in the form of sponsorships or brand collaborations.[33–49] Athletes are expected to follow media rules at both the national and international level regarding freedom of speech and display of an athlete's own values.[50] The IOC Rule 50 guidelines developed by the IOC Athletes' Commission, last updated for the 2020 Tokyo Olympics, gives athletes permission to express their personal and political views during press conferences, interviews, at team meetings, and on digital media platforms in accordance with local laws; players are restricted from voicing these views on the field of play or on the award podium.[50]

ATHLETES AND SOCIAL MEDIA

It is difficult to understate the popularity of social media worldwide, with estimates that of the world's 7.81 billion people, 4.74 billion use social media as of 2022.[51] Of the major social media platforms, Facebook is the largest, with an estimated 2.9 billion users.[51] It is estimated that 90% of Americans interact with social media.[51]

There is a large body of research that explores the associations between social media and mental health in the general population. Since the emergence of social media in the early 2000's, rates of anxiety, depression, and suicidality among all age groups have increased dramatically.[52–55] One systematic review of 13 studies found that time spent on social media, social media activity, social media addiction, and social media investment were all positively correlated with "depression, anxiety, and psychological distress."[56] In addition, there is an alarming link between eating disorders and social media use, which was identified by Facebook's own internal research and leaked to the United States government.[57] Independent research studies align with Facebook's findings, and one meta-analysis found a small but statistically significant relationship between body image disturbance and social media use, with video-based platforms posing an even higher risk.[58] Another study of 996 adolescents found that time spent on Instagram was positively correlated with higher Eating Disorder Examination-Questionnaire scores.[3] The relationship between eating disorders and social media use amongst athletes specifically is an area that deserves further investigation and possible intervention.

Compared to the average social media user, athletes have additional incentives to use social media, including self-promotion, recruitment, and industry networking that may ultimately lead to sponsorships and financial support. Athletes also often use their wide reach on social media to express personal beliefs, educate followers, promote social change and social justice, and bring attention to world events. In 2021, the Name, Image and Likeness (NIL) agreement passed, allowing NCAA collegiate athletes to profit off their name, which further motivates athletes to utilize social media for monetary gains.[59,60] While this change may lead to positive financial gains for collegiate athletes, some fear that this added pressure may have harmful long-term effects on one's mental health.[60] There are currently no major studies that specifically address the effect of social media use on the different aspect of an athletes' mental health. Thus, this area will require further investigation, as social media continues to play a prominent role in athletics at all levels.

TRADITIONAL MEDIA COVERAGE OF FEMALE ATHLETES

The number of female athletes participating in sports has increased tremendously over the past decade. At the 2020 Tokyo Olympics and 2022 Beijing Olympics, females made up 48% and 45% of participants, respectively.[33,34] However, media coverage has not reflected this progress, as research has consistently shown that female athletes receive less media coverage compared to their male counterparts at all levels of sports.[34–45] In fact, several longitudinal studies have shown that media coverage of female athletes and women's sport has even declined over the years.[34,37,44,46–49]

Despite females participating in sports in record numbers and exhibiting record setting performances, they continue to experience disproportionate and trivializing media coverage that can negatively impact perceptions of their athleticism.[34] Extensive qualitative literature has demonstrated that coverage of female athletes in sports media often focuses on their attractiveness rather than their athleticism.[43,61–64] Unfortunately, athletes whose coverage focuses on their attractiveness may be perceived as less talented and viewed less favorably compared to athletes whose coverage focuses on their athletic ability.[61]

Substantial research in the area of eating disorders suggests that media exposure to the "thin ideal" is related to increases in disordered eating among the adolescent female population.[61] A smaller body of emerging research evaluates exposure to sports media specifically and its effects on athletes' body image.[65] In one study, researchers surveyed Division 1 female collegiate athletes on their exposures to entertainment and sports media.[65] The study disturbingly found that neither participation in a competitive sport nor sports media exposure mitigated the harmful messages found in entertainment media, with the athletes demonstrating surprisingly high levels of eating disordered behaviors.[65] This research suggests that even indirect interactions with media can have profound negative effects on athletes, especially females.

MEDIA AND ATHLETES OF MINORITIZED BACKGROUNDS

Ethnically & racially diverse athletes are often exposed to interpersonal and institutional racism, which can negatively impact mental health.[66,67] Recognizing that student athletes of minoritized backgrounds endure racial inequities and systemic marginalization placing them at higher risk of poor mental health, the NCAA's Summit on Diverse Student-Athlete Mental Health and Well-Being released a consensus statement addressing the mental health needs of student-athletes of color.[67–69] This statement acknowledged that individuals experiencing more stress related to their minority racial identity tend to have significantly more depressive symptoms.[67,70]

Stress experienced by individuals who identify as coming from a minoritized background–whether due to race, sexual identity, sexual orientation, or disability– can be magnified by media coverage. Media can be highly influential in framing ideas about race, on one hand, celebrating the achievements of these individuals, and on the other hand, reinforcing racist, sexist or discriminatory stereotypes.[71] Although media portrayals of individuals from minoritized backgrounds have been shown to influence viewers' perception of these groups,[72] the consequences of racial stereotypes perpetuated by sport media may be underrecognized or under-acknowledged. Given that sport media reaches a large and broad audience, one can argue that it plays an influential and critical role in disseminating, maintaining, or dismantling racial stereotypes.

By analyzing verbal content of traditional sports media, researchers have found differences in sports commentary between athletes of different races or ethnicities.[71] One early study found that football commentators gave white athletes more play-related praise and portrayed them in a more positive light than black athletes.[71,73] Although overtly racist messages have largely disappeared from sport broadcasts, multiple content analysis studies of sports commentary have found that more covert ethnic and racial biases still occur.[71] For instance, a Detroit Tigers television analyst was suspended for mocking Los Angeles Angels player Shohei Ohtani by using an offensive accent while discussing his performance on air.[74]

Furthermore, studies have found that black athletes are often portrayed as 'naturally' athletic, whereas white athletes are often portrayed as being harder-working or equipped with better decision-making skills.[71,75–80]

Although social media platforms enable athletes to interact with their fans, they can also expose athletes, especially athletes of minoritized backgrounds, to online abuse. Online environments provide an anonymity that allows for an abandonment of social restrictions and thus serves as a space for abuse targeted at high-profile individuals, such as athletes.[81] One study analyzing the online abuse of athletes on Facebook and Twitter during the 2015 Wimbledon Tennis Championships found that of the top five seeded athletes, Serena Williams received an overwhelming number of abusive posts.[81] Serena Williams was subject to severe sexualized threats of violence and racially charged hostility,[81] perhaps, because as Adjepong and Carrington explain, 'black sportswomen exist at the intersections of racial, gendered, sexual, and classed oppression'.[82]

However, social media also gives ethnically diverse athletes backgrounds a platform, and possibly power to fight back against and raise awareness about social injustices, although not always free of negative consequences.[83,84] Social media platforms enable athletes to participate in activism and advocacy efforts and spur collective action in response to social injustices.[83,84] Given that high-profile athletes often receive much attention on social media, they can spearhead and bring awareness to important social issues in front of large audiences.[83,84] For instance, in response to the murder of George Floyd, an unarmed Black man by a white police officer during Summer 2020, several NFL players not only utilized their social media platforms to protest police brutality, but also publicly criticized the NFL's delayed and vague response.[83] The day after several NFL athletes participated in a video demanding a statement of support from the NFL, the NFL's Commissioner responded by releasing a statement condemning systematic racism and police brutality.[83]

MEDIA ATTENTION AND THE MALE ATHLETE

Male athletes generally experience more media exposure and are not immune to the effects of the increased scrutiny. Studies evaluating the media most frequently consumed by male athletes found the outlets consistently portrayed male athletes as "strong, tough, aggressive, and above all, a winner," even willing to compromise long term health for athletic performance.[85] Media portrayals of the male "ideal" body type and gender role expectations are correlated with a rise in the prevalence of eating disorders and body dysmorphic disorders in males; a recent study found that males may represent up to 25% of all patients with eating disorders.[86] Elite male soccer players reported that social media, especially the expression of dissatisfaction with a player or the team by supporters is a powerful source of stress and anxiety.[87] A study of Australian elite athletes showed that experiencing financial hardship and social media abuse were uniquely associated with poorer mental health outcomes in men compared with women athletes.[88]

THE PRESSURES OF MEDIA ATTENTION

Elite athletes cope with a number of unique 'workplace' stressors, including injuries that can prematurely end careers, limited interpersonal support due to schedules, training and relocation, and intense public scrutiny through media.[89] Both traditional and digital media play a significant role in high-level sports, and given widespread access to the internet, even a local story can escalate to national or international media coverage.[90] The combination of intense mental and physical demands can make elite athletes more susceptible to mental health issues.[89,91]

Even professional athletes who have demonstrated considerable success in their sport feel the pressures of media scrutiny. Simone Biles, who was portrayed as the face of USA Gymnastics for the 2020 Tokyo Olympics and favored to win multiple medals, withdrew from the competition due to mental health reasons.[2] She later returned to compete, winning a bronze medal on the balance beam.[2] In one study, researchers interviewed four male elite athletes and six female elite athletes who had won at least two gold medals at separate Olympics or World Championships.[92] This study identified media attention as a source of stress surrounding high-profile events, leading to athletes isolating themselves from reporters to focus on competing; one athlete even contemplated ending his career after he became Olympic champion due to pressure and demands of media.[92] Another study investigated sources of stress experienced by seventeen U.S. national champion figure skaters and found that those who experienced more stress after winning their title attributed it to increased media attention, among other factors.[93] The constant public scrutiny athletes face in their day-to-day life is a prominent source of tension that can be magnified by media attention.[94]

From a team dynamics standpoint, media attention can also be damaging; it has the potential create or fuel problems within a team, most often after difficult losses.[90] In a study published in 2008, researchers interviewed four Norwegian female and four Norwegian male elite wrestlers on their perceptions of media coverage; the wrestlers' described media coverage as often focusing on sensationalism and scandals.[95] When a team has several "star" athletes competing for media attention, the competitive climate may also be exacerbated, sometimes to a team's detriment.[96]

Collegiate student athletes may also face greater pressure to engage in media attention due to the NIL policy change issued by the NCAA in 2021. Previously, student athletes were classified as amateurs, and thus not permitted to monetize their NIL.[97] Although the NIL policy change gives student athletes the potential to achieve monetization benefits, the financial incentive may also introduce substantial pressure for student athletes to invest in media attention and build their online presence through social media, possibly without proper media training.[97]

SUMMARY

Media comprises an essential, highly visible, and potentially lucrative component of collegiate, elite, professional and Olympic sports. At the professional and Olympic level, athletes are required by written agreements to engage with the media, ultimately increasing revenue by both increasing interest amongst sports fans and generating new fans. However, disparities among male and female athletes exist in both traditional media coverage and social media visibility. Likewise, discrepancies are apparent in the media coverage of athletes from minoritized or marginalized backgrounds.

Social media has created a far-reaching impact in the world and continues to gain traction. The widespread adoption of social media amongst high school, collegiate, elite, and professional athletes allow for interaction and dialogue between players, fans, and members of traditional media. Athletes who participate in sports less often covered by traditional media have utilized social media to expand their financial opportunities and increase athlete visibility to a much wider audience than what was previously achievable.

In all its forms, media places additional pressure on athletes. Proper interaction with traditional media is a skill that must be learned and developed, and the use of social media also requires thoughtful navigation. Educational and training courses designed to prepare athletes for traditional media interaction and social media use are being offered to athletes at both the collegiate, professional and Olympic levels.[23,24,27,32] Despite this, the challenges media presents to athletes can potentially be detrimental to mental health, as demonstrated by investigational studies. Social media presents different challenges and pressures that also may be harmful to athlete mental health, as evidenced by high-profile athlete commentary. Despite a wealth of studies that assess the effects of social media on the general public, there is a paucity of literature specifically addressing athlete mental health and social media use. This is an area of much needed additional research and may play a unique role in improving the overall well-being of athletes during their time of participation in athletics and beyond.

REFERENCES

1. Castaldelli-Maia JM, Gallinaro JGdMe, Falcão RS, et al. Mental health symptoms and disorders in elite athletes: a systematic review on cultural influencers and barriers to athletes seeking treatment. Br J Sports Med 2019;53(11):707–21.
2. Faustin M, Burton M, Callender S, et al. Effect of media on the mental health of elite athletes. Br J Sports Med 2022;56(3):123–4.
3. Wilksch SM, O'Shea A, Ho P, et al. The relationship between social media use and disordered eating in young adolescents. Int J Eat Disord 2020;53(1):96–106.
4. Chang CJ, Putukian M, Aerni G, et al. American medical society for sports medicine position statement: mental health issues and psychological factors in athletes: detection, management, effect on performance, and prevention—executive summary. Clin J Sport Med 2020;30(2):91–5.
5. Reardon CL, Hainline B, Aron CM, et al. Mental health in elite athletes: International olympic committee consensus statement (2019). Br J Sports Med 2019; 53(11):667–99.

6. Van Slingerland KJ, Durand-Bush N, Bradley L, et al. Canadian centre for mental health and sport (CCMHS) position statement: principles of mental health in competitive and high-performance sport. Clin J Sport Med 2019;29(3):173–80.

7. Gouttebarge V, Bindra A, Blauwet C, et al. International olympic committee (IOC) sport mental health assessment tool 1 (SMHAT-1) and sport mental health recognition Tool 1 (SMHRT-1): towards better support of athletes' mental health. Br J Sports Med 2021;55(1):30–7.

8. Henriksen K, Schinke R, Moesch K, et al. Consensus statement on improving the mental health of high performance athletes. Int J Sport Exerc Psychol 2020;18(5):553–60.

9. Vella SA, Schweickle MJ, Sutcliffe JT, et al. A systematic review and meta-synthesis of mental health position statements in sport: Scope, quality and future directions. Psychol Sport Exerc 2021;55:101946.

10. Force NMHT. Inter-Association Consensus Document: Best Practices for Understanding and Supporting Student-Athlete Mental Wellness. 2016. Available at: https://ncaaorg.s3.amazonaws.com/ssi/mental/SSI_MentalHealthBestPractices.pdf. Accessed February 20, 2023.

11. Downward P, Rasciute S. Does sport make you happy? An analysis of the well-being derived from sports participation. Int Rev Appl Econ 2011;25(3):331–48.

12. Jewett R, Sabiston CM, Brunet J, et al. School sport participation during adolescence and mental health in early adulthood. J Adolesc Health 2014;55(5):640–4.

13. Graupensperger S, Sutcliffe J, Vella SA. Prospective associations between sport participation and indices of mental health across adolescence. J Youth Adolesc 2021;50(7):1450–63.

14. Slutzky CB, Simpkins SD. The link between children's sport participation and self-esteem: exploring the mediating role of sport self-concept. Psychol Sport Exerc 2009;10(3):381–9.

15. Taipale S, Oinas T, Karhinen J. Heterogeneity of traditional and digital media use among older adults: a six-country comparison. Technol Soc 2021;66:101642.

16. Reid Chassiakos YL, Radesky J, Christakis D, et al. Children and adolescents and digital media. Pediatrics 2016;138(5). https://doi.org/10.1542/peds.2016-2593.

17. Fisher C. News Sources and Journalist/Source Interaction. In Communication (pp. 1). (Oxford Research Encyclopedia of Communication). Oxford University Press. 2018. https://doi.org/10.1093/acrefore/9780190228613.013.849.

18. Aichner T, Grunfelder M, Maurer O, et al. Twenty-five years of social media: a review of social media applications and definitions from 1994 to 2019. Cyberpsychol, Behav Soc Netw 2021;24(4):215–22.

19. Moritz B. What is sports media's role when it comes to mental health? Global Sport Matters 2022.

20. Reid J. For Some, Attention Is Too Hot To Handle: Coverage: Young athletes, eager to be cooperative and advance their careers, reveal items of a personal nature they later regret. Los Angeles Times. Available at: https://www.latimes.com/archives/la-xpm-1993-01-24-sp-2681-story.html. Accessed 17 February 2023.

21. Reid J. High School Sports and the Media: Coverage Gets Bigger, Imprint Turns Bolder: Overview: Prep reporters widening their scope to include girls' sports and off-the-field activities. Los Angeles Times. 1993. Available at: https://www.latimes.com/archives/la-xpm-1993-01-21-sp-2037-story.html.

22. LoMonte F. Universities Continue to Block Athletes from Talking to the Media. That's got to stop. Available at: https://www.jou.ufl.edu/insights/universities-continue-to-

block-athletes-from-talking-to-the-media-thats-got-to-stop/. Accessed 17 December 2022.

23. Karam T. Media Training. Available at: https://acsa.lsu.edu/sports/2013/11/1/ mediatraining.aspx?path=lifeskills. Accessed 23 January 2023.

24. 2021 NFL Media Access Policy. 2021. Available at: https://www.profootballwriters. org/wp-content/uploads/2021/09/21NFLMediaAccessPolicy.pdf.

25. Regular Season Club/Media Regulations.

26. NBA announces media availability and access policies for 2022-23 season. 2022. Available at: https://pr.nba.com/nba-media-availability-access-policies-2022-23-season/#:~:text=In%20order%20to%20qualify%20for,the%20teams'%20press %20conference%20rooms. Accessed 17 December 2022.

27. Support for players, on and off the field. Available at: https://operations.nfl.com/ inside-football-ops/players-legends/nfl-player-engagement/support-for-players-on-and-off-the-field/. Accessed 20 February, 2023.

28. Newport K. Marshawn Lynch at Super Bowl Media Day: 'I'm Just Here so I Won't Get Fined'. bleacherreport.com2015. https://bleacherreport.com/articles/2344416-marshawn-lynch-at-super-bowl-media-day-im-here-so-i-wont-get-fined.

29. Conway T. Kyrie Irving, Nets Fined $35K Each for Violating NBA's Media Access Rules. 2021. 5 May 2021. Available at: https://bleacherreport.com/articles/10002 109-kyrie-irving-nets-fined-35k-each-for-violating-nbas-media-access-rules. Accessed 20 February 2023.

30. Marnin J. WTA Says Athletes Have 'Responsibility' to Speak to Media After Naomi Osaka Forgoes French Open Press. Newsweek. Available at: https://www. newsweek.com/wta-says-athletes-have-responsibility-speak-media-after-naomi-osaka-forgoes-french-open-press-1595969.

31. Jackson R. Venus Williams hit with $5,000 fine for skipping post-match press conference. The Guardian. 2016. Available at: https://www.theguardian.com/sport/ 2016/jan/20/venus-williams-hit-with-5000-fine-for-skipping-post-match-press-conference. Accessed 23 January 2023.

32. Grow Your Brand Authentically. Available at: https://olympics.com/athlete365/ courses/sports-media/. Accessed 23 January, 2023.

33. Wilson A. The State of Women in College Sports. 2022:18. Title IX 50th Anniversary Report. Available at: https://www.ncaa.org/news/2022/6/23/media-center-title-ix-report-shows-gains-in-female-participation-though-rates-lag-increases-by-men. aspx.

34. Fink JS. Female athletes, women's sport, and the sport media commercial complex: have we really "come a long way, baby". Sport Manag Rev 2015;18(3):331–42.

35. Bishop R. Missing in action - Feature coverage of women's sports in Sports Illustrated. J Sport Soc Issues 2003;27(2):184–94.

36. Kian EM, Vincent J, Mondello M. Masculine hegemonic hoops: an analysis of media coverage of march madness. Sociol Sport J 2008;25(2):223–42.

37. Lumpkin A. Female representation in feature articles published by sports illustrated in the 1990s. Women Sport Phys Activ J 2009;18(2):38–51.

38. Pratt J, Grappendorf K, Grundvig A, et al. Gender differences in print media coverage of the 2004 summer Olympics in Athens, Greece. Women Sport Phys Activ J 2008;17(2):34–41.

39. Billings AC. From diving boards to pole vaults: gendered athlete portrayals in the "big four" sports at the 2004 athens summer Olympics. South Commun J 2007; 72(4):329–44.

40. Billings AC, Eastman ST. Gender, ethnicity, and nationality: formation of identity in NBC's 2000 Olympic coverage. Article. Int Rev Sociol Sport 2002;37(3):349–68.

41. Billings AC, Eastman ST. Framing identities: gender, ethnic, and national parity in network announcing of the 2002 Winter Olympics. Article. J Commun 2003;53: 369–86.

42. Caple H, Greenwood K, Lumby C. What league? the representation of female athletes in Australian television sports coverage. Article. Media Int Aust 2011;140: 137–46.

43. Clavio G, Eagleman AN. Gender and sexually suggestive images in sports blogs. J Sport Manag 2011 2011;25(4):295–304.

44. Cooky C, Messner M, Hextrum R. Women play sport, but not on TV a longitudinal study of televised news media. Commun Sport 2013;1:203–30.

45. Kian ETM, Mondello M, Vincent J. ESPN—The women's sports network? A content analysis of internet coverage of March madness. J Broadcast Electron Media 2009;53(3):477–95.

46. Billings AC, Angelini JR, Duke AH. Gendered Profiles of Olympic History: Sportscaster Dialogue in the 2008 Beijing Olympics. J Broadcast Electron Media 2010; 54(1):9–23.

47. Eagleman AN, Pedersen PM, Wharton B. Coverage by gender in ESPN the magazine: an examination of articles and photographs. Article. International Journal of Sport Management 2009;10(2):226–42.

48. Kane M. The Better sportswomen get, the more the media ignore them. Commun Sport 2013;1:231–6.

49. Weber J, Carini R. Where are the female athletes in sports illustrated? A content analysis of covers (2000–2011). Int Rev Sociol Sport 2013;48:196–203.

50. International Olympic Committee Athlete's Commission's recommendations on Rule 50 and Athlete Expression at the Olympic Games fully endorsed by the IOC Executive Board. 2020. Available at: https://olympics.com/ioc/news/ioc-athletes-commission-s-recommendations-on-rule-50-and-athlete-expression-at-the-olympic-games. Accessed February 20, 2023.

51. Ruby D. Social Media Users - How Many People Use Social Media in 2023. Available at: https://www.demandsage.com/social-media-users/. Accessed 22 December 2022.

52. Karim F, Oyewande AA, Abdalla LF, et al. Social media use and its connection to mental health: a systematic review. Cureus 2020;12(6):e8627.

53. Naslund JA, Bondre A, Torous J, et al. Social media and mental health: benefits, risks, and opportunities for research and practice. J Technol Behav Sci 2020;5(3): 245–57.

54. Thygesen H, Bonsaksen T, Schoultz M, et al. Social Media use and its associations with mental health 9 months after the COVID-19 outbreak: a cross-national study. Front Public Health 2021;9:752004.

55. Edosomwan S, Prakasan SK, Kouame D, et al. The history of social media and its impact on business. J Appl Manag Enterpren 2011;16(3):79.

56. Keles B, McCrae N, Grealish A. A systematic review: the influence of social media on depression, anxiety and psychological distress in adolescents. Int J Adolesc Youth 2020;25(1):79–93.

57. Keith M. Facebook's internal research found its Instagram platform contributes to eating disorders and suicidal thoughts in teenage girls, whistleblower says. Businessinsider.com 2021. https://www.businessinsider.com/facebook-knows-data-instagram-eating-disorders-suicidal-thoughts-whistleblower-2021-10.

58. Saiphoo AN, Vahedi Z. A meta-analytic review of the relationship between social media use and body image disturbance. Comput Hum Behav 2019;101:259–75.

59. Smith M. Social media dominates NIL activity, latest data shows. Sports Business Journal. 2022. 17 February 2022. Available at: https://www.sportsbusiness journal.com/Daily/Issues/2022/02/17/Marketing-and-Sponsorship/NIL-data.aspx. Accessed 20 February 2023.
60. Harris H, Brison NT, Dixon MA. Hidden consequences: examining the impact of NIL on athlete well-being. J Appl Sport Manag 2021;13(2):7.
61. Knight JL, Giuliano TA. He's a laker; she's a "looker": the consequences of gender-stereotypical portrayals of male and female athletes by the print media. Sex Roles 2001;45(3):217–29.
62. Daddario G. Gendered sports programming: 1992 summer olympic coverage and the feminine narrative form. Sociol Sport J 1997 1997;14(2):103–20. https://doi.org/10.1123/ssj.14.2.103.
63. Kane MJ. Media coverage of the female athlete before, during, and after Title IX: sports illustrated revisited. J Sport Manag 1988 1988;2(2):87–99.
64. Kane MJ. The post title IX female athlete in the media. J Phys Educ Recreat Dance 1989;60(3):58–62.
65. Bissell KL. Sports model/sports mind: the relationship between entertainment and sports media exposure, sports participation, and body image distortion in division i female athletes. Mass Commun Soc 2004;7(4):453–73.
66. Williams DR, Lawrence JA, Davis BA. Racism and health: evidence and needed research. Annu Rev Public Health 2019;40(1):105–25.
67. Kroshus E, Coakley S, Conway D, et al. Addressing mental health needs of NCAA student-athletes of colour: foundational concepts from the NCAA summit on diverse student-athlete mental health and well-being. Br J Sports Med 2023;57(3):137–45.
68. Betancourt JR, Green AR, Carrillo JE. Defining cultural competence: a practical framework for addressing racial/ethnic disparities in health and health care. Public health reports 2003;118(4):293.
69. New evidence regarding racial and ethnic disparities in mental health: policy implications. Health Aff 2008;27(2):393–403.
70. Sadberry S, Mobley M. Sociocultural and mental health adjustment of black student-athletes: within-group differences and institutional setting. J Clin Sport Psychol 2013 2013;7(1):1–21.
71. Van Sterkenburg J, Knoppers A, De Leeuw S. Race, ethnicity, and content analysis of the sports media: a critical reflection. Media Cult Soc 2010;32(5):819–39.
72. Morawitz E. and Ortiz M., Race, ethnicity, and the media, 2013, The Oxford Handbook of Media Psychology, 252–266.
73. Rainville RE, McCormick E. Extent of covert racial prejudice in pro football announcers' speech. Journal Q 1977;54(1):20–6.
74. Silva C. Baseball announcer Jack Morris suspended indefinitely for racist remark about Shohei Ohtani. NBC Asian American. 2023. Available at: https://www.nbcnews.com/news/asian-america/baseball-announcer-jack-morris-suspended-indefinitely-racist-remark-sh-rcna1707. Accessed March 4, 2023.
75. Maguire J. Sport, racism and British society: a sociological study of England's elite male Afro/Caribbean soccer and rugby union players. Basingstoke: Falmer Press; 1991. p. 94–123.
76. Maguire JA. Race and position assignment in english soccer: a preliminary analysis of ethnicity and sport in Britain. Sociol Sport J 1988;5(3):257–69.
77. Long J, Carrington B, Spracklen K. 'Asians cannot wear turbans in the scrum': explorations of racist discourse within professional rugby league. Leisure Stud 1997;16(4):249–59.

78. Davis LR, Harris O. Race and ethnicity in US sports media. In: MediaSport. 1st edition. Issue: 9780203014059; 1998. p. 154–69.
79. Rada JA, Wulfemeyer KT. Color coded: racial descriptors in television coverage of intercollegiate sports. J Broadcast Electron Media 2005;49(1):65–85.
80. Tyler Eastman ACBS. Biased voices of sports: racial and gender stereotyping in college basketball announcing. Howard J Commun 2001;12(4):183–201.
81. Litchfield C, Kavanagh E, Osborne J, et al. Social media and the politics of gender, race and identity: the case of Serena Williams. European Journal for Sport and Society 2018;15(2):154–70.
82. Adjepong L.A. and Carrington B., Black female athletes as space invaders. Routledge handbook of sport, gender and sexuality, 2014, Routledge, 189–198.
83. Brown-Devlin N. Examining the role of social media, employee voice, and the National Football League's organizational response to NFL athlete racial justice protests. Public Relat Inq 2023;12(1):71–91.
84. Sanderson J, Frederick E, Stocz M. When athlete activism clashes with group values: social identity threat management via social media. Mass Commun Soc 2016;19(3):301–22.
85. Madill L, Hopper TF. The best of the best discourse on health: Poetic insights on how professional sport socializes a family of men into hegemonic masculinity and physical inactivity. Am J Men's Health 2007;1(1):44–59.
86. Eichstadt M, Luzier J, Cho D, et al. Eating disorders in male athletes. Sports Health 2020;12(4):327–33.
87. Kvillemo P, Nilsson A, Strandberg AK, et al. Mental health problems, health risk behaviors, and prevention: a qualitative interview study on perceptions and attitudes among elite male soccer players. Front Public Health 2023;10:1044601.
88. Walton CC, Rice S, Gao CX, et al. Gender differences in mental health symptoms and risk factors in Australian elite athletes. BMJ open sport & exercise medicine 2021;7(1):e000984.
89. Rice SM, Purcell R, De Silva S, et al. The mental health of elite athletes: a narrative systematic review. Sports Med 2016;46(9):1333–53.
90. Dosil J. The sport psychologist's handbook: a guide for sport-specific performance enhancement. Wiley; 2005.
91. Hughes L, Leavey G. Setting the bar: athletes and vulnerability to mental illness. Br J Psychiatry 2012;200(2):95–6.
92. Durand-Bush N, Salmela JH. The development and maintenance of expert athletic performance: perceptions of world and Olympic Champions. J Appl Sport Psychol 2002;14(3):154–71.
93. Gould D, Jackson S, Finch L. Sources of stress in national champion figure skaters. J Sport Exerc Psychol 1993;15:134–59.
94. Noblet AJ, Gifford SM. The sources of stress experienced by professional australian footballers. J Appl Sport Psychol 2002;14(1):1–13.
95. Sisjord MK, Kristiansen E. Serious athletes or media clowns? Female and male wrestlers' perceptions of media constructions. Sociol Sport J 2008 2008;25(3):350–68.
96. Kristiansen E, Halvari H, Roberts GC. Organizational and media stress among professional football players: testing an achievement goal theory model. Scand J Med Sci Sports 2012;22(4):569–79.
97. Kunkel T, Baker BJ, Baker TA, et al. There is no nil in NIL: examining the social media value of student-athletes' names, images, and likeness. Sport Manag Rev 2021;24(5):839–61.

Mental Health of Elite Sport Coaches and Entourage

Rosemary Purcell, MPsych, PhD[a,b,*], Joshua Frost, BSc, MSc[a,b],
Vita Pilkington, BA (Hons)[a,b]

KEYWORDS

- Mental health • Wellbeing • Elite sport • Coach • Entourage • Support staff

KEY POINTS

- The mental health of elite coaches and entourage staff has been understudied, particularly in comparison to the mental health of elite athletes.
- Elite coaching and entourage staff are subject to similar sport-related stressors and mental health risk factors as elite athletes, such as performance demands, scrutiny, and travel away from home for sport.
- Available evidence, while scarce, shows that elite coaches and entourage experience depression, anxiety, and psychological distress at similar levels to elite athlete samples.
- Additional research is needed to strengthen understanding of the extent of mental ill-health and mental health needs among individuals working in elite-level sport alongside athletes.
- Based on the extant literature, mental health screening and interventions for elite athletes should be extended to the coaches and entourage staff working in the same high-performance environments.

INTRODUCTION

Research indicates that a range of sport-specific and general stressors are associated with mental health symptoms in elite athletes.[1,2] Sport-specific stressors include performance decline,[3] serious injury,[4–6] competing for selection, deselection,[7] and maladaptive perfectionism (characterized by setting unrealistic standards or seeking a high degree of control within the sport setting).[8,9] General risk indicators that may or may not be related to the sporting role include adverse life events, inadequate social support, unhelpful coping style (eg, avoidance), and sleep dysregulation.[10,11]

While elite athlete mental health has gained significant attention, the mental health of others within elite sports settings has received considerably less attention in the sports psychology literature. Although a small evidence base is developing regarding mental health among elite-level coaches, mental health among high-performance

[a] The Centre for Youth Mental Health, The University of Melbourne, Melbourne, Australia;
[b] Elite Sports and Mental Health, Orygen, 35 Poplar Road, Parkville, Victoria 3052, Australia
* Corresponding author.
E-mail address: rpurcell@unimelb.edu.au

Clin Sports Med 43 (2024) 199–211
https://doi.org/10.1016/j.csm.2023.06.005
0278-5919/24/© 2023 Elsevier Inc. All rights reserved.

support staff (HPSS; referred to throughout this article as "entourage") has been neglected. Entourage members include physiotherapists, strength and conditioning coaches, athletic trainers, and other allied health practitioners, such as nutritionists, sport psychologists, sports medicine physicians, player development managers, and athlete wellbeing advisors. Coaches and sports entourage staff operate within the broader "ecology" of elite sporting environments[12] and have critical roles to play in supporting the mental health of elite athletes.

Ecological systems can be used to conceptualize the relationship between the aspects or experiences of an individual and the broader socio-cultural contexts in which they work or operate.[13] Coaches and entourage (along with teammates and parents/family where appropriate) function as the core "microsystem" to support and enable elite athletes. Coaches and entourage interact with athletes in the daily training and competitive environments and therefore are often best placed (along with family or loved ones) to observe changes in an athlete's behavior, mental state, or demeanour (or in the case of some health staff, non-observable signs such as changes in muscle/body tension). Given the leadership and support roles that they occupy (in terms of supporting athletes' health, functioning, and performance), coaches and entourage can be critical to the early detection of mental ill-health and encouraging and supporting athletes to seek professional help.[12,14]

In comparison to the literature of elite athlete mental health, there has been a paucity of attention to the mental health of elite coaches and entourage despite them operating in the same high-performance environments and being subject to high expectations regarding individual or team performance outcomes. We speculate that elite coaches may be more susceptible to mental health challenges than their elite athletes because they encounter additional potential stressors in their roles, such as organisational responsibilities (including reporting to executives and boards); acting as the "public face" or spokesperson for their sport/team; educating, mentoring, and motivating their staff and athletes; long working hours; insecure employment; feeling undervalued in their role; and intense media scrutiny.[15–19] These are in addition to their key roles as technical and strategic experts. Finally, coaches and entourage also may have to contend with various personal stressors (often exacerbated by long work hours or role stress and scrutiny), such as social isolation and relationship difficulties.[17,20–23] Given the confluence of factors potentially impacting elite coaches, the lack of research consideration directed toward their mental health is surprising.

Prevalence and Risk Factors for Mental Health Symptoms in Elite Coaches

Several reviews have explored stressors and psychological health among elite coaches; however, most have focused on the constructs of wellbeing, coping, and burnout,[24–28] rather than mental health symptoms or disorders. The handful of studies that have considered common forms of mental ill-health—such as anxiety, depression, psychological distress, and alcohol use—are reviewed in the following sections. We provide the caveat that most participants in these research studies (over 70%) are men, rather than women. The overrepresentation of men in the literature is consistent with the broader gender imbalance observed in sports psychology literature[29] but also reflects the greater representation of men among elite coaching ranks.[30] Future research examining the mental health experiences of elite women coaches is a priority.

Anxiety and depression

A handful of studies have examined the prevalence of anxiety and depressive symptoms in elite coaching cohorts, with mixed results. Kegelaers and colleagues[22] reported that 39.5% of a large sample of Dutch and Flemish coaches ($n = 119$) reported anxiety and depression symptoms (assessed using the 12-item General Health Questionnaire), whereas in a smaller sample of New Zealand coaches ($n = 69$), Kim and colleagues[31] found that only 14.1% met the threshold for at least moderate depressive symptoms (assessed using the Center for Epidemiologic Studies Depression Scale-Revised). Among coaches seeking treatment for mental ill-health ($n = 34$), Åkesdotter and colleagues[32] found that the vast majority (93%) were experiencing clinical levels of anxiety, while 28% met diagnostic criteria for major depression.

Based on available research, known correlates of anxiety and depression symptoms among elite coaches include goal incongruence, poor coping effectiveness, contemplating retirement, family history of mood disorder, and increased frequency of daily hassles.[31,33] Burnout is also associated with mental ill-health among elite coaches and was found in two studies to be the strongest predictor of anxiety and depression,[34,35] although we note that burnout can be both a predictor and a consequence of mental ill-health.

General psychological distress

Rates of "high" psychological distress (eg, broadly defined as feelings of emotional pressure, anxiety, and/or reduced ability to cope with life) range from 10.3% to 19.3% in elite coaches,[22,23,34–36] although we note that different measures of psychological distress have been used across studies, which limits comparisons. Protective factors associated with reduced psychological distress among elite coaches include satisfaction with life balance, satisfaction with social support, and older age,[23] whereas one longitudinal study indicated that psychological distress was found to peak during the competitive mid-season in comparison to preseason.[35]

Substance use

Two studies have examined risky alcohol consumption in elite coaches using the same measurement tool (the Alcohol Use Disorder Identification Test-Concise); however, different cut-off scores were applied, resulting in discrepant results. The reported rate of risky alcohol consumption was 19.3% in the study by Kegelaers and colleagues[22] versus 48.3% in the study by Pilkington and colleagues.[23] The study by Åkesdotter and colleagues using a sample of mental health help-seeking coaches found that 17% met the diagnostic criteria for a substance-use disorder.[32] Most other research related to substance use in elite sport has largely focused on athletes' substance use, including reported alcohol consumption and doping behaviors and attitudes.

Other forms of mental ill-health

One study found that risk of eating disorder in a small cohort of National Collegiate Athletics Association Division I coaches ($n = 21$) was 38.1%.[37] Although the study by Åkesdotter and colleagues[32] also assessed eating disorder symptomatology among elite coaches (who were seeking outpatient mental health support), the number of coaches meeting eating disorder criteria was too small to report. However, Åkesdotter's study did find a high prevalence of stress and adjustment disorders among elite coaches, with 72% of coaches presenting to the service meeting criteria for stress-related disorders (including acute stress reactions, adjustment disorder, post-traumatic stress, other reactions to severe stress), relative to only 25% of elite athletes meeting criteria for stress-related disorders at the same service.

Sleep disturbance

While not a diagnosable mental disorder, sleep disturbance is recognized as both an antecedent and a consequence of mental ill-health.[38] Two studies reported similar prevalence rates of sleep disturbance in elite coaches (23.4% and 25.2%, respectively).[22,23] Several studies have reported an association between sleep disturbance and burnout.[39–41]

Burnout
Burnout is also not a mental health disorder but is one of the most frequently studied health outcomes in elite coaches and has been shown to act as a key correlate of mental ill-health in a number of studies. According to the World Health Organization, burnout refers to chronic workplace stress characterized by; 3 domains: emotional and physical exhaustion increased feelings of negativity or cynicism or mental distance from one's role: and a decrease in professional efficacy or accomplishment.

Studies that have investigated burnout in elite coaches report heterogeneous results, ranging from low,[42–47] through moderate,[42,46,48,49] and high[49] levels of burnout. In a large cohort of Finnish elite-level coaches ($n = 499$), 22% met criteria for mild burnout symptoms and 2% for severe symptoms.[44]- Correlates of high exhaustion in coaches at risk of burnout include negative perceptions of the sport organization's management and leadership, high workload, and performance outcomes (athlete win or loss records).[39]

Summary
While a growing interest in elite coach mental health is apparent, mental health among elite coaching staff remains poorly characterized, particularly relative to the elite athletes they support and mentor. Available data show significant variation in the reported rates of mental health symptoms among elite-level coaches, reflecting differences in sampling and measurement across studies. These methodological inconsistencies can be remediated by future studies consistently employing validated measures to assess mental health and wellbeing outcomes in sporting contexts (see Gouttebarge et al, [50]). To date, entourage staff have rarely been included in mental health literature.

AN EMPIRICAL STUDY OF MENTAL HEALTH IN ELITE COACHES AND SPORTS ENTOURAGE STAFF

The burgeoning research attention to the mental health of elite coaches has not been matched by consideration of other staff working within high-performance sport, despite the fact that elite coaches and entourage share many role-related stressors, including high workloads, competitive performance expectations, role insecurity, travel away from home, and social isolation.[51] To our knowledge, no empirical study has examined the prevalence of mental ill-health in HPSS and directly compared this to elite coaches, prior to our 2022 study.[23]

We surveyed a cohort of coaches ($n = 78$; mean age 46 years, 24% female) and HPSS ($n = 174$: mean age 40 years, 57% female) working in Australia's high-performance sports system to understand the prevalence and correlates of mental health symptoms and to explore similarities and differences in the mental health profiles between groups. The survey was conducted between March and May of 2020 and, therefore, coincided with the COVID-19 pandemic and associated lockdowns and interruptions to competitive sport. Key outcome measures included psychological distress, "caseness" (defined as symptoms of depression and anxiety at a level that would usually warrant treatment by a health professional), alcohol consumption, and sleep dysregulation. In addition to assessing the prevalence of mental health symptoms and wellbeing outcomes, we examined a range of possible correlates of these mental health and wellbeing outcomes. Possible correlates included demographic variables (eg, age, gender, relationship status, duration working in high-performance sport), adverse life events, overall satisfaction with life, satisfaction with social support, satisfaction with life balance, quality of life, and level of concern about COVID-19.

As shown in **Table 1**, the rates of mental health symptoms were consistent between elite level coaches and entourage/HPSS, with no statistically significant differences between groups across all outcome measures.

In addition to reporting similar levels of mental health symptoms, coaches and entourage also endorsed similar adverse life events, including almost half who reported feeling undervalued or underpaid (across the lifetime). The most robust correlates of coach and entourage mental health outcomes were satisfaction with life balance and satisfaction with social support. Life balance emerged as a widespread issue among the sample, with just over half the sample reporting they felt satisfied with their life balance at the time of the survey and others reporting the need for greater life balance.

The only demographic variable associated with a mental health outcome (in this instance, psychological distress) was age, with younger coaches and entourage reporting elevated levels of distress. Interestingly, no gender differences were found in this survey, which contrasts with the findings among elite athlete samples, where elevated rates of mental health symptoms are observed in female athletes.[52] This suggests a differential role of gender between athletes and members of the daily training environment that warrants further research attention.

The results of this study also demonstrate the relative consistency between the rates of mental health symptoms in coaches and entourage and those of the elite athletes with whom they work alongside. Reported rates were similar across probable caseness (43.6% of coaches, 40.1% of entourage, 35% of athletes[10]), psychological distress (10.3% of coaches, 15.5% of entourage, 17.7% of athletes[10]), and sleep disturbance (23.4% of coaches, 15.1% of support staff, 16.0% of athletes[53]), although risky drinking was reported at higher rates among coaches (48.1%) and entourage (39.0%), relative to published athlete samples (25.8%[54]). This reinforces the notion that stressors encountered within elite sports settings contribute to mental health difficulties among those regularly operating within these systems.[12]

Table 1		
Prevalence of reported mental health symptoms among coaches and sports entourage staff from Pilkington et al[23]		
Measure	**Coaches (%)**	**Entourage (%)**
Probable caseness	43.6	40.1
High to very high psychological distress	10.3	15.5
Moderate to severe sleep disturbance	23.4	15.1
Risky alcohol consumption	48.1	39.0

"Probable caseness" refers to the proportion of participants reporting mental health symptoms at levels that usually warrant psychological support and was measured by the General Health Questionnaire-28 item version (GHQ-28). Scores of 5 or higher (with binary coding) indicated probable caseness. Psychological distress was measured by the Kessler-10 item version (K-10). Scores between 22 and 50 indicated "high to very high" psychological distress. Sleep disturbance was assessed using the Athlete Sleep Screening Questionnaire (ASSQ). Scores between 8 and 17 indicated moderate to severe sleep disturbance. Alcohol consumption was assessed using the Alcohol Use Disorders Identification Test-Condensed version (AUDIT-C). Scores of 4 or more for female staff and 5 or more for male staff indicated risky alcohol consumption.

CASE EXAMPLE: TOM

Tom was a 37-year-old sports medicine physician working for a major national professional sport. He was married with 2 elementary-school-aged children. His role required significant travel, nationally and occasionally internationally, and he was often away from home for more than 5 months of the year. In addition to his clinical role, Tom held an academic appointment, supervised junior sports medicine practitioners, and maintained a small private practice.

Tom described his sports medicine career as "busy but for the most part completely fulfilling." He thrived in the high-performance environment and enjoyed the deep connections and comradery he established with his colleagues and the national team players with whom he traveled extensively. He was mindful of maintaining boundaries in his role and so rarely socialized outside the team environment (eg, only celebrating wins in the locker room after games) or consumed alcohol, which, in his opinion, was a highly problematic aspect of the sporting culture. Tom exercised regularly and communicated daily with his wife and children (and his aging parents) when traveling. He described feeling guilty about missing family events, such as his children's birthdays and wedding anniversaries, due to travel, but felt he was contributing to his family by providing an income that supported a comfortable lifestyle for his wife and children.

According to Tom, engaging in robust discussions with team management, coaches, and players about the fitness of players to compete was a regular element of his role. He took his ethical responsibilities to protect player health seriously and was relaxed that he occasionally had to make unpopular calls about players' availability due to injury and/or incomplete recovery. Tom felt he had earned the trust and respect of his colleagues after more than 6 years working with the national team. This shifted, however, when Tom experienced an unsettling event in which he was verbally abused on field by a player forcefully resisting leaving play for a mandatory assessment following a heavy collision. The abuse was brief, but personal and intense, and televised. Tom felt shocked and humiliated by the encounter, which was exacerbated by the player's subsequent refusal to apologize, believing that Tom cost the team the game by removing him from play at a crucial stage. Tom complained about the abuse to the coach and team manager (citing workplace safety rules), but not only were his concerns dismissed, the coach and manager sided with the player's views that Tom's actions probably cost them the game. Tom was deeply troubled that his decision-making and ethical responsibilities were questioned. He described this being the start of "the sleepness nights" and second guessing his value to the team. He acknowledged that he ruminated about the encounter long after the player, coach, and manager had moved on from it.

Tom continued to travel with the team but felt somewhat "disconnected" from the players and coaching staff. He started to "lose the love" for the sport and increasingly spent time in his hotel room or local cafes. He neglected exercising and gained a few pounds for the first time. Tom began to take sleeping tablets to fall asleep but woke early each morning (around 4 AM) unable to get back to sleep. His wife complained about his being "even more remote than usual," which triggered an argument in which Tom was blindsided by his wife's resentment at having to "functionally raise the kids alone!", when, from his perspective, he was "busting a gut" to financially establish his family's future. That night, Tom described sitting in the backyard, uncharacteristically drinking whiskey, until the early hours of the morning "wondering whether it was all worth it anymore." When his wife came down to find him, she was shocked to find Tom silently crying. The next morning, with his wife's and dad's encouragement, Tom spoke to a sport psychiatrist he knew outside of his sport. Tom knew that he was struggling and felt that he was probably burned out, but he was surprised that he scored in the "severe" range of the depression measure that the psychiatrist administered. Tom subsequently spoke confidentially to the team manager about needing to take some time away for health reasons and was supported to do so.

RISK AND PROTECTIVE FACTORS FOR MENTAL HEALTH IN ELITE COACHES AND ENTOURAGE
Workload and Recovery

Given the myriad of responsibilities for which coaches and HPSS are accountable (including managing athlete performance, condition, and leading tactical strategies), individuals within these roles commonly report highly demanding workloads.[51] Excessive workloads can emerge from role overload,[41] role conflict or ambiguity,[55] or attempts to compensate for a lack of role-based experience or resources.[39] Research indicates that as workloads intensify, coaches and entourage may be susceptible to lower wellbeing, poor mental health, and symptoms of burnout.[43,56]

Despite the demanding workloads, there is evidence to suggest that recovery processes (eg, psychological, physical, social) may play a leading role in shaping the mental health of high-performance entourages.[57,58] For example, Kellmann and colleagues found in a cohort of professional Australian football coaches that although stress levels remained relatively stable over the course of a season, recovery levels decreased throughout the competition.[58] This finding indicates that members of the sporting entourage should be provided with opportunities to psychologically detach and physically recuperate from their roles, as a lack of recovery time may contribute toward the onset of burnout.[40,41,43]

Psychological Skills and Coping Strategies

A range of individual-level characteristics have been found to influence the mental health of high-performance coaches and entourage. Several psychological characteristics have been found to protect entourage members from experiencing mental ill-health, including traits such as hardiness and resilience, which have been found to negatively predict symptoms associated with burnout, anxiety, and depression.[22,59] Conversely, entourage who possess low emotional intelligence or traits associated with maladaptive perfectionism may be at greater risk of experiencing mental ill-health.[40,41,60] Given that psychological skills can be shaped and nurtured over time, it is critical that coaches and support staff are offered opportunities to expand upon their repertoire of skills. When provided with training, mindfulness-based interventions have shown promise in significantly reducing negative affective states and symptoms of anxiety.[61] Hägglund and colleagues, for instance, found that mindful self-reflection cultivated greater levels of self-awareness in elite-level coaches.[62] Participants also reported that self-awareness helped to manage daily stressors more effectively. Because current evidence suggests that effective coping can enhance hedonic and eudaimonic wellbeing,[21,42] while ineffective coping may lead to the development of emotional exhaustion or the proliferation of symptoms associated with anxiety,[33,42] it is imperative that elite-level coaches and HPSS possess appropriate psychological tools that can be employed to manage the plethora of performance, organizational, and personal stressors that persist.

Social Support

The presence of robust social support is a key protective factor in mitigating poor mental health among elite coaches and entourage. An entourage member's support network may comprise both formal (eg, mentors) and informal (eg, friends and family) sources of social support.[51] Satisfaction with one's social support has been negatively associated with a range of mental health outcomes, including symptoms of anxiety, depression, psychological distress, sleep disturbance, and burnout.[23,33,41,46,59] Considering the link between insufficient social support and the onset or development of mental ill-health,[46,59] it is important for sporting organizations to be mindful of the social supports available to their high-performance employees. This support is invaluable in safeguarding the mental health of a coach or staff member not only throughout their tenure but also after employment or competition.[63] For example, Bentzen and colleagues[64] and Kenttä and colleagues[65] reported the pivotal role social support plays in preserving the mental wellbeing of elite-level coaches who have been dismissed from their role. These supports have been found to assist coaches with reflecting, recovering, and experiencing positive emotions during this transitional phase. Given the value of maintaining robust social networks both during and outside of one's involvement in elite sport, quality social supports should be considered sacrosanct in safeguarding the mental health of high-performance coaches and support staff.

Organizational Support

Organizations and governing bodies are integral to supporting the mental health of elite-level coaches and entourage. Given organizational demands have been found to significantly predict symptoms of anxiety and depression in elite-level coaches (unlike performance and personal stressors),[22] organizations should be cognisant of the role they play in alleviating or exacerbating symptoms of mental ill-health. Research has shown that the perceived satisfaction from upper management,[48] autonomy-supportive environments,[56] and sufficient financial resources[49] can operate as protective factors for elite-level coaches. Hill and colleagues also found that organizations which promote together and belonginess, cultivate a challenging yet supportive environment, and possess a clear organizational vision or philosophy are more likely to protect the mental health and wellbeing of high-performance staff.[51] Organizations should subsequently seek to define and establish these core values, to ensure role-based expectations are realistic and understood and that coaches and support staff feel part of a cohesive and supportive working environment which fosters psychological protection via relatedness.[66]

SUPPORTING ELITE-LEVEL COACH AND ENTOURAGE MENTAL HEALTH

Mrazek and Haggerty proposed that mental health support can be classified into three broad stages of intervention—prevention, treatment, and maintenance.[67] Considering these foci, Frost and colleagues explored several potential measures that could be implemented when developing an early intervention framework for elite-level coaches.[68] It is proposed that mental health screening and monitoring, mental health literacy, psychological safety, and pathways to mental health supports warrant consideration. These measures should be equally applied to elite coaches and support staff as they encounter similar stressors (eg, high workloads, job insecurity, lack of role clarity)[23,63] and report similar rates of mental health symptoms.

Despite the utility and applicability of these strategies, at present, a greater body of evidence is needed to design and adapt these measures to specifically accommodate elite-level entourages. At the Canadian intercollegiate level, Sullivan and colleagues found no significant differences in mental health literacy between coaches and athletic therapists.[69] Results indicated, however, that female professionals possessed significantly higher levels of mental health literacy than their male counterparts and that a significant negative correlation was identified between mental health literacy and total coaching experience. Future research should replicate similar procedures to evaluate mental health literacy levels and specific demographic and background-related variations among individuals operating within elite sport. This evidence may help inform organizations with tailoring mental health literacy programs to meet the specific needs of coaches and support staff.

Finally, psychological safety is increasingly recognized as critical to creating mentally healthy elite sporting environments.[70] Psychometric tools such as the Sport Psychological Safety Inventory could be used to measure psychological safety in high-performance environments,[71] including among elite-level coaches and HPSS with whom the tool was validated. This information can potentially shed light upon a coach's or support staff's sense of security in sharing sensitive information or raising issues with management,[72] subsequently providing partial insights into the degree to which these individuals feel supported by their organization. Further research is ultimately needed, however, to evaluate the perceived support that high-performance coaches and support staff receive with regard to their mental health.

SUMMARY

Elite sporting coaches and entourage operate in the same high-performance environments as elite athletes and, therefore, encounter similar risk factors for mental health as the athletes that they coach, train, and support. Despite this, there has been less research attention to the mental health of elite coaches and entourage, beyond studies examining burnout and wellbeing. A greater focus on understanding the prevalence of a range of mental health symptoms in these cohorts and the factors that contribute to vulnerability or exert a protective influence on mental health is necessary to support best-practice prevention and early intervention strategies.

CLINICS CARE POINTS

- A range of dynamic risk and protective factors have been identified that can be addressed to improve the mental health of elite coaches and entourage.
- Mindfulness based interventions and psychological skills training show promise for supporting mental welbeing among elite coaches.

DISCLOSURE

The authors have nothing to disclose.

REFERENCES

1. Reardon CL, Hainline B, Aron CM, et al. Mental health in elite athletes: International Olympic Committee consensus statement (2019). Br J Sports Med 2019; 53(11):667–99.
2. Küttel A, Larsen CH. Risk and protective factors for mental health in elite athletes: a scoping review. Int Rev Sport Exerc Psychol 2020;13(1):231–65.
3. Hammond T, Gialloreto C, Kubas H, et al. The prevalence of failure-based depression among elite athletes. Clin J Sport Med 2013;23(4):273–7.
4. Gulliver A, Griffiths KM, Mackinnon A, et al. The mental health of Australian elite athletes. J Sci Med Sport 2015;18(3):255–61.

5. Rice SM, Gwyther K, Santesteban-Echarri O, et al. Determinants of anxiety in elite athletes: a systematic review and meta-analysis. Br J Sports Med 2019;53(11): 722–30.

6. Peluso MAM, Andrade LHSGd. Physical activity and mental health: the association between exercise and mood. Clinics 2005;60(1):61–70.

7. Blakelock DJ, Chen MA, Prescott T. Psychological distress in elite adolescent soccer players following deselection. J Clin Sport Psychol 2016;10(1):59–77.

8. Jensen SN, Ivarsson A, Fallby J, et al. Depression in Danish and Swedish elite football players and its relation to perfectionism and anxiety. Psychol Sport Exerc 2018;36:147–55.

9. Jordana A, Ramis Y, Chamorro JL, et al. Ready for Failure? Irrational Beliefs, Perfectionism and Mental Health in Male Soccer Academy Players. J Ration Emot Cogn Behav Ther 2022;41:1–24.

10. Purcell R, Rice S, Butterworth M, et al. Rates and correlates of mental health symptoms in currently competing elite athletes from the Australian National high-performance sports system. Sports Med 2020;50(9):1683–94.

11. Gouttebarge V, Castaldelli-Maia JM, Gorczynski P, et al. Occurrence of mental health symptoms and disorders in current and former elite athletes: a systematic review and meta-analysis. Br J Sports Med 2019;53(11):700–6.

12. Purcell R, Gwyther K, Rice SM. Mental health in elite athletes: increased awareness requires an early intervention framework to respond to athlete needs. Sports medicine-open 2019;5(1):1–8.

13. Bronfenbrenner U. Ecological systems theory. London, England: Jessica Kingsley Publishers; 1992.

14. Chang C, Putukian M, Aerni G, et al. Mental health issues and psychological factors in athletes: detection, management, effect on performance and prevention: American Medical Society for Sports Medicine Position Statement—Executive Summary. Br J Sports Med 2020;54(4):216–20.

15. Didymus FF. Olympic and international level sports coaches' experiences of stressors, appraisals, and coping. Qualitative Research in Sport, Exercise and Health 2017;9(2):214–32.

16. Knights S, Ruddock-Hudson M. Experiences of occupational stress and social support in Australian Football League senior coaches. Int J Sports Sci Coach 2016;11(2):162–71.

17. Thelwell RC, Weston NJV, Greenlees IA, et al. Stressors in elite sport: A coach perspective. J Sports Sci 2008;26(9):905–18.

18. Rhind DJ, Scott M, Fletcher D. Organizational stress in professional soccer coaches. Int J Sport Psychol 2013;44(1):1–16.

19. Srem-Sai M, Hagan JE, Ogum PN, et al. Assessing the prevalence, sources and selective antecedents of organizational stressors among elite football players and coaches in the Ghana premier league: Empirical evidence for applied practice. Frontiers in Sports and Active Living 2022;4:938619.

20. Olusoga P, Butt J, Hays K, et al. Stress in Elite Sports Coaching: Identifying Stressors. J Appl Sport Psychol 2009;21(4):442–59.

21. Baldock L, Cropley B, Neil R, et al. Stress and Mental Well-Being Experiences of Professional Football Coaches. Sport Psychol 2021;35(2):108–22.

22. Kegelaers J, Wylleman P, van Bree INA, et al. Mental Health in Elite-Level Coaches: Prevalence Rates and Associated Impact of Coach Stressors and Psychological Resilience. International Sport Coaching Journal 2021;8(3):338–47.

23. Pilkington V, Rice SM, Walton CC, et al. Prevalence and correlates of mental health symptoms and well-being among elite sport coaches and high-performance support staff. Sports Medicine-Open 2022;8(1):89.
24. Fletcher D, Scott M. Psychological stress in sports coaches: A review of concepts, research, and practice. J Sports Sci 2010;28(2):127–37.
25. Norris LA, Didymus FF, Kaiseler M. Stressors, coping, and well-being among sports coaches: A systematic review. Psychol Sport Exerc 2017;33:93–112.
26. Potts AJ, Didymus FF, Kaiseler M. Psychological stress and psychological well-being among sports coaches: a meta-synthesis of the qualitative research evidence. Int Rev Sport Exerc Psychol 2021;1–30.
27. Olsen MG, Haugan JA, Hrozanova M, et al. Coping Amongst Elite-Level Sports Coaches: A Systematic Review. International Sport Coaching Journal 2021; 8(1):34–47.
28. Olusoga P, Bentzen M, Kentta G. Coach Burnout: A Scoping Review. International Sport Coaching Journal 2019;6(1):42–62.
29. Walton CC, Gwyther K, Gao CX, et al. Evidence of gender imbalance across samples in sport and exercise psychology. Int Rev Sport Exerc Psychol 2022;1–19.
30. Serpell BG, Harrison D, Dower R, et al. The under representation of women coaches in high-performance sport. Int J Sports Sci Coach 2023;0(0):1–13.
31. Kim SSY, Hamiliton B, Beable S, et al. Elite coaches have a similar prevalence of depressive symptoms to the general population and lower rates than elite athletes. BMJ open sport & exercise medicine 2020;6(1):e000719.
32. Åkesdotter C, Kenttä G, Eloranta S, et al. Prevalence and comorbidity of psychiatric disorders among treatment-seeking elite athletes and high-performance coaches. BMJ Open Sport & Exercise Medicine 2022;8(1):e001264.
33. Lee YH. The Roles of Different Appraisals in Anxiety and Emotional Exhaustion: A Case of NCAA Division I Head Coaches. Am J Psychol 2021;134(3):269–83.
34. Ruddock S, Ruddock-Hudson M, Rahimi-Golkhandan S. The impact of job-burnout on Australian Football League coaches: Mental health and well-being. J Sci Med Sport 2017;20:S73–4.
35. Ruddock S, Ruddock-Hudson M, Rahimi-Golkhandan S. Examining within-season change of job-burnout and psychological distress for Australian Rules Football coaches. J Sci Med Sport 2018;21:S41–2.
36. Ruddock S, Rahimi-Golkhanden S, Ruddock-Hudson M, et al. Tracking the mental health outcomes of occupational burnout with Australian Rules Football coaches: A 2-year longitudinal study. J Sci Med Sport 2019;22:S52.
37. Smith A, Torres-McGehee T, Monsma E, et al. Prevalence of Eating Disorder Risk and Body Image Perceptions of Collegiate Cheerleading Coaches. Journal of Sports Medicine & Allied Health Sciences: Official Journal of the Ohio Athletic Trainers' Association 2018;4(1):1–2.
38. Gwyther K, Rice S, Purcell R, et al. Sleep interventions for performance, mood and sleep outcomes in athletes: A systematic review and meta-analysis. Psychol Sport Exerc 2022;58:102094.
39. Bentzen M, Lemyre P-N, Kenttä G. The process of burnout among professional sport coaches through the lens of self-determination theory: a qualitative approach. Sports Coaching Review 2014;3(2):101–16.
40. Lundkvist E, Gustafsson H, Hjälm S, et al. An interpretative phenomenological analysis of burnout and recovery in elite soccer coaches. Qualitiative Research in Sport, Exercise and Health 2012;4(3):400–19.
41. Olusoga P, Kenttä G. Desperate to Quit: A Narrative Analysis of Burnout and Recovery in High-Performance Sports Coaching. Sport Psychol 2017;31(3):237–48.

42. Baldock L, Cropley B, Mellalieu SD, et al. A Longitudinal Examination of Stress and Mental Ill-/Well-Being in Elite Football Coaches. Sport Psychol 2022;36(3): 171–82.
43. Bentzen M, Lemyre P-N, Kenttä G. Development of exhaustion for high-performance coaches in association with workload and motivation: A person-centered approach. Psychol Sport Exerc 2016;22:10–9.
44. Kaski SS, Kinnunen U. Work-related ill- and well-being among Finnish sport coaches: Exploring the relationships between job demands, job resources, burnout and work engagement. International Journal of Sport Science & Coaching 2021;16(2):262–71.
45. Lundkvist E, Gustafsson H, Madigan D, et al. The Prevalence of Emotional Exhaustion in Professional and Semiprofessional Coaches. J Clin Sport Psychol 2022;12:1–14.
46. Nikolaos A. An examination of a burnout model in basketball coaches. Journal of Physical Education & Sport 2012;12(2):171–9.
47. Ryska TA. Multivariate Analysis of Program Goals, Leadership Style, and Occupational Burnout Among Intercollegiate Sport Coaches. J Sport Behav 2009; 32(4):476–88.
48. Gencay S, Gencay OA. Burnout among Judo Coaches in Turkey. J Occup Health 2011;53(5):365–70.
49. Hjälm S, Kenttä G, Hassmén P, et al. Burnout among elite soccer coaches. J Sport Behav 2007;30(4):415–27.
50. Gouttebarge V, Bindra A, Blauwet C, et al. International Olympic Committee (IOC) Sport Mental Health Assessment Tool 1 (SMHAT-1) and Sport Mental Health Recognition Tool 1 (SMHRT-1): towards better support of athletes' mental health. Br J Sports Med 2021;55(1):30–7.
51. Hill DM, Brown G, Lambert T-L, et al. Factors perceived to affect the wellbeing and mental health of coaches and practitioners working within elite sport. Sport, Exercise, and Performance Psychology 2021;10(4):504–18.
52. Walton CC, Rice S, Gao CX, et al. Gender differences in mental health symptoms and risk factors in Australian elite athletes. BMJ open sport & exercise medicine 2021;7(1):e000984.
53. Biggins M, Purtill H, Fowler P, et al. Sleep in elite multi-sport athletes: Implications for athlete health and wellbeing. Phys Ther Sport 2019;39:136–42.
54. Åkesdotter C, Kenttä G, Eloranta S, et al. The prevalence of mental health problems in elite athletes. J Sci Med Sport 2020;23(4):329–35.
55. Hassmén P, Kenttä G, Hjälm S, et al. Burnout symptoms and recovery processes in eight elite soccer coaches over 10 years. Int J Sports Sci Coach 2019;14(4): 431–43.
56. Bentzen M, Lemyre P, Kenttä G. Changes in Motivation and Burnout Indices in High-Performance Coaches Over the Course of a Competitive Season. J Appl Sport Psychol 2016;28(1):28–48.
57. de Sousa Pinheiro G, Túlio de Mello M, Gustavo dos Santos F, et al. Analysis of stress level and recovery of formative football coaches. Case studies. Retos: Nuevas Perspectivas de Educación Física. Deporte y Recreación 2021;41: 345–53.
58. Kellmann M, Altfeld S, Mallett CJ. Recovery–stress imbalance in Australian Football League coaches: A pilot longitudinal study. Int J Sport Exerc Psychol 2016; 14(3):240–9.

59. Georgios K, Nikolaos A. An Investigation of a Model of Personal-Situational Factors, Stress and Burnout in Track and Field Coaches. Journal of Physical Education & Sport 2012;12(3):343–9.
60. Lee YH, Chelladurai P. Affectivity, Emotional Labor, Emotional Exhaustion, and Emotional Intelligence in Coaching. J Appl Sport Psychol 2016;28(2):170–84.
61. Longshore K, Sachs M. Mindfulness Training for Coaches: A Mixed-Method Exploratory Study 2015;9(2):116–37.
62. Hägglund K, Kenttä G, Thelwell R, et al. Mindful self-reflection to support sustainable high-performance coaching: A process evaluation of a novel method development in elite sport. J Appl Sport Psychol 2021;34:1–24.
63. DeWolfe CEJ, Dithurbide L. Beware of the blues: Wellbeing of coaches and support staff throughout the Olympic Games. Int J Sports Sci Coach 2022;17(6): 1243–57.
64. Bentzen M, Kenttä G, Lemyre P-N. Elite Football Coaches Experiences and Sensemaking about Being Fired: An Interpretative Phenomenological Analysis. Int J Environ Res Publ Health 2020;17(14):5196.
65. Kenttä G, Mellalieu S, Roberts C-M. Are Career Termination Concerns Only for Athletes? A Case Study of the Career Termination of an Elite Female Coach. Sport Psychol 2016;30(4):314–26.
66. Ng JYY, Ntoumanis N, Thøgersen-Ntoumani C, et al. Self-Determination Theory Applied to Health Contexts: A Meta-Analysis. Perspect Psychol Sci 2012;7(4): 325–40.
67. Mrazek PJ, Haggerty RJ. Reducing risks for mental disorders: Frontiers for preventive intervention research. Washington, DC, US: National Academy Press; 1994.
68. Frost J, Walton CC, Purcell R, et al. Supporting the mental health of elite-level coaches through early intervention. Arthroscopy, Sports Medicine, and Rehabilitation 2023. https://doi.org/10.1016/j.asmr.2023.04.017.
69. Sullivan P, Murphy J, Blacker M. The Level of Mental Health Literacy Among Athletic Staff in Intercollegiate Sport. J Clin Sport Psychol 2019;13(3):440–50.
70. Purcell R, Pilkington V, Carberry S, et al. An Evidence-Informed Framework to Promote Mental Wellbeing in Elite Sport. Front Psychol 2022;13:780359.
71. Rice S, Walton CC, Pilkington V, et al. Psychological safety in elite sport settings: a psychometric study of the Sport Psychological Safety Inventory. BMJ Open Sport and Exercise Medicine 2022;8(2):e001251.
72. Vella SA, Mayland E, Schweickle MJ, et al. Psychological safety in sport: a systematic review and concept analysis. Int Rev Sport Exerc Psychol 2022;1–24.

Moving?

Make sure your subscription moves with you!

To notify us of your new address, find your **Clinics Account Number** (located on your mailing label above your name), and contact customer service at:

Email: journalscustomerservice-usa@elsevier.com

800-654-2452 (subscribers in the U.S. & Canada)
314-447-8871 (subscribers outside of the U.S. & Canada)

Fax number: 314-447-8029

Elsevier Health Sciences Division
Subscription Customer Service
3251 Riverport Lane
Maryland Heights, MO 63043

*To ensure uninterrupted delivery of your subscription, please notify us at least 4 weeks in advance of move.